Security in the Health Care Environment

David H. Sells, Jr. MC/CJ, CPP, CHPA, CSE

AN ASPEN PUBLICATION®

Security in the Health Care Environment

David H. Sells, Jr. MC/CJ, CPP, CHPA, CSE
President
Sells & Company
Charlotte, North Carolina

AN ASPEN PUBLICATION®
Aspen Publishers, Inc.
Gaithersburg, Maryland
2000

Library of Congress Cataloging-in-Publication Data
Sells, David H.
Security in the health care environment/ David H. Sells.
p. cm.
Includes bibliographical references and index.
ISBN 0-8342-1225-0
1. Health facilities—Security measures. I. Title.

RA969.95.S44 1999
362.1′068′4—dc21   99-0051847

Orders: (800) 638-8437
Customer Service: (800) 234-1660

Editorial Services: Kate Hawker
Library of Congress Catalog Card Number: 99-0051847
ISBN: 0-8342-1225-0

Printed in the United States of America

1 2 3 4 5

List of Contributors

James P. Finn, CHPA, CSE, CHSE
Manager, Safety and Security Services
Gaston Memorial Hospital
Gastonia, North Carolina

Rick J. Flinn, RN, MSN
Executive Director, Emergency and Trauma Services
North Broward Hospital District
Fort Lauderdale, Florida

William P. Gibbons III
Sales Engineer
SFI Electronics, Inc.
Charlotte, North Carolina

John B. Rabun, Jr., BA, MSSW
Vice President and Chief Operating Officer
National Center for Missing and Exploited Children
Alexandria, Virginia

John Thomas Readling, BA
Special Agent
North Carolina State Bureau of Investigation
North Carolina Department of Justice
Raleigh, North Carolina

David H. Sells, Jr., MC/CJ, CPP, CHPA, CSE
President
Sells & Company
Charlotte, North Carolina

Table of Contents

Preface

I was often asked during the past year why I decided to undertake such an enormous task as writing this book. To be honest, I am not sure. I have written or co-authored four other books, so one might think I would remember just how much work is involved. When you write a book, you start off with unlimited enthusiasm. Midway through the project, you resemble a tired football player in the fourth quarter: it doesn't matter whether you are winning or losing, you just want the game to be over.

I was fortunate in having some very supportive cheerleaders to encourage me to "stay in the game." One of these cheerleaders was my editor, Sandy Cannon, who I know grew tired of my Friday afternoon phone calls but who was always nice enough to give me the support I needed. The other cheerleader, my wonderful wife Pamela, understood and accepted the fact that no matter what time it was, if I felt the urge to write, I had to write. For the many missed dinners I do apologize, and for her encouragement I am deeply appreciative.

I realized early in this project that the book would be more balanced and provide better information if I invited other authors to contribute. Some of these authors had never written before, so writing a chapter was quite an undertaking for them. They were very patient with my nagging them to keep on schedule. Their contributions are excellent and add to the overall quality of the book. The book is a good example of six heads being better than one.

When I began my career in health care security, I told the CEO who hired me, Byron Bullard, that I knew a great deal about security but not much about hospitals. Mr. Bullard smiled and said, "That's okay—I know hospitals, so we'll make a great team." I owe Mr. Bullard a debt of gratitude. He allowed me to grow immensely as a professional and was always very supportive.

There are other books on the market about security in a health care facility, but I have tried to fashion this work to serve two specific audiences. The first is the new health care security director or the manager of an ancillary department who also has security as an area of responsibility. These managers need guidance and an overview of the complex workings of the health care security industry. The second audience is the veteran health care security director. All professionals know that they must constantly be learning. This book can help experienced security professionals re-think various areas of their operation and explore new options for accomplishing their tasks.

There is no doubt that health care in general and health care security specifically will change dramatically in the next few years. As a consultant who has health care clients of various sizes in the United States and six foreign countries, I find that everyone is facing the same problems: not enough time and money and fear of litigation. These challenges will not disappear, and budgetary constraints will probably become even tougher in the future. The health care security director of tomorrow must be willing not only to work harder but, more important, to work smarter. This book was written to offer assistance and guidance in these endeavors.

In closing, I ask all who enter this profession to keep one thing in mind: always do what is best for the patient. These people have come to us to cure their ills and make them whole again. They are the reason hospitals and health care workers exist; they are the people we serve. When you are faced with a decision, always ask yourself, "If I were the patient, what would I want done?" If you do this, you will always make the right decision.

Chapter 1

Introduction to Security in the Health Care Environment

CHAPTER OBJECTIVES

1. Be introduced to the health care environment.
2. Be exposed to an overview of the various types of health care facilities and their particular security problems.
3. Learn the process of accreditation for hospitals and other health care facilities and organizations.

INTRODUCTION

In writing an introductory chapter, the author must determine who the targeted readers are and what they should learn from the material. In fact, the introductory chapter is by far the most difficult to write because a variety of people will read the chapter—and the book—for a variety of reasons.

For the experienced security director, most of this material will be a review. However, the book may help these experienced professionals reexamine their programs and gain some insight into possible solutions to their problems. For the novice security director, or someone whose main focus is not security but who has security as an added responsibility, the book can provide an outline for setting up a successful program.

To determine how security interacts with and functions in the health care environment, it is necessary to briefly discuss that environment and how it has significantly changed over the past few years. The term "health care facility" has changed to mean several different types of facilities. The first part of our review will focus on the typical hospital; the second part, on the health care facilities that make up an integrated system; and the third part, on accreditation.

A TYPICAL HOSPITAL

Most hospitals can be divided into two categories, on the basis of (1) the geographic region the hospital serves and (2) the ownership structure of the hospital.

Geographic Region Served

Most hospitals can be classified as being in an urban (i.e., inner-city), suburban, or rural environment. The actual location of the facility is the primary indicator of the determination, although the type of patients seen and the ownership of the facility can help determine the category of the facility. For example, if the facility is located in the suburbs but is county owned and operated, it could be considered an inner-city facility in terms of its security problems, because it will be treating the same kinds of patients and experiencing the same problems as an urban facility. Likewise, if the facility is a privately owned hospital in a suburban area of a sparsely populated county, it might be considered a rural facility. These geographic "labels" help to determine the kinds of security problems hospitals will encounter.

Ownership

Before the coming of integrated systems, hospital ownership fell into three main classifications: (1) nonprofit, (2) for profit, and (3) government owned and operated. Most privately owned hospitals were in the first category. However, nonprofit does not mean that the hospitals did not make money; in fact, they usually had higher profit margins than most other companies. The difference was that they had to reinvest their profits into the facility, unlike the for-profit hospitals, which could distribute their profits in bonuses and dividends to shareholders.

Government-owned facilities, as the name implies, were owned and operated by a government agency. The Veterans Administration hospitals are a prime example. These facilities received their operating budgets from the appropriate government agency and all operated under the same charter, regardless of their location.

In recent years, there has been an interesting integration of these three categories. For example, a nonprofit hospital may be located on government land (usually county land) and may be operating as the county hospital. Going back to the geographic region determination, this hospital may be in a suburban setting, but the security professional may view the facility as "urban" because of the kinds of security risks associated with a county hospital.

Hospital Population

The hospital population is also worthy of a review. By looking at the population mix we can see that a hospital is truly a small town unto itself. The employees of a hospital range from entry level to the highest possible skill level; this makes for a wide range of education and income levels. The hospital population includes the following categories:

Physicians

In the past, most physicians were not part of the hospital. They were independent contractors who owned and operated their practices alone or with a small group of professionals. Today, more and more physicians are hospital employees. Most hospitals have a chief of staff who acts as the chief medical executive for the hospital. The chiefs of all the specialties (oncology, family practice, surgery, etc.) report to this executive.

Medical Staff

Most of the medical support staff in the hospital are hospital employees. Their role is to help evaluate and treat patients (for example, radiology) and to provide care for patients in the hospital (for example, the nurse). The archaic view was that all medical staff worked for the physician, carrying out his or her orders without question. The modern concept is that all medical staff work together to provide the best care for the patient. This is especially true in view of the fact that the physician probably spends less time with the patient than any of the other caregivers.

Administration

Hospital administrators have executive-level decision-making authority. Most have a master's degree in hospital administration, business, or finance, and most also have earned the certification of Fellow, American College of Healthcare Executives (FACHE).

Department Heads/Managers

Department heads and managers usually have at least a bachelor's degree in their field. They are charged with managing and coordinating a particular function and integrating the function into the overall goals of the facility. They are considered in most cases to be middle management; however, most serve on committees with administrators to assist in decision making.

Hospital Staff and Others

The staff includes all other hospital employees, from entry-level workers to highly skilled professionals. **In addition to its employees, the hospital population includes many other people:**

- Sales representatives—people employed by the various companies from which the hospital buys goods and services.
- Consultants—outside specialists who have contracted with the hospital for a specific project.
- Construction workers—Has anyone seen a hospital that is NOT under some type of renovation or construction?
- Auxiliary/volunteer staff—These wonderful people give countless hours of service to the hospital in a variety of roles.
- Visitors—Most inpatients have at least two or three visitors a day. Visitors can be problematic for the security director, because they are often under stress and may not act rationally.

And last, but by far most important,

- The patient—These are the people for whose benefit the hospital exists. It is the place where we treat and, we hope, heal our fellow citizens who need medical care. They may be inpatients (admitted and staying overnight) or outpatients (coming in for an appointment or same-day surgery). Keeping patients safe can present many challenges to the security director; for example, the overdose patient who must be kept from injuring him- or herself or others, or the suicidal patient who tries to escape from the psychiatric unit. These and all other patients deserve the highest degree of professionalism and service.

So—how many security officers would be needed for a 350-bed hospital? It all depends . . . on the geographic location, type of ownership, probability of certain kinds of security problems, and also on the kinds of patients the hospital serves.

OTHER KINDS OF HEALTH CARE FACILITIES

In the past, the term "health care facility" usually has referred to hospitals; however, in the changing environment of health care, other kinds of facilities are becoming more prevalent and are coming together to form integrated systems. The security director must be familiar with these entities and with the risks associated with them. Most of the information in this book concerns hospital security, but it is applicable to other facility types as well. For example, many of the safeguards used in a hospital can also be used in a clinic. **The following are the main kinds of health care facilities and their associated security risks.**

Private Physician's Office

The physician operating as a sole proprietor is almost a thing of the past. Most physicians' offices today consist of physicians in partnership—from 4 to 5 physicians to as many as 75 to 100—and their support staff. Regardless of the size of the office, three main areas should be reviewed by a security director.

Cash Handling

Most physicians' offices receive cash from one primary source: payment for office visits. The security of the cash must be ensured at the cashier's area, while it is being moved from the business office, and while it is stored in the safe. In addition, the cash control method should be periodically audited, comparing billing records with cash receipts. If a loss is detected or something suspicious occurs, security would work with the auditors to fully audit the office and interview office staff as well. In a four-physician practice, a cashier was able to embezzle over $20,000 by falsifying co-payment receipts and stealing the money paid by patients. This may not seem like a large sum, but the theft occurred over a period of only three months!

The security director must ensure that sound cash security practices are in place. Many of the cash-handling practices outlined in Chapter 17 can be adapted for physicians' offices and other medical practices.

Sample Drugs

Pharmaceutical representatives supply many drug samples to physicians' offices. This is a common practice that benefits both the patient and the physician, but care must be observed. In one instance, a new analgesic was promoted by drug representatives as safe and nonaddictive. In reality, the drug could become addictive. More than 500 sample units of this medication were stolen by an employee over a three-month period. Her accomplice was selling the drugs on the street.

Prescription Pads and Controlled Substances

In many physicians' offices, prescription pads are left in each examination room. The problem is that most of the pads contain the physician's name, address, Drug Enforcement Administration (DEA) number, and phone number. Anyone who possesses even a passing knowledge of medicine could easily steal the pad and forge prescriptions. The physician should carry the pad, and extras should be stored under lock and key.

Many physicians' offices have very poor security practices regarding Schedule II or III drugs. They may be stored in a small case or left setting on a shelf. Rarely are the drugs audited or tested to verify that another drug has not been substituted.

Urgent Care Facilities

These freestanding urgent care facilities, often called "doc-in-the-box" facilities, have the same risks as a physician's office, and some others as well. Most are sparsely staffed, with only one physician on duty, and they often have extended hours—until late at night or even 24 hours a day. The hours alone make them vulnerable to street crime. The risk of armed robberies for cash or drugs is higher than for a "normal" physician's office. Staff safety is another concern, with people walking to their vehicles late at night.

These facilities resemble emergency department in the long waits to see a physician and the high percentage of minor trauma cases. As in the emergency department, communication between the medical staff and the waiting family is important, to keep people from becoming fearful and agitated.

Some of these facilities hire contract security companies or employ individuals to provide late-night security, especially if they are located in areas where gang-related crimes occur.

Nursing Homes

The nursing home industry has long been plagued by two main security problems: patient abuse and wandering patients.

Patient Abuse

Patient abuse can occur in a number of ways, from theft of personal items up to physical abuse. In Chapter 26, we discuss patient abuse claims. The issue to be addressed here is screening of prospective staff. Since 1996, federal legislation has required nursing homes to conduct criminal background checks on new employees. Some states also require that Certified Nursing Assistants (CNAs) be registered with the state and that employers check with the CNA licensing body to see if any complaints of abuse have been registered against the applicant.

Most nursing homes comply with the regulations, but criminal background checks take time. It is not uncommon to wait 4 to 12 weeks for a check to be completed, so applicants often are hired on a conditional basis. Nursing homes experience an extremely high employee turnover rate; thus, the new employee might already have left by the time the background check is completed. A person could apply, start working, and leave one nursing home after another and never have a criminal record catch up!

In addition, many states require that the criminal record check for nursing home employees be conducted through the state's criminal repository. In most states, counties are required to report only felony convictions, and sometimes violent misdemeanors, to the repository. So a person could have a lengthy arrest and conviction record in several counties that would not be reported to the state repository.

Security directors should consider using an on-line service to conduct their own criminal record checks, in addition to those required by statute. All states and counties where the applicant has lived or worked for the past five years should be checked, and any gaps in employment should be investigated.

Wandering Patients

A major security issue in nursing homes is that of patients simply wandering away from the facility. These patients, often suffering from dementia or early Alzheimer's disease, may not be able to find their way back to the facility. The following are two steps the security director can take to prevent wandering.

First, alarm all exit doors. In most states, the fire code will allow you to install a delayed opening system. (Be sure to check local regulations.) With these devices the doors will not open for a set time, usually 15 seconds, during which an alarm sounds to alert staff. Another way to protect wandering patients is to use an electronic tagging system. These systems are similar to the devices used in department stores to tag high-theft merchandise. They can be attached around the wrist or ankle or worn on a small chain, like a pendent. The device sets off an alarm if the patient passes through a control point, such as an elevator or stairwell door.

Outpatient Surgery Centers

These centers are becoming more popular as inpatient reimbursement rates decline. In most cases, they have most of the security risks of a hospital, with additional threats in the following areas:

Burglaries

Because these centers are usually in freestanding buildings and are closed at night, the likelihood of burglaries exists. The most common way to secure the building is with an alarm system; however, controlling the system may be a problem. In most of these facilities, surgeries are finished and staff leaves between 5:00 and 7:00 p.m. Housekeeping usually cleans after the staff leaves, which means that someone must be responsible for setting the alarm. Some facilities have experienced break-ins between the time the staff leaves and the time housekeeping arrives.

Theft

Theft of patients' personal property is a concern for outpatient surgery centers. Most patients are driven to the center by a friend or relative, but they usually carry a purse or wallet. Although most facilities tell patients to give their valuables to the person who brought them to the center, in actual practice this does not always happen. Installation of patient lockers can solve the problem of patient property theft.

Narcotics

As in hospitals, narcotic control is a concern in outpatient surgery centers, many of which have a pharmacy on-site. From this pharmacy, anesthesia carts are stocked or case packs are prepared. Many facilities have adopted the policy that anesthesiologists may not "waste" any narcotic. The unused portions of the carpujects are returned to the pharmacy. The pharmacy then performs a random quality assurance check to make sure that the liquid in the syringe is, for example, morphine and not saline.

Day Psychiatric Units

These units often care for patients who, while they are mentally or emotionally troubled, do not need to be confined. One of the main security problems at these facilities is communication between the medical staff and security. If the medical staff asks security to prevent certain patients from leaving the facility, security needs to know how much—if any—force should be used. A coding system should be in place to convey the level of force to be used.

The coding system for determining the amount of force to be used includes the following levels:

- Level 1—This code is used if a patient is under the influence of alcohol and/or drugs but is still within the functional range. It tells security that only verbal restraints should be used.
- Level 2—This code is used if a patient has been given medication by the physician and is clearly impaired. It tells security that verbal and "soft hands" can be used. Soft hands is defined as gently placing your hands on a patient's arm or shoulder to walk them in a given direction.
- Level 3—This code is used if a physician has dictated an order that the patient is a clear threat to themselves or others or if the patient has had legal commitment papers issued. Reasonable force, including restraints, can be used to restrain the patient.

This coding system helps the medical staff and security staff work better together because they understand the expectations of both departments.

Another security risk is the possibility that weapons or drugs could be brought into the facility. The facility must have a strict consent-to-search policy, with a form for the patient to sign at the time of admission. Either freestanding or handheld metal detectors can be used to check for weapons.

Part of the treatment for many of these patients is to take them on walks or other outings. The accompanying staff should make sure that they can reach the facility and/or the security/police department quickly in case of a mishap. Cell phones that are preprogrammed for these numbers work well.

Animal Research Centers and Abortion Clinics

Obviously, these two facilities have nothing to do with each other, except that they share some of the same security risks. Both are targets of highly zealous groups that oppose their work. Both may face protests that range from peaceful demonstrations to bombings and (in the case of abortion clinics) even assassinations. The security director should network through professional associations and contacts and learn which groups are protesting and the methods they use. Armed with this information, the security director can meet with law enforcement officials and ascertain the local activity level of these groups.

Medical Office Buildings

These structures have become commonplace in today's health care environment; in fact, many are built by a hospital or its corporate parent, and often they are actually connected to the hospital by a walkway of some sort. In most cases the tenants are not hospital departments but individual physicians' commercial offices. This makes for a difficult security situation. The hospital administrator may assure a prospective tenant that the hospital security department will provide assistance if necessary. However, in most states, the security department would have to be licensed as a contract security company to provide security inside these offices. (They can, of course, provide security in the common areas and in offices owned and operated by their hospital or corporate holding company.) The security director must make the administrator aware of the proper licensing requirements for this service.

Security must have clear guidelines on its areas of responsibility. The walkway can present additional security problems. What time is it locked? Do tenants in the medical office building have card access to the building and, via the skywalk, to the hospital after hours? If the hospital has contracted with a local pharmacy to operate in the office building, what security arrangements have been made for this unit? How are deliveries handled to the various tenants, especially after normal business hours ? Is security responsible for signing for and accepting these deliveries? What about storage areas for nuclear medicine or blood?

These are just some of the questions that occur when a medical office building is added into the hospital system. The challenge is even greater if the hospital is a fully integrated system that includes many kinds of health facilities—in other words, a medical center.

SECURITY FOR INTEGRATED SYSTEMS

The biggest security problem with integrated systems is establishing clear guidelines for the role security plays in the various components. Will they patrol all the components of the system? Will they be on-call consultants to handle problems on a case-by-case basis? How are security costs distributed among the various components of the system—by square foot? calls for service? Will there be different security protocols for the facilities that are not on the medical center's main campus? For example, in the hospital, the security department may be called to handle all security incidents and the local police used as a backup. In off-campus properties, the roles may be reversed.

Most important, all decisions on security issues must be communicated to everyone concerned. When a problem occurs is not the time to formulate policies and procedures.

ACCREDITATION

An important aspect of the health care environment is accreditation. Most hospitals in the United States strive to be accredited by the Joint Commission on Accreditation of Healthcare Organizations, although this is not mandatory. The Joint Commission is neither a government licensing agency nor a mandatory regulating body. It is an industry group that oversees and promotes quality patient care by means of a standardized accreditation process. The Joint Commission was originally composed of representatives from four organizations: the American College of Surgeons, the American Medical Association, the American Hospital Association, and the American College of Physicians. Later, the American Dental Association was added. These organizations elect the commissioners, and hospitals and other health care organizations request and pay to have them visit and survey their facilities. **The Joint Commission has standards for the following health care entities:**

- hospitals
- non-hospital-based psychiatric and substance abuse organizations
- long-term care facilities
- home care organizations
- ambulatory care organizations
- pathology and clinical laboratory services
- health care networks

The Joint Commission inspection team usually consists of a hospital administrator, a registered nurse, a physician, and either an ambulatory care director or a plant engineer. The team uses the *Comprehensive Accreditation Manual for Hospitals,* which is published annually by the Joint Commission. This manual sets forth the standards against which the facility is measured.

The Joint Commission normally accredits hospitals for a three-year period. It may conduct random, unannounced surveys on accredited organizations, and reserves the right to conduct unannounced visits whenever it has reason to believe that there has been a substantial deterioration in clinical care, that there is an immediate threat to patient care or safety, or that the inspection team was given false information.

At the end of the accreditation survey, the inspection team holds an exit conference with the chief executive officer of the hospital to inform him or her of any and all deficiencies it has noted. The chief operating officer, nurse administrator, and chief of the medical staff should also attend this conference. Within 60 days of this conference, the Joint Commission will issue one of the accreditation decisions listed below.

- Accreditation with commendation—the organization has displayed exemplary adherence to the standards.
- Accreditation—the organization meets the overall compliance standards.
- Accreditation with a type 1 recommendation—the organization must resolve a problem or improve an area that does not meet the standard within a specific period of time or risk losing accreditation.
- Conditional accreditation—the organization does not meet the standards in a number of areas and must correct these deficiencies to be considered for full accreditation. A follow-up survey will be conducted to review the improvements.
- Provisional accreditation—the organization is new but has demonstrated substantial compliance with the standards in surveys that were conducted under the Early Survey Policy. This provisional status remains until the organization successfully completes its second full survey.
- Not accredited—the organization does not meet standards, and accreditation is denied or withdrawn.

KEY POINTS

- Hospitals can be categorized in several ways.
  - –by geographic location (urban, suburban, rural)
  - –by ownership (nonprofit, for profit, government)
- The hospital population comprises many groups: physicians, medical staff, administration, department heads/managers, hospital staff, sales representatives, consultants, construction workers, volunteers, visitors, and—most important—patients.
- There are many kinds of health care facilities and organizations besides hospitals: private physician offices, urgent care facilities, nursing homes, outpatient surgery centers, day psychiatric units, animal research centers, abortion clinics, medical office buildings.
- Many of these facilities and organizations are coming together to form integrated systems.
- Hospitals and other health care facilities and organizations seek accreditation from the Joint Commission on Accreditation of Healthcare Organizations.
  - –Accreditation surveys are usually conducted every three years.
  - –Results of a Joint Commission survey may be Accreditation with Commendation, Accreditation, Conditional Accreditation, Provisional Accreditation, or Not Accredited.

Chapter 2

The Security Program: Form and Structure

CHAPTER OBJECTIVES

1. The role of security in the health care environment.
2. The various staffing options.
3. The role of security management and the types of management systems.
4. Professional development programs available to the security director.

INTRODUCTION

As we head into the new millennium, the role of health care security—like health care itself—is rapidly changing. As a result of corporate mergers and downsizing, security is reverting in many ways to the form it had in the late 1970s. At that time, especially in small and mid-sized facilities, security was usually an add-on function under the plant manager, along with plant engineering, safety, groundskeeping, and construction management. As hospitals grew and expanded in the 1980s, many of the mid-sized and larger ones created a separate department for safety and security. But as the Joint Commission on Accreditation of Healthcare Organizations (Joint Commission) developed more standards for hospital safety, safety and security were separated; in many cases, safety merged with risk management and quality assurance.

By the late 1980s and early 1990s, even smaller hospitals had separated the security function into an entity of its own. During this time, most hospitals were experiencing tremendous growth. The growth occurred not only on the hospital campus but in the profusion of medical office buildings, physicians' offices, home health agencies, and outpatient services. The drive for market share dictated that a hospital be "new and improved," and hospitals were evolving as a true American business type. No longer could a hospital exist by itself; it had to be a "regional medical system," with a full line of services and alliances with other hospitals and physicians. With these new complexities, administrators understood the need for an effective security program.

However, as we moved into the mid-1990s, with managed care and tighter budgets, the growth in security departments started to reverse itself. As a cost- and not a revenue-producing center, security was the target of staffing reductions and downsizing of security man-

11

ager/director jobs. The larger hospital systems began to merge the safety and security management function, and in smaller and mid-sized facilities, these functions once again moved under the plant manager.

As these changes occurred in security management, the role of security also changed. In the earlier days, security meant guards—very little more than a fire-watch and turnkey function. As the crime rate in the United States increased and health care facilities expanded, the security department took on more of an enforcement role. Administrators often hired retired law enforcement officers as managers, and although their law enforcement expertise was valuable, most of these managers did not have the education and training necessary to develop the security department into anything more than a mini–police department. As the functions of the security department became more complex, we saw the emergence of professional security directors and proactive security departments. To continue to survive, security must develop a philosophy of service, assistance, and protection.

THE MISSION OF SECURITY

Any institution must have a mission, and the security department is no different. Security departments may differ in many ways, but their overall mission should resemble that expressed in the following statement.

The mission of the department of security services is to

- assist the medical staff in rendering quality medical care
- provide a safe and secure campus
- assist administration in the enforcement of corporate policies
- maintain peace and enforce the law

ASSISTING THE MEDICAL STAFF

Everyone who works in a hospital should remember that they are there for one reason and one reason only: to take care of patients. Even though security officers may have limited direct patient contact, they play an important role in supporting those who render care.

The most obvious support lies in maintaining a safe and secure campus, but more personal interaction occurs on a daily basis. Whether it is providing an escort for a staff member to her car or helping to restrain an unruly patient, security officers must be professional and knowledgeable in their endeavors. The following are some of the ways security assists the medical staff: on-call procedures, patient restraints, courtesy services, education on current security incident trends, maintaining security control in the emergency department, fire safety inspection, employee-requested visitor restriction, traffic control, and visitor restrictions for patients.

PROVIDING A SAFE AND SECURE CAMPUS

Physically securing the campus is the most obvious function of the security department, and there are various aspects of this task.

High-Visibility Patrol

High-visibility patrol, either on foot or in a marked patrol car, is one of the best deterrents against crime. A highly visible security officer sends the message to potential perpetrators that the institution takes security seriously and makes the staff feel safer, especially late at night and early in the morning.

The patrol officer should concentrate his or her efforts on different parts of the campus, depending on the time of day. During the high-traffic daytime hours, the officer may want to concentrate the patrol in and around the entrance/exit areas and inside the building, with less attention to parking lots/decks during night hours (security may want to increase the patrol in parking lots/decks). Inside the hospital, the officer should be an obvious presence in such areas as the emergency department (an officer may need to be posted full time in the ED, depending on the facility), the maternity center, and the pharmacy, especially if it has a retail function.

Access Control

Access to the facility fluctuates according to the time of day. A health care facility typically has numerous entrances and exits that are usually unlocked and unattended. As the facility begins to close down for the day, the doors should either be on self-locking timers or be physically locked by security. After hours, access should be restricted to one public door (typically at the ED) and one employee entrance that is controlled by card access.

Several areas of the facility are normally considered "sensitive areas" and should receive special consideration in reviewing access control: the pharmacy, the nursery, and the psychiatric unit. These areas should remain in a locked-down mode at all times, accessible only with special cards. The treatment areas of the ED should also be controlled. The Joint Commission requires that facilities review their sensitive areas annually.

ENFORCING CORPORATE POLICIES

Unlike the police, who have clear authority to act under given circumstances, the security department is mandated to assist administration in the enforcement of corporate policies that may include many "gray" areas. Remember that a security officer is the only employee vested with the authority to enforce a corporate rule or policy among peers in other departments. The enforcement of the policies must be tempered with sound judgment and a professional attitude. Some of the policies the security officer must enforce on a daily basis are parking/traffic control, administrative inspections, access control, and regulatory issues such as Joint Commission standards, Occupational Safety and Health Administration (OSHA) guidelines, and fire prevention standards.

MAINTAINING PEACE AND ENFORCING THE LAW

Although service and administrative functions take up most of the officers' time, the security department must remember that its image is formed when it is maintaining peace and performing law enforcement functions. If officers can be relied upon to react in a calm, professional manner in crisis situations, the reputation they earn will be positive. The areas in which their professionalism will be publicly tested are mediating in potentially hostile situations, conducting investigations, and preventing crimes.

Mediating Hostile Situations

All officers should keep in mind that, except for the people who have chosen to work in the health care field, no one wants to be in a hospital. When people are there, they are under stress, from pain, fear, or anxiety over a loved one's condition. Even the joyous occasion of the birth of a child is stressful, especially if there are complications.

The security department receives most of its calls for service from the ED, intensive care unit (ICU), cardiac care unit (CCU), maternity center, psychiatric units, and business office.

In the emergency department, all the components for an explosive situation are present. Not only must patients and visitors deal with the stress of an unexpected medical emergency, but many times the event that caused the injury carries over into the ED. Victims of domestic violence, gang wars, bar fights, and drug deals gone bad present themselves on a regular basis to EDs, and the original attackers may arrive at the ED to "finish what they started."

Even when a patient is not a victim of violence, the family or friends may become violent in their fear or grief. An officer trained to handle verbal aggression can deescalate the situation.

The maternity center offers many challenges for security. Conflicts regarding abortion, child custody, and unwanted visits by spouses are just a few of the circumstances that, if not handled properly, can lead to a violent outcome. The possibility of an infant's being abducted, while small, is a profoundly serious matter for the new parents and the facility.

In the business office, the officer may be called upon to assist with a distraught family member or patient who, after a prolonged medical episode, may be faced with a medical bill that will wipe out his or her life savings. In addition, the threat of robbery is always present.

Investigations

The security officer will be called upon to investigate a wide range of incidents, from petty theft, to assaults, to drug diversions. As more and more hospitals become self-insured, the security department is called upon to handle a wide variety of cases. In most facilities, the security department is the "investigative division" for the risk management department. Investigations may involve malpractice suits, workers' compensation, preemployment background checks, fraud, embezzlement, and internal audits.

Crime Prevention

This is one area where private security can really make a difference. The ability to prevent a crime has long been the primary area of expertise of private security. Police departments are generally reactive by nature, while professional security departments are proactive.

Two concepts that the public sector is now using—community watch and community policing—have proved to reduce crime. Both of these concepts work well in a hospital, too. A "hospital watch" program can draw on hundreds, if not thousands, of eyes and ears to alert security to possible criminal events. A security liaison program—in which security officers are assigned to certain departments of the hospital, to educate and assist in reducing crime—is most effective.

THE SECURITY DIRECTOR'S RESPONSIBILITIES

The security director of today is not just the "company cop." They are professional managers, handling budgets that may be in the millions of dollars and charged with the responsibility of maintaining a secure environment for thousands of patients, visitors, and staff. It is a challenge they cannot meet alone. They must integrate themselves into the mainstream of the organization. They must be professional in appearance and demeanor. They must earn the respect of the administration and their fellow managers, as well as rank-and-file employees. The best way to accomplish this is to educate everyone in how security can help them with their day-to-day activities.

As health care budgets shrink, the security department, in order to survive, must become more integrated into the mainstream of hospital operations. The department must take on more tasks. A "leaner and meaner" approach to budgeting is necessary. Now is the time to rethink old assumptions: if we are doing a task because "that's the way we've always done it," maybe we are not doing it the best way. Challenge the line security officers to rethink the processes of protection: can we provide the same outcome—a safe and secure campus—using more efficient and effective methods?

More and more, security directors must start viewing themselves as in-house consultants. They are paid and recognized for their knowledge and ability to accomplish goals and objectives. If they do only what is necessary to maintain the status quo, they are doomed to failure. The director must use the facility as a "laboratory" to experiment with new techniques and methods of protection. The constant challenge must be "How can I accomplish the same objective in a more efficient and effective method?" Of course, this challenge is always tempered by the commitment to serve the patient, who is the most important person in the facility.

HOSPITAL SECURITY TODAY

The current challenges in hospital security are defined by the concerns of CEOs, the standards developed by the Joint Commission, and OSHA guidelines.

CEOs and Security Issues

In 1990, the American Hospital Association, recognizing that hospital security issues were becoming more and more important, published *CEO Briefing on Key Security Issues*.[1] **The following primary security issues for hospitals were identified:**

- employee screening
- security staffing and training
- violence
- drug theft/tampering
- theft
- infant kidnapping
- outside threats

More and more CEOs are realizing that security is not just another non-revenue-producing department, costing the hospital money. They realize that, as public budgets shrink and crime increases, the private sector must provide its own security. In fact, a well-managed security department can even add to the bottom line through a reduction in theft losses, less turnover because of higher employee morale, and fewer negligence-related lawsuits.

Joint Commission Standards

In 1995, the Joint Commission on the Accreditation of Healthcare Organizations began implementing security standards under a new Environment of Care category, EC 1.4.[2] In response to these new standards, administrators started to review the need for an effective security program. The key word is "program." The accreditation criteria are based on outcomes, and while the security department is an important part of the security program, it is only part of the program. Building working relationships within a facility to reach a common goal is more vital than ever before.

OSHA Guidelines

The Occupational Safety and Health Administration recently established guidelines for the prevention of violence in health care facilities.[3] Failure to follow these guidelines can lead to a fine under the General Duty clause of the OSHA regulations, for failure to maintain a safe and healthful workplace. The security director is responsible for ensuring that the facility adheres to these guidelines.

ORGANIZATIONAL MODELS FOR THE SECURITY DEPARTMENT

As we can see, there are numerous challenges facing the health care security director today, including accrediting criteria, federal legislation, and budget reductions. How can we meet these challenges and continually do more with less? Part of the answer lies in the organizational structure of the security department.

The security function can be performed via several different models. In the traditional model, all the employees of the security department were hospital employees. The Joint Commission requires only that the facility maintain a security program that meets its needs. In its accreditation standards, the Joint Commission outlines the basic concepts it considers to be minimal under the OSHA guidelines. The fulfillment of these standards is in many ways up to the facility. With this in mind, let's examine several organizational models.

Small Facilities (Fewer than 250 Beds)

In a small rural facility, the security function may be performed by members of the plant engineering staff. The staff's primary responsibilities would be to lock and unlock the facility at designated times, and perhaps to help the nursing staff restrain an unruly patient in the emergency department. In most cases, the plant engineering employees would receive no training in security practices and procedures. One step up from this arrangement would be to add a contract security officer to patrol the facility at night. Again, in most cases, the contract officer would not have received any formal training, and his or her primary responsibility might be to provide a security presence in the parking areas at shift change.

The same organizational model can be seen in many smaller urban and suburban hospitals, with one addition: in many cases, these facilities may also employ an off-duty law enforcement officer to be stationed in the emergency department during peak hours. This organizational model is shown in Figure 2–1.

Mid-Sized Facilities (250–450 Beds)

Depending on the location, most mid-sized facilities have at least one security officer on duty 24 hours a day, with some overlapping coverage during the late evening and nighttime hours. There is usually a security manager as well. In smaller facilities, this person may report to the plant manager; in larger facilities, the security manager usually reports to an assistant administrator. Smaller facilities often use a contract service for security officers, while the larger facilities tend to use in-house security officers. An off-duty law enforcement officer may be employed in the ED during peak hours.

In addition to having a security officer on each shift, facilities in this size range usually have a closed-circuit television (CCTV) system, and someone is designated to watch the screens and serve as a central dispatch for security service. These two organizational models are shown in Figure 2–2 and Figure 2–3.

Large Facilities (More than 450 Beds)

Most large facilities have a formal security program managed by a security director. Facilities with more than 450 beds tend to be located in larger urban areas, which normally dictate a comprehensive security program. In large teaching hospitals, it is not uncommon for the security department to resemble a small police department, and the security officers may indeed be sworn police officers with the authority to make arrests for crimes committed on the grounds of the facility. In addition, the department may have plainclothes investigators. Designated personnel are responsible for dispatch, CCTV, and any alarm functions.

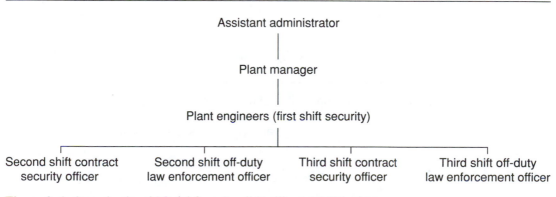

Figure 2–1 Organizational Model for a Small Facility (< 250 beds).

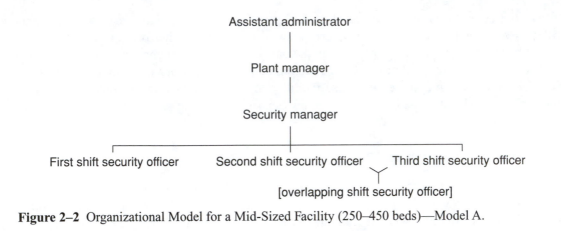

Figure 2–2 Organizational Model for a Mid-Sized Facility (250–450 beds)—Model A.

In many large departments, the director is also be responsible for the parking and transportation functions at the hospital. In large urban facilities, parking is not only a key function but may also be the source of a special set of security problems. The director may also supervise the hospital's safety officer. The organizational model for security in a large facility is shown in Figure 2–4.

OFF-DUTY LAW ENFORCEMENT

Many facilities use off-duty police officers in their security programs, especially in the emergency department. Some facilities even contract with these officers to, in essence, *be* their security department. In an urban medical center in a high crime area, it may be necessary to have an off-duty law enforcement officer in the ED; however, this level of security is not always required. In addition, most law enforcement officers are not trained to handle patient-related security issues. When there is a problem, they may react as they would on the street, and this response may not be appropriate or in the best interest of the facility or the patient. If it is extreme, it may make the facility vulnerable to a lawsuit.

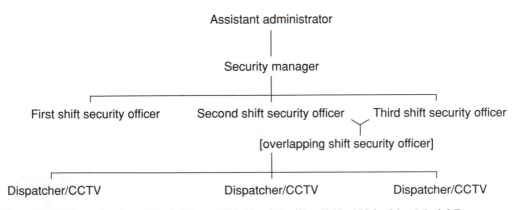

Figure 2–3 Organizational Model for a Mid-Sized Facility (250–450 beds)—Model B.

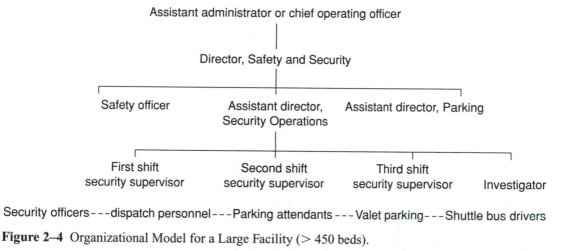

Figure 2–4 Organizational Model for a Large Facility (> 450 beds).

Another problem is inconsistent staffing. In most jurisdictions, off-duty law enforcement work is scheduled by a liaison officer who works for the law enforcement agency. The shifts are often filled on a rotating basis, which means the facility may have a different officer on every shift. All of these officers may not meet the orientation and safety training requirements of the Joint Commission.

If it is necessary to have a sworn officer in the ED, the company police option may serve the facility better.

COMPANY POLICE

Most states have a mechanism whereby the security department at a medical facility can apply to the state for a charter to become sworn law enforcement officers, with full arrest authority on the facility's property. This can be a lengthy process, and usually the security department must meet the state's hiring qualifications and process for sworn officers. This process may include a polygraph, lengthy background investigation, physical fitness test, and psychological screening. Once hired, the officer must complete a course at the law enforcement academy. The states vary greatly in the length of the academy, from three weeks to over six months. Thus, the investment in hiring and training a sworn officer can be substantial. And if the facility does not have a competitive pay scale, it will just become a training ground for the surrounding municipal law enforcement agencies: as soon as an officer finishes training, he or she will be hired by one of these agencies.

Again, the facility's management, along with its attorney, should determine whether the legal risks associated with having sworn officers outweigh the benefits.

IN-HOUSE VERSUS CONTRACT SECURITY

The debate over which is better—in-house or contract security—has been going on for many years, and there is no definitive answer. The facility must weigh many factors before deciding whether to develop an in-house program or turn to a vendor. Even in the current environment of cost containment, cost should not be the deciding or even the most important factor. However, since cost must be considered, the following can serve as a guide to compare the true costs of in-house and contract security.

In-House Security

Hiring: recruitment, advertising, interviewing, health screening, orientation.

Wages: salaries, yearly evaluations, merit increases, bonuses.

Uniforms: uniform and security patch design costs, costs of officers' uniforms. If the officers are responsible for purchasing their own uniforms, consider setting up an account with a local uniform shop so they can purchase the uniforms on a payroll deduction plan. The cost of a uniform can range from $200 to $350. The average starting wage for an in-house security officer is $7.50–$9.50 an hour, so asking someone to spend that amount at one time may turn a potentially good employee away.

Training: Who will train the officers? How much in wages and time will that cost you? (See Chapter 6 for more information on training.)

Management and supervision: Who will manage and supervise the officers? Who will write the policies and procedures? Who will follow up on their reports and investigate incidents? How will the department be structured and how many levels of supervision are needed?

Labor market: What is the current condition of the local labor market? Can you find quality staff? Can you realistically hire the part-time people you need, or will you be forced into overstaffing just to fill the necessary positions?

Contract Security

Hourly rate: What is the true hourly rate? For example, are you paying hidden charges such as overtime for "call-outs" (scheduled employees calling in sick)? Are you paying extra administrative charges to hire and train the contract officers? What is the premium (overtime) pay rate for holidays? Is there an add-on for emergency extra staff, and will they be trained to your specifications?

Officer pay rate: How much will the officers themselves be paid? Is it sufficient to attract and keep qualified officers? What is the average merit increase for the officers? Is the increase factored into the contract price in a multiyear contract?

Officer benefits: Is the contractor offering the officers a benefit program? If so, is it attractive enough to keep qualified officers?

Officer turnover rate: What has been the average turnover rate on comparable contracts? If an officer leaves, will you be charged overtime to fill the position until another candidate is hired and trained? If the expected turnover is higher than that of the facility, how will this affect the relationship between security and the rest of the organization?

Uniforms: Will the officer wear the contractor's uniform, or do you want the officer to wear your facility's uniform? If the latter, is there an extra charge for purchasing these uniforms? Some states have laws that prohibit contract officers from wearing any uniform other than that of the contractor, so be sure to clarify this point.

Guaranteed rate increases: Is there a guaranteed rate increase in subsequent years of a multiyear contract? If so, is this justified if the turnover is such that all or most of the officers are new? Will you be required to pay an increased hourly wage in the second year for officers who are recently hired and should be paid on the first-year scale?

OTHER FACTORS TO CONSIDER

As you can see, comparing the true cost differences between in-house and contract security, and factoring in the use of off-duty law enforcement officers or company police, is a complicated exercise. And remember, cost should not be the deciding factor.

For example, assume that a facility reviewed the costs of in-house and contract security, and chose the less expensive option, without regard for any other criteria. In security, as in most businesses, you get what you pay for. What happens if the facility is sued because of a negligent action of one of the officers or because of inadequate security (one of the fastest growing areas of litigation today), and the plaintiff's attorney asks, "On what basis did the facility choose its security program?" If the answer is, "We picked the cheapest one," how do you think the jury will vote?

You must consider other factors besides cost when you set up a security program.

Security Survey

A good place to start is with a security survey. As the facility exists today, what security threats are present? What is the current level of security? A comprehensive survey can help determine the level of security the facility needs (see Chapter 3 for further discussion).

Expectations for Security

Do you want the security staff to be a professionally trained department, able to serve as a deterrent and trained to respond to critical situations? Or do you want the department to simply be a set of eyes and ears whose job is to call the local police for each and every incident? Do you want a security department that is a public relations department at heart? Or do you want a security department that can be of greater value to the organization by not only protecting patients, visitors, and staff but also helping to investigate thefts and tort actions, deal with employee misconduct, and conduct background investigations? Security can only function at its highest level of competence if the goals and objectives of the department are clarified by top management. The administration's expectations for security should be set down in writing before any decisions are made concerning the structure of the department.

Type of Security

Is the facility going to depend on a large complement of security officers and very little electronic equipment to assist them? Or will the facility install a state-of-the-art security system and depend on a minimal number of officers? While electronics should be part of the security program, the presence of a well-trained, physically fit, professional security officer makes employees feel safest and is the best deterrent to crime.

Uniform Type

Should the officers wear a military-style uniform or should they adopt a "softer" look, such as a blazer and slacks? This may depend on the crime rate in and around the facility. If the officers will encounter many confrontational situations, the military look may be better; if they will be working mainly inside the facility and functioning primarily in a public relations mode, then the blazer is better. What are the year-round weather conditions? If the climate is extreme—either very hot or very cold most of the year—and the officers will be outside, the blazer will probably not work.

COMBINATION SYSTEMS

We have reviewed the traditional models of the security department. Historically, facilities have either been exclusively in-house or exclusively contract. However, in recent years, several spin-off concepts have appeared and are gaining favor. The idea of integrating in-house and contract staff, while not a new one in most other fields, is fairly new in health care security. Combination systems can function in several different ways.

In-House Manager and Supervisors, Contract Staff

In this model, manager of the security function (either the plant manager or the security manager) and his or her assistants are in-house employees. They set the training standards, review officer performance, and determine work schedules. The contract company simply furnishes the officers. In some cases, the facility installs a separate time clock for the officers to use, thereby eliminating the need for them to contact the contractor for time and attendance purposes. In this model, the contract officers may even wear the facility uniform, badge, and security patch.

The officers are responsible to their in-house supervisors on a daily basis. The supervisors—with input from the facility's in-house manager—evaluate the performance of the officers and make recommendations for their wage increases. These increases are reviewed by the security manager and the contract liaison manager to determine how much the increases will affect the hourly billing rate. If the increases are within the predetermined contract price, no further review is necessary. In most cases, the officers can receive the increase without any difficulty.

If the wage increase is outside the limits of the contract, three things may occur: (1) the increase is reduced so it is within the contract limits; (2) the contract company agrees to the increase and accepts a lower profit margin to cover it; (3) the facility agrees to raise the contract rate to accommodate the pay increase. If the facility has received good service from the contract, it will usually agree to cover the increase; however, if the contractor has performed poorly, the facility may elect to rebid the contract.

In-House Manager, Contract Supervisors and Staff

This concept is similar to the previous one, with one critical difference: the supervisors of the officers are employees of the contract service. This arrangement frees the facility from daily supervision, but there is a trade-off. During normal business hours, the in-house manager of the security function is in charge, but after hours, the facility is relying on contract supervisors to maintain quality control of the security program and, indirectly, of the image and reputation of the facility itself. Unfortunately, some contractors fall short. The desire to increase the vendor's profit sometimes pushes contract supervisors to work with unskilled officers or to "let things slide" after hours. While this is not always the case, a strong in-house security manager is required to stay on top of the program. The manager should be in close contact with other after-hours in-house managers and supervisors who can keep him or her informed of situations in the security program that may need attention.

Mix of In-House and Contract Officers

Some facilities have tried to blend in-house and contract officers in the same department. Unless there is a clear difference in job functions and uniforms, these mixed programs do not work. The in-house officers are likely to receive more training, higher wages, and better benefits than the contract officers. This scenario usually leads to tension in the department, which can have demoralizing effects.

The concept is feasible if the officers work at separate facilities; for example, the in-house officers patrol the hospital and the contract officers are assigned to a medical office building. Still, strict guidelines must be in place that define the role of each officer. Should the contract officers serve as eyes and ears only and call the in-house officers to handle situations, or should the contract officers function as a stand-alone unit? Questions like this one must be answered before you attempt to use the combination model.

In-House Manager, Outside Consultant

This concept is gaining favor among small and some mid-sized facilities that cannot afford to hire a professional security director. In many cases, these facilities delegate the management of the security function to the plant manager or a security manager, which may be sufficient for managing the day-to-day activity of the department. However, these people may be managing several other departments as well, giving the security function only a fraction of their time, and in most cases they are not security professionals. This is a situation in which retaining a professional health care security consultant can have a major effect on the quality of the department, at a relatively low cost.

Typically, the consultant is used to help establish the department. He or she can help the facility decide on the best type of program. If a contract service is to be used, the consultant can draft the request for proposals (RFP) and review the submitted proposals. This is an extremely valuable function. The facility will not only save time in the bidding and review process, but it will know that an experienced professional is protecting its interests and ensuring that the contract bidders adhere to the RFP.

The consultant should oversee the implementation process, too. The contractor may agree to the terms of the RFP, but may make changes during implementation. The most common change is in training. The industry standard for training health care security officers is the Security Officer Basic Training Program offered by the International Association for Health Care Security and Safety (IAHSS). Most consultants will write this into the RFP, and the contractor will agree. However, many vendors are not familiar with the program or cannot fulfill the requirement because they do not have a qualified staff trainer. A consultant can handle this situation and ensure that the officers receive proper training.

After the program is implemented, the consultant should visit the facility on at least a quarterly basis to check on the program. The consultant should always be available by telephone to help resolve operational issues, draft policies and procedures, and act as a professional resource on health care security.

By using a consultant, the facility can tap into a higher level of professional expertise without the expense of employing a professional security director. The following example shows the cost savings in this model.

Professional security director

Salary $55,000–$75,000
Benefits (28%) $15,400–$19,600
Total first year cost $70,400–$94,600

(Remember, this is only the first year; the cost will increase each year with salary increases.)

Security manager

Salary $35,000–$45,000
Benefits (28%) $9,800–$12,600
Total first year cost $43,800–$57,600

Add to this the cost of a consultant, at an average of $1,200 per day for 20 days and expenses of $150 per day.

Consultant costs $27,000
Cost of consultant and security manager, first year $70,800–$84,600

As the program develops and the security manager gains experience, the consultant's time on-site can be reduced. At this point the facility will save at least $10,000–$15,000 per year and still be able to maintain a professional security program. It is not surprising that this concept is gaining in popularity.

STAFF SIZE

This subject is always an issue. Security directors/managers and administrators inevitably struggle with the question of how many security officers the facility needs. The answer to the question is as varied as the facilities. Some managers attempt to use the number of beds (for example, one security officer per shift for every 200 beds); some use the size (square feet) of the facility; and some use the number of employees. None of these gives a true picture of security needs. **Professional security experts recommend that a comprehensive security survey be completed to determine the correct staffing level for a facility. The survey would include the following key indicators:**

- *Bed size:* average census per day and number of visitors per day.
- *Facility size:* number of square feet, not only inside the facility but in the parking areas as well. (If parking decks are used, calculate all levels of deck and driveways, because these areas must be patrolled also.)
- *Security history:* How many and what kinds of incidents have occurred at the facility within the past 24 months? Is there a pattern as to when they occurred? Has the number of incidents increased?
- *Emergency department visits:* Is the hospital a trauma center or a community hospital, and, if so, how does this affect the types of cases seen in the ED? How busy is the ED, and what are the peak patient load times? What kinds of incidents have occurred in the ED in the past?
- *Outpatient procedures:* peak time for these procedures, including times that patients are admitted and discharged.
- *Crime rate:* What is the crime rate by type within a 1½-mile radius of the facility?
- *Gang activity:* Does the area have a gang problem?
- *Local police response time:* How quickly do the local police respond? Does it vary by time of day?
- *Parameters/comprehensiveness of the security program:* What type of program does the facility expect? What is the mission statement of the security department? What level of protection is needed to maintain a reasonably safe environment? What are the community and national norms for a similar facility?

PROFESSIONAL GROWTH

The only way to be effective and survive in the changing environment of health care security is with a highly educated, well-trained staff. The security officers of today are not high school dropouts who have chosen security because they cannot get a job doing anything else. An officer must be able to communicate effectively with people from all levels of society and work efficiently with little or no supervision. This is only possible if the officer is educated and properly trained. The IAHSS has excellent basic security, safety, and security supervisory training programs. The Professional Security Television Network offers basic and monthly training programs specifically designed for health care facilities.

Not only must today's security directors possess technical skills, they must have a background in management. Most directors have at least a bachelor's degree, and many have graduate degrees. The security director must continue to learn and keep abreast of new developments. The IAHSS has an excellent professional credential program leading to the designation Certified Healthcare Protection Administrator.[5] The American Society for Industrial Security offers a Certified Protection Professional program that has long been recognized as a security industry standard of excellence.[6] And the Security Management Institute (SMI) has a unique credentialing service that allows the security director to take certification examinations any time, anywhere in the world. In addition, SMI offers specialization exams in many areas, including one leading to the designation Certified Healthcare Security Executive.[7]

These are challenging times for anyone with the responsibility for security in the health care environment. Today's security managers will find themselves inventing new methods and practices and becoming truly part of the health care management team. To fulfill this role effectively, they must stay up to date on the ever-changing environment of health care security.

KEY POINTS

- The mission statement of the security department should be consistent with that of the facility: assist medical staff, provide a safe and secure environment, enforce corporate policies, maintain peace.
- The security director's job has changed: he or she must be a professional manager and must become integrated into the mainstream of the organization.
- Hospital CEOs are becoming more concerned about security issues.
- The Joint Commission and OSHA address security in standards and guidelines.
- The security department can be structured in a variety of ways: in-house, contract, or a combination.
- A comprehensive security survey is necessary to determine security program functions and staff size.
- An outside consultant can save money for a facility by developing the security program and being available to resolve problems.
- The security professional must continue to learn and earn professional certification.

REFERENCES

1. American Hospital Association, CEO Briefing on Key Security Issues (Chicago: AHA, 1990).
2. Joint Commission on the Accreditation of Healthcare Organizations, Comprehensive Accreditation Manual for Hospital (Oakbrook Terrace, IL: Joint Commission, 1996), EC 1.4.
3. Occupational Safety and Health Administration.
4. Joint Commission, 1996.
5. International Association for Healthcare Security and Safety, P.O. Box 637, Lombard, IL 60148.
6. American Society for Industrial Security, 1625 Prince Street, Alexandria, VA 22314.
7. Security Management Institute, 11706 Battery Place, Charlotte, NC 28273.

Chapter 3

The Security Audit

CHAPTER OBJECTIVES

1. Understand the difference between a security survey and a security audit.
2. Know the why, when, who, what, and how of audits.

INTRODUCTION

Consider the following situations:

- The 1999 Environment of Care standard EC 1.4 of the Joint Commission on the Accreditation of Healthcare Organizations[1] states that the facility, in its security management plan, must control access to "sensitive areas" and provide a security orientation and education program that addresses processes for minimizing security risks for personnel in these areas. How does a facility determine which areas should be designed as sensitive? The standard also states that "The objectives, scope, performance, and effectiveness of the security management plan are evaluated annually." How is this appraisal completed?
- A hospital staff member was raped in the parking deck. She alleges that when she was preparing to get off work she called security and asked for an escort to her vehicle. She was told that, because of a downsize in staffing, there was not an officer available to escort her to her vehicle at that time. She was told that an officer would be available in approximately 45 minutes. She decided to walk to her car alone, since the campus was covered by a closed-circuit television (CCTV) system. She did not know that the monitors were not being scanned by a person; they were just videotaped. What is the liability of the hospital?
- A charge nurse tells the security director that her unit frequently has trouble balancing the narcotic inventory at shift change and asks for help with this problem.

Each of these situations calls for a security survey or audit. They are not the same thing. A survey is an overview of the existing security program based on current industry norms. An audit uses the same standards as a survey but goes into much more detail. An audit is more operationally oriented and more comprehensive.

For example, a survey may determine that the facility has 2.8 full-time equivalents (FTEs) assigned to security per shift. The person or organization conducting the survey reviews security-related incidents and crime statistics in the area and talks with security personnel at other hospitals of similar size. The survey determines that this staffing level is correct for the facility.

An audit would include a task analysis of the duties of the officers, their educational and experience backgrounds, and the facility training program. In the example above, 1.4 FTEs were posted in the emergency department, with strict orders not to leave the area. The other 1.4 FTEs also served as part-time maintenance workers for the facility. Of the 2.8 FTEs allotted per shift, the task analysis showed that one officer was posted at the ED and therefore unable to patrol the facility, while the other 1.4 FTE assigned to the shift spent 50 percent of her time conducting engineering control (boiler, chiller) checks. Therefore, at any given time on the shift, security was proactively patrolling the facility no more than 25 percent of the time. The security audit shows that the staffing level is too low for the facility if 50 percent of the security officers are posted in a fixed location and the other 50 percent spend half of their time doing nonsecurity tasks.

Surveys and audits are both valuable tools. If a cursory view will provide the information needed to make a decision, a survey will probably suffice. If more details are required—for example, for such things as security program evaluation, litigation, or new program assessment—then an audit is needed. **The following questions will help you determine whether you need an audit, who should perform it, and how it should be done.**

- WHY conduct an audit?
- WHEN should an audit be performed?
- WHO should conduct the audit?
- WHAT areas should be reviewed?
- HOW will the audit be performed?

WHY CONDUCT AN AUDIT?

Regulation

The Joint Commission requires that an audit be conducted annually to assess the effectiveness of the security program. In the first or baseline audit, answer all questions in a straightforward manner. This is no time to hide any flaws in the system. Likewise, expand on the positive aspects of the program. After the original audit has been completed, the security director, with input from the Environment of Care Committee (formerly the Safety Committee), can measure performance every year as required by the standard. However, the Joint Commission requirement is only one reason to conduct an audit.

Litigation

A serious security incident and/or the possibility of a lawsuit signals the need for an audit. In the case of the staff member who was raped in the parking deck, staffing levels would be reviewed, a task analysis would be conducted, and a review would be conducted of the incident management process, officer hiring requirements, orientation and ongoing training programs, level of supervision of officers, and competence of the supervisors.

New Program Needs

The initiation of a new program at the facility also should trigger an audit. Does the new program have special security requirements? For example, after-hours Lamaze classes may require special parking arrangements. Will security unlock and relock classrooms? All new programs should be reviewed for security needs in the developmental stages, so that input from the security director can help the new program director decide on locations and make informed decisions about operational and supervision concerns. A tragic example of what can happen if security's input is not received was the case of a hospital in the Midwest that began new prenatal classes in an older, seldom-used office building owned by the hospital. On the first evening of classes, one of the couples attending was robbed and the husband shot. Had the prenatal program director checked with security, she would have learned that the reason the building was seldom used was because it was in an extremely high crime area, where drug selling and robbery were common.

All programs should be reviewed at least annually to ensure that their security needs are being met. Processes may have changed, hours of service altered . . . there are many factors that can change the security requirements of a program.

Changes in the Environment

Any time that the facility becomes aware of a specific threat to patients, visitors, staff, or property, an audit should be conducted of the affected area. For example, if the emergency department has recently begun seeing an increase in the number of gang-related injuries, this situation should prompt an audit of the emergency department and security staffing.

WHEN SHOULD AN AUDIT BE CONDUCTED?

Security Incidents

Any time there is a significant security incident, or a "near miss," an audit should be conducted. For example, a gang member who has been shot is brought by ambulance to the ED. While he is being treated, rival gang members arrive and demand to "see" the patient. Security intercedes and the rival gang members leave. Although the incident was handled, the situation could easily have became violent. This kind of near miss would necessitate an audit.

Specific Urgent Needs

Another situation that would trigger an audit is when the facility becomes aware of a possible threat. Suppose a supervisor calls security and tells them that one of her employees is having domestic problems. She explains that the employee's spouse has threatened to come to the facility and kill the employee. The supervisor tells security that she believes the employee has brought a gun to work and has it in her locker. After security handles the problem, an audit should be conducted of security support policies. Does the facility have a resource for threatened employees, such as an Employee Assistance Program? Does the facility have a policy that allows security to search employees' lockers with or without their permission? Is there a violence-in-the-workplace policy and procedure?

WHO SHOULD CONDUCT THE AUDIT?

There are basically three options for who should conduct the security audit: (1) the facility's security director, (2) an outside consultant, or (3) a combination, with the consultant directing the overall audit, assisted by the security director and other key members of the organization. **The following are the pros and cons of each option.**

Security Director Conducts Audit

Pros

- Low cost.
- Knows the layout of the facility.
- Knows the culture of the facility.
- Has experience handling incidents at the facility and knows where they occur.
- Knows the strengths and weaknesses of the security staff and the level of cooperation they receive from other departments.

Cons

- May not be able to "see the forest for the trees."
- Operational security problems may have been caused by the director.
- May not be candid about the weaknesses of the security department.
- May not be experienced enough to know how to conduct an operational audit.
- May tend to focus blame on other departments rather than analyzing data and solving problems.

Outside Consultant Conducts Audit

The "outside consultant" may be a fellow security director at another facility or a professional health care security consultant. The key is to get a set of "fresh eyes" to look at your facility, someone with knowledge and experience and whose opinion can stand the test of legal scrutiny if necessary.

Pros

- Has the experience to conduct the audit in a complete, unbiased manner.
- Has had experience with many facilities and can suggest solutions that have already worked elsewhere.
- Has a resource file of policies and procedures that can be adjusted to fit the particular needs of your facility.

- Is a certified security professional: Certified Protection Professional (CPP), Certified Security Executive (CSE), or Certified Healthcare Protection Administrator (CHPA); these certifications give the findings of the audit more validity; they would be considered the opinion of an expert in court.
- Can conduct the audit in a truly objective manner, because he or she is not involved with facility politics in any of the departments that might be involved.
- Is not offended if suggestions are not adopted, is there to gather and analyze data and to suggest solutions to problems.
- Serves the facility without particular alliances. For example, one facility that used contract security officers wanted to add CCTV in its parking areas. The plant engineer, who supervised security, asked the contract security company to secure bids for the job. All the bids were in the $150,000–$175,000 range. Later, the plant engineer contacted a professional security consultant to conduct an audit of the security department. The consultant also was asked to review the CCTV bids. The consultant was able to design a system of CCTV and audio security for $30,000 less than the lowest bid, a savings that more than paid for the consultant.

Cons

- Higher cost. Most professional security consultants charge from $1,200 to $1,500 per day plus expenses. The facility will pay $5,000–$7,000 for an audit, plus ordinary travel expenses.
- The consultant may not be experienced enough to conduct the audit. Check for certifications!
- The consultant may be proficient only in the management of a security department, not a security program. When you interview consultants, ask operational questions and listen to the answers. Ask consultants about innovative programs they initiated or have seen in other facilities.
- If the consultant is working alone, the audit may take longer to complete, which means a higher consulting charge.
- The consultant may have a hidden agenda. Many sales representatives for security companies that sell guard and patrol services or electronic security systems call themselves "consultants." In fact, they are simply looking for ways to sell services and/or equipment.

Combination Audit

This kind of arrangement—in which the consultant, security director, and other department managers take active roles in the audit—can be both effective and efficient. The consultant provides a series of self-audit questionnaires to the facility. The consultant should allow at least two weeks for the departments to complete the questionnaire and should emphasize that the answers should accurately describe what is being done in the department, even if that conflicts with existing policy. The facility completes the questionnaires and returns them to the consultant, who reviews them before he or she visits the facility. This gives the consultant a better idea of what to focus on.

The consultant should take a tour of the overall facility and visit each department that completed an audit questionnaire. Visits should also be made during the second and third shifts to look for any discrepancies in policies and procedures that may affect the security of the facility. After the on-site visits are completed, the consultant should hold a roundtable discussion with the affected departments. At the roundtable, each department should receive a copy of the consultant's recommendations. A date should be set to reaudit the facility to review progress.

Pros

- Less expensive than having the consultant complete the audit questionnaires.
- More input from the organization, therefore increasing awareness.
- Participation increases security awareness throughout the facility.
- Less disruptive to the organization, because the consultant would probably be on-site only one to three days.

Cons

- The departments may be less than candid in completing the audit forms. However, an experienced consultant should be able to spot inconsistencies and vague answers.
- While less expensive than having the consultant conduct the audit alone, this method still costs more than an in-house audit.
- Completing the self-audit forms at the departmental level takes time away from patient care.

WHAT SHOULD BE AUDITED?

In addition to the examples given earlier in the "WHY" section of this chapter, additional audits should be preformed at least annually, including the following:

- Any department that shows a significant increase in security-related incidents should be audited. Has there been a change in the patient population? Has there been a change in supervision or staffing levels?
- Critical or sensitive areas should be reviewed at least every six months. Keep in mind that sensitive areas are determined by the overall facility audit and may change from time to time.
- Whenever new construction or renovation takes place, the areas affected should be audited.

HOW SHOULD THE AUDIT BE CONDUCTED AND THE INFORMATION USED?

Once the decision is made to conduct an audit, the decision should be communicated throughout the facility. Stress the fact that completing an audit is a proactive way to preventing security-related problems. Publishing the upcoming audit will also increase security awareness.

The audit process should employ some form of checklist or key point indicators similar to the Joint Commission survey. In addition to reviewing the completed audit form, the auditor(s) should interview staff. Ask how they complete a function and check to see what the written policy is on the subject. In many cases, there will be a variance. Remember, what is actually done IS the policy, regardless of what is written.

During the audit, make sure to include a thorough review of key policies and procedures. When was the last time a policy/procedure was reviewed? Is the policy still correct? Are new policies needed? Make sure that local as well as industry standards are reviewed in relationship to what is done at the facility. If there is a difference (for example, lower standard of care), can the facility defend its position? Lack of money is not a defense.

CONCLUSION

Conducting a comprehensive security audit is not a simple task. Determining who will conduct the audit is critical. The person in charge of the audit should be considered an expert in the field. In smaller facilities, where the plant engineer also manages security, this expertise is even more important. The facility is going to be held to the same standard of care as a facility with a full-time security director. In this case, the facility would be wise to consider an outside consultant's assistance.

Once the audit is completed, the recommendations must be distributed, reviewed, and discussed, and a time line for improvement established. At the end of that period, the facility should conduct another audit, closely reviewing the areas needing attention as established in the first audit. Have all deficiencies been corrected? If not, is there a valid reason? (Being busy is not a reason.) For uncorrected deficiencies, is there a plan for correction and a time line for completion?

Conducting a security audit can be the first step in ensuring a secure environment for all concerned. It can be time-consuming and costly, but it can help the facility identify and correct weaknesses. Done correctly, the security audit is the best method of establishing a quality security program.

KEY POINTS

- Security audits are more detailed than security surveys.
- A security audit should always be conducted
  –after a major security incident
  –after a near miss
  –when a new program is established
  –as soon as the facility becomes aware of a specific problem
- A professional security consultant should either perform the audit or work in conjunction with the on-site security director/manager.
- The entire facility should be audited annually to identify security problems.
- Sensitive areas are determined by the audit.

REFERENCE

1. Joint Commission on the Accreditation of Healthcare Organizations, *Comprehensive Accreditation Manual for Hospitals* (Oakbrook Terrace, IL: Joint Commission, 1996), EC 1.4.

Chapter 4

The Security Management Plan

CHAPTER OBJECTIVES

1. Understand the emergence of standards for security.
2. Know where to locate the Joint Commission on Accreditation of Healthcare Organizations standards for security.
3. Know the requirements for security under the Joint Commission standards.
4. Understand the various components of a security management plan.
5. Have reviewed several different types of security management plans.

INTRODUCTION

Despite its critical role in safeguarding patients, visitors, staff, and facility assets, security has been largely unregulated in the health care industry. In the past, the standards for the security program were pretty much left up to the individual administrator of the facility. If the administrator was pro-safety/security, the facility usually had a good program; if the administrator viewed security as a necessary evil, something the insurance carriers required, the program was usually little more than a night watchman. Even administrators who were very security conscious did not have a clear set of guidelines describing what was needed in a security program. In most cases, the administrator would hire a retired police officer as the chief of security, assuming that the person's previous employment provided the necessary understanding to develop and manage a successful department.

In some cases this worked, but in many cases the security department fell short in being able to integrate security principles into the health care setting. Even if the chief understood the dynamics of health care security, it was often difficult to get enough support from the organization to implement a good program. Part of the problem was that, before 1995, no regulatory body stated that a health care facility must have an active security department and a plan to address security issues. In such a highly regulated industry as health care, administrators tend to wait for a regulation (or a lawsuit) before they address an issue. As the need to protect patients, visitors, and staff grew more obvious, standards emerged.

In 1995, the Joint Commission issued a very weak standard on security in health care facilities. The standard basically stated that the facility should have a security program that met its

35

needs. What did that mean? It was anyone's guess. In 1996, with the assistance of the International Association for Healthcare Security and Safety (IAHSS), the Joint Commission adopted more specific standards for security. These standards are found in the Environment of Care section of the *Comprehensive Accreditation Manual for Hospitals.*[1] This section is reprinted in its entirety below, after which each standard is discussed.

Standard EC 1.4: A management plan addresses security.*

Intent of EC 1.4

A security management plan describes how the organization will establish and maintain a security management program to protect staff, patients, and visitors from harm. The plan provides processes for:

a. leadership's designation of personnel responsible for developing, implementing, and monitoring the security management plan;
b. addressing security issues concerning patients, visitors, personnel, and property;
c. reporting and investigating all security incidents involving patients, visitors, personnel, or property;
d. providing identification, as appropriate, for all patients, visitors, and staff;
e. controlling access to and egress from sensitive areas, as determined by the organization; and
f. providing vehicular access to urgent care areas.

In addition, the plan establishes

g. a security orientation and education program that addresses:
  1. processes for minimizing security risks for personnel in security sensitive areas;
  2. emergency procedures followed during security incidents; and
  3. processes for reporting security incidents involving patients, visitors, personnel, and property.
h. performance improvement standards that address one or more of the following:
  –Staff security management knowledge and skills;
  –Level of staff participation in security management activities;
  –Monitoring and inspection activities;
  –Emergency and incident reporting; or
  –Inspection, preventive maintenance, and testing of equipment.
i. emergency security procedures that address
  1. actions taken in the event of a security incident or failure,
  2. handling of civil disturbances,
  3. handling of situations involving VIPs or the media, and
  4. provision of additional staff to control human and vehicular traffic in and around the environment of care during disasters; and
j. how an annual evaluation of the security management plan's objectives, scope, performance, and effectiveness will occur.

---

*Source: © Comprehensive Accreditation Manual for Hospitals. Oakbrook Terrace, IL: Joint Commission on Accreditation of Healthcare Organizations, 1996, pp. 12–13 and 346. Reprinted with permission.

ANALYSIS OF EC 1.4

Intent of EC 1.4

A security management plan describes how the organization will establish and maintain a security management program to protect staff, patients, and visitors from harm.

The language provides us with some of the words necessary to write the security department's mission statement: "establish," "maintain," "program to protect." In addition, the word "processes" indicates that security must be a systems approach: security does not mean only the security department, it is the responsibility of everyone in the organization.

a. leadership's designation of personnel responsible for developing, implementing, and monitoring the security management plan.

The CEO or chief operating officer (COO) must designate the security function to a particular entity. This entity can be a person or a department, but the organizational structure should show a line of authority from the entity in charge of security to the CEO or COO. This designation is usually handled through an executive order issued to all departments in the organization.

b. addressing security issues concerning patients, visitors, personnel, and property.

What is a "security issue"? In most facilities, security issues are more than just criminal offenses. While protection is one of the key components of the security mission statement, there are other service issues as well, such as traffic control, lost and found, and courier services. Additional security issues, in both the protection and service areas, are usually discovered during the security audit.

c. reporting and investigating all security incidents involving patients, visitors, personnel, or property.

An educational and procedural process must be in place to let staff know how to report security problems and incidents. Staff should be made aware that they need to report potential as well as actual incidents. For example, the fact that some of the lights in the parking deck are out could create a security problem.

In addition, the standard means that security incidents must be investigated. The types of security incidents, their frequency, and any follow-up must be reported to the Environment of Care Committee (formerly the Safety Committee) at least quarterly.

d. providing identification, as appropriate, for all patients, visitors, and staff.

Facilities should issue photo name badges to all employees. All patients should wear identifying name bracelets.

In addition, a process should be in place to identify all other personnel who are frequently on the property for business purposes. For example, vendors should be required to check in at the materials management department and be issued a vendor pass, good only for the day stamped. Contractors should require all laborers to wear their company name badges. Most facilities identify visitors as all others who are not identified in some manner.

e. controlling access to and egress from sensitive areas, as determined by the organization.

"Sensitive areas" are determined by the security audit, but the designation is one that may change often. Certain departments are usually considered sensitive by virtue of their activity and inherent security threats; for example, the pharmacy, maternity center, emergency department, and psychiatric unit. Or an area may become sensitive if security problems occur; for example, a sudden rash of vehicle break-ins would make a parking lot a sensitive area.

How does the facility manage pedestrian, vehicular, visitor, or staff flow into and out of the sensitive areas? What is used—a card access system, lock and key, signs, gates on the parking lots?

f. providing vehicular access to urgent care areas.

Is there a mechanism in place for routing both public and emergency vehicles into and out of the emergency department?

What is included in this mechanism—gates, signs, road striping?

In addition, the plan establishes

g. a security orientation and education program that addresses:

1. processes for minimizing security risks for personnel in security sensitive areas:

All employees should be introduced to the facility's security department function during employee orientation. Employees who work in sensitive areas should receive additional orientation to the possible security risks, as well as updates at least every six months on how to prevent security incidents and how to respond to them if they occur.

2. emergency procedures followed during security incidents;

What should an employee do during a bomb threat or hostage situation? What happens if there is severe civil disturbance? These are some of the types of policies and procedures that must be addressed.

3. processes for reporting security incidents involving patients, visitors, personnel, and property.

Staff, patients, and visitors must know how to report incidents. The patient information booklet should include the telephone number of the security department, and signs with this number should be posted throughout the facility. If the facility has outside security alarm callboxes, they should be obvious to visitors and staff.

h. performance improvement standards that address one or more of the following:

–Staff security management knowledge and skills;

–Level of staff participation in security management activities;

Demonstrate that the person in charge of security is keeping up with the many changes in the industry. Who provides the security training, and are they qualified? How often are required training sessions held? Do staff members understand the security plan and the part they play?

–Monitoring and inspection of activities;

Most facilities rely on patrols and the use of closed-circuit television (CCTV) and access control systems to monitor security activities. In addition, monthly, quarterly, and annual security reports should be used to monitor trends in the security field.

–Emergency and incident reporting;

–Inspection, preventive maintenance, and testing of equipment;

How often are the emergency alarms tested? Are the burglar alarms tested frequently? Is there a preventive maintenance plan for the CCTV and access control systems? Are security officers tested frequently on the use of emergency equipment? (This means everything from firearms, if they are armed, to patient restraint devices, if they are called upon to assist in patient restraints.)

i. emergency security procedures that address
1. actions taken in the event of a security incident or failure,

Does the security department have a policies and procedures manual that addresses the actions to be taken not only for "normal" security incidents, such as petty theft, but in the event that some component of the security system fails? For example, the access control system in the nursery did not work and an infant was abducted. Is there a plan to coordinate activities to work with law enforcement in the investigation?

2. handling of civil disturbances,

Is there a plan for placing extra security officers on duty in the case of a civil disturbance? How will they be summoned? If the facility has only a small number of security officers, how will additional help be obtained? What precautions are in place to protect staff, such as home care workers, who are on duty in the community when the disturbance begins?

3. handling of situations involving VIPs or the media,

The facility should predetermine the inpatient rooms that can be used as VIP rooms. These rooms should be in an area where access can be easily controlled and should have adjacent rooms available for the use of the VIP's family and staff.

Is security always told when and where media briefings will occur? In the event of heavy media coverage, is security increased to ensure patient confidentiality and safety?

4. provision for additional staff to control human and vehicular traffic in and around the environment of care during disasters,

Can staff other than security be trained to help control the human traffic inside the facility? What part will the public relations department play in controlling the movement of the media? If a natural disaster occurs, where will the large number of visitors to the emergency department be kept? Is a procedure in place to secure the use of off-duty law enforcement officers to help control traffic and parking areas?

j. how an annual evaluation of the security management plan's objectives, scope, performance, and effectiveness will occur.

The security department must be able to show that standards have been established and that performance has been measured to those standards. The performance rating for each standard should also be noted. For example,

Standard: All security panic alarms are checked weekly.

Performance measurement: Review the weekly security activity log to see whether the alarms were checked.

If they were checked 26 times during the year, the performance rating for this standard is 50 percent.

Standard: All victims of crimes will receive a 24-hour and a 72-hour follow-up call after the incident to see if more information can be obtained or to further advise the victims of actions they need to take, such as canceling credit cards that were stolen.

Performance measurement: Check all victim-of-crime reports for follow-up. If the department has had 500 cases and the 24/72 follow-up was conducted on 450, the performance rating for this standard is 90 percent.

An annual security audit should be conducted to discover any new security risks and to follow up on the recommendations of the previous year's audit.

WRITING THE SECURITY MANAGEMENT PLAN

No specific format is required for the security management plan; however, the plan must cover all the sections mentioned above. **In summary, the plan should include the following elements:**

1. mission statement
2. assignment of responsibility for the security function
3. comprehensive policies and procedures to address the areas noted in standard EC 1.4
4. procedures for completion of a security audit
5. procedures for reporting security incidents
6. designation of sensitive areas and plan for controlling access
7. procedures for training and education of all staff, with special training for those working in sensitive areas
8. procedures for evaluating the security program, including performance improvement criteria

Mission Statement

The key to the security management plan is the mission statement. These statements vary in length, from a single sentence to several paragraphs. The security director should review the facility's overall mission statement and use it as a model for the security department statement. A typical security management plan would note that the role of the department is:

1. to assist the medical staff in rendering quality patient care
2. to provide a safe and secure environment
3. to enforce all applicable corporate policies and local, state, and federal laws

The key roles are listed in the proper order: (1) service, (2) prevention, and (3) enforcement.

Policies and Procedures

In establishing the plan, the security director should turn to existing policies and procedures. In many cases there will be policies/procedures already in place that sufficiently address the Joint Commission standards. These may be security department policies, other departmental policies, or facility policies. If they meet the Joint Commission standards, the director need only note, "See XXX policy, dated XX/XX/XX," and attach a copy of the policy in the appendix of the security management plan.

If existing policies and procedures are used in the security management plan, the security director must be sure that they are current. Too often the Joint Commission survey finds that that a policy was changed or deleted months, or even years, ago. **Make sure all policies and procedures used in the plan are current, especially those that address the security standards in EC 1.4.**

Scoring

In addition to EC 1.4, the security management plan should take special note of standard EC 2.3,[2] which reads as follows:

Scoring for EC 2.3

Has the organization implemented the security management plan described in EC 1.4?

Score 1   Yes
Score 2   The identified performance standards are not measured.
Score 3   Some
Score 5   No

Other Standards

Depending on the scope of the security department's service, it may need to address other Joint Commission standards, such as those for prisoner patients and life safety and fire drills.

Sample Security Management Plans

Appendixes 4–A, 4–B, 4–C, and 4–D show how some facilities have written their security management plans.

REFERENCES

1. Joint Commission on the Accreditation of Healthcare Organizations, *Comprehensive Accreditation Manual for Hospitals* (Oakbrook Terrace, IL: Joint Commission, 1996), EC 1.4.
2. Joint Commission, 1996, EC 2.3.

Appendix 4-A

Security Management Plan A

Hospital Name:

Subject: Security Management Plan   **Issued Date:**

Distribution: Environment of Care Manual

Originated by: Safety Officer   **Approved by:** Safety Committee

1.0 Introduction

The Security Management Program at _____ Hospital involves the coordinated efforts of the Safety Committee, the Security Department, the Engineering and Maintenance Department and all other departments within the hospital. Together, they strive to provide a safe and secure environment of care for all patients, staff, and visitors.

2.0 Mission

The life safety management program is designed to help ensure that the overall mission of _____ Hospital is achieved. This program ensures that the patients, visitors, and staff have a safe and secure setting for the provision of care.

3.0 Organization and Scope

The Safety Committee has the ultimate responsibility for the success of this program, which is administered by the director of engineering. The program's policies and procedures are designed to provide a method for protecting patients, personnel, visitors, and property from harm by including the following:

A. leadership's designation of personnel responsibility for developing, implementing, and monitoring the security management program
   (SEE POLICY #___)

B. addressing security issues concerning patients, visitors, personnel, and property
   (SEE POLICY #___)

C. reporting and investigating all security incidents involving patients, visitors, personnel, or property (SEE SECTION # 4.0 Security Incidents)

D. providing indentification, as appropriate, for all patients, visitors, and staff
(SEE POLICY #___)
E. controlling access to sensitive areas, as determined by the organization
(SEE POLICY #___)
F. providing vehicular access to urgent care areas
(SEE POLICY #___)
G. a security orientation and education
(SEE POLICY #___)
H. performance standards
(SEE POLICY #___)
I. emergency security procedures
(SEE POLICY #___)
J. requiring an annual evaluation of the objectives, scope, performance, and effectiveness
of the documented life safety management plan (SEE SECTION # 8.0 Annual Evalua-
tion)

4.0 Security Incidents

To ensure that the security status of this facility remains at the highest level possible, the
hospital has in place a mechanism for investigating and reporting all security incidents.

4.1 Investigating

An on-going life safety inspection and surveillance plan will be maintained. Any noted deficiencies will be fully investigated and an appropriate action plan developed. Any items that
require corrective action will be entered into the hospital's security plan for improvement
database (SEE TAB # _____ Hazard Surveillance).

4.2 Reporting

All life security deficiencies and actions taken will be reported to the Security Subcom-
mittee of the Safety Committee.

5.0 Orientation and Education

To ensure that the employees, medical staff, students, and volunteers are adequately prepared for dealing with security issues, the Safety Committee, in conjunction with other departments, provides initial and annual education programs to all agents of the hospital.
At a minimum, this educational program shall address the following:

A. processes for minimizing security risks for personnel in security-sensitive areas,
B. emergency procedures followed during security incidents, and
C. processes for reporting security incidents involving patients, visitors, personnel, and
property
(SEE TAB # ___ Orientation and Education).

6.0 Performance Standards

Performance improvement for the security management program is accomplished using data gathered through the hospital's hazard surveillance inspections and occurrence reports. The Safety Committee established one or more of the following as performance standards:

A. staff security management knowledge and skill
B level of staff participation in security management activities
C. monitoring and inspection activities
D. emergency and incident reporting procedures that specify when and to whom reports are communicated
E. inspection, preventive maintenance, and testing of security equipment

The Safety Officer analyzes these data and presents suggestions for improvement to the Safety Committee for approval (SEE TAB # ___ Performance Standards).

7.0 Emergency Procedures

_____ Hospital's security management program shall address as a minimum the following:

A. actions taken in the event of a security incident or failure
B. handling of civil disturbances
C. handling of situations involving VIPs or the media
D. provision of additional staff to control human and vehicle traffic in and around the environment of care during disasters

8.0 Annual Evaluation

To assist in the process of continuously improving and monitoring the security management plan, there will be an annual evaluation of the objectives, scope, performance, and effectiveness of the plan. The process is as follows:

A. The goal for the new year will be set during the annual review.
B. Participants in this review will include but are not limited to the director of engineering, the security director, the safety director, and key members of the Safety Committee.
C. The findings will be reported to the entire Safety Committee at its first scheduled meeting of the new year.
D. The evaluation will determine
   1. How the life safety management program has met its goals and objectives for the year (by comparing accomplishments with goals).
E. Whether the scope of the program should be expanded or diminished, including recommendation for changes (evaluation of accomplishments and potential).
F. Whether the monitoring of each performance indicator should be continued, changed, or deleted and a new indicator used (validity of current indicators).
G. Whether anything should be changed to enhance the effectiveness of the program (effectiveness of the program based on the performance indicators and in comparison with the previous year).

(SEE TAB # ___ Annual Evaluation)

Appendix 4-B

Security Management Plan B

I. MISSION STATEMENT

It is the mission of the security department of _____ Hospital system to provide for a safe and secure environment for employees, visitors, and patients. Toward this objective, it will be the goal of the security department and the responsibility of the director of security to provide not only for the protection of employees, visitors, and patients but also for the protection of their property and the property of the hospital.

II. AUTHORITY

The security department receives its authority from the Administrative Council of _____ Hospital System. The Administrative Council reports to the chief executive officer. The security department is given the authority to enforce hospital rules and regulations that provide for the safety and security of all personnel on hospital property.

III. ORGANIZATION

Security personnel patrol three primary _____ Hospital System campuses. The first campus is _____, which includes three office buildings, Professional Centers #1, #2, and #3. These professional centers house hospital administration, the education department, the marketing department, and numerous physicians' offices. _____ campus also includes a resident retirement home called _____ and an exercise and rehabilitation facility called _____.

The second campus is _____. This campus includes three office buildings, Professional Centers #4, #5, and #6, which house physicians' offices, the hospital human resources department, the billing collection department, the finance department, and the information systems department. The magnetic resonance imaging (MRI) facility is also located on this campus.

The third campus is called _____. This campus houses physicians' offices, the hospital newborn nursery, and women patient rooms and treatment facilities. It includes a three-story medical office building called Professional Center #7. It is also the site of the new hospital, which is under construction.

Security personnel perform mobile patrols of all three campuses 24 hours a day, seven days a week. Security officers staff the _____ 5:00 p.m. to 8:00 a.m., seven days a week.

These patrols are documented on security check log sheets, which include the date, time, and any observations the officer may have. This documentation includes but is not limited to those areas determined to be sensitive: the pharmacy, health information management (medical records), the emergency department (urgent care), ICU/CCU, nuclear medicine, and the operating/surgical areas. Access is controlled by staff assigned to the area. Security assistance is called when needed, in addition to regular checks. The security program includes access control policies and procedures for these sensitive areas.

In conjunction with and with the assistance of the City of _____ Police Department, security personnel also provide a response capability to those hospital facilities that are located off the three main campuses.

Security personnel report to their respective on shift/campus supervisors, who report to the director of security.

The security department reports to the coordinator of administrative services, who is a member of the Administrative Council, which reports to the chief operating officer and the chief executive officer. Between the coordinator of administrative services and the Environment of Care Committee, all security needs are addressed.

IV. RESPONSIBILITIES

It is the responsibility of the coordinator of administrative services to provide direct oversight of the security department. Oversight may also originate from the Administrative Council or the Environment of Care Committee.

The director of security reports on a regular basis to the coordinator of administrative services regarding security-related issues and concerns, and on a monthly basis to the hospital Environment of Care Committee.

The director of security and the three campus security supervisors meet on a regular basis to discuss issues and concerns relating to the uniformed security force.

The security officers on shift on all three campuses provide a number of services in addition to those basic to their primary responsibility of protecting life and property. Those services are outlined in campus security post instructions and security internal operating procedures.

Security officers, campus security supervisors, and the director of security meet on a regular basis to conduct training sessions and exchange information regarding security issues as they relate to the hospital. This is also an opportunity for officers and supervisors to discuss internal security issues with the security director.

It is the responsibility of all security personnel to ensure that their equipment is in good working order. Some equipment, such as the golf cart, is maintained by outside contractors. Other equipment is maintained on an as-needed basis by vendors. If equipment fails, the campus supervisor notifies the director of security, who coordinates repair with the appropriate vendor or the maintenance department.

V. IMPORTANT FUNCTIONS

Incident reporting and incident response are the primary functions of the security department. The management system revolves around these functions to accomplish the goal of protecting the hospital. Security patrols, building checks, routine investigations, and crime prevention methods are all employed by the security department. Security officers document all requests for service. Security officers perform initial investigations. Further investigatory functions are performed by the director of security and, when necessary, supplemented by the City of _____ Police Department.

Security incident reports are used to document significant events at the hospital, such as criminal activity.

Reporting of all criminal activity and other ancillary activity is done on a monthly basis to the Environment of Care Committee. Trends are identified to the committee and measures are taken when appropriate to prevent recurrence.

Trends are also monitored to compare them with the security department's annual performance improvement standards, goals, and objectives.

The escort service is also a major function that enhances the security of the hospital. The security escort service is conducted upon request 24 hours a day for patients, visitors, and employees. Its goal is to reduce victimization by creating a safe mode of travel on campus to those who feel threatened for any reason.

Another important security function is the immediate response to criminal activity and to potentially threatening situations. Supplementing security's response is the quick response of the City of _____ Police Department. Immediate responses by the security department and the police department help to achieve a safe environment.

In addition to security's response and incident reporting functions, it is responsible for opening and closing hospital facilities in the morning and evening, with checks in between. Security performs a variety of other services to employees, visitors, and patients.

Security officers offer to jump-start vehicles that owners cannot start. Officers provide a door-opening service for people who have locked their keys in their vehicle. Officers can also inflate flat tires so the driver can get to a service facility to get the tire repaired.

Security officers make frequent visits to the hospital pharmacies and laboratory facilities at the request of employees. Officers provide for the transportation of patients and employees upon request.

Officers on day shift perform parking enforcement based on administrative policy.

Officers assigned to the _____ on night shifts, when not performing patrol duties, are assigned to the emergency department. These officers maintain a safe and secure environment for the patients, visitors, and employees. The officers work closely with hospital personnel to monitor the security aspects of the ED areas. A key role for these officers is controlling violent, assaultive, and abusive patients or visitors. Radio communications are available to ED personnel when security officers are not physically present.

Officers assigned to the Women's Center on night shifts also perform receptionist duties when not actively performing building and door checks.

The security director offers personal safety classes to employees, designed to raise the level of security awareness while they are on hospital property. Crime prevention literature and classes are available on request. The security director is a regular contributor to the hospital employee newsletter, writing about security and crime prevention–related subjects. Incidents occurring at other health care facilities, both locally and nationally, are transmitted to employees as Security Briefs via the hospital LAN computer system. These briefs maintain the employees' security awareness.

The security director provides input on security-related concerns to nurse managers, department directors, and coordinators in various disciplines. This input is generally in procedure review or in the form of security surveys of a particular work area or facility.

Other areas of importance and concern to security are:

1. Patient valuables: The protection of patients' property is accomplished through the hospital's administrative policies and procedures. These measures afford protection for valuables brought into the environment of care by patients.

2. Providing identification: Identification is an integral part of the policies and procedures for security, and it is provided by several means at _____ Hospital System. All identification policies and procedures are contained in the security program.

Hospital personnel are provided either nametags or photographic identification, depending on their work assignment. Hospital human resources policies and procedures require that hospital-issued badges, regardless of type, be worn at all times while the hospital personnel are on duty.

Depending on the work area, the identification is enhanced to include certain prescribed clothing to differentiate employees in that area from other employees in the hospital. Identification may also include supplemental badging requirements, as in the case of the labor and delivery room and the nursery at the Women's Center.

Patients are provided with wristbands as part of their admission process into the hospital.

Visitors are not provided with any type of identification.

Vendors and contractors are provided with identification by the materials management and maintenance departments while they are on hospital property.

3. Providing access control: Access control is accomplished with designated procedures for the hospital on the three main campuses and its freestanding facilities.

Administrative policies and procedures provide for the control of access and egress between the hours of 9:00 a.m. and 6:00 p.m. Access to sensitive areas—such as the pharmacy, health information management, the emergency department, ICU/CCU, nuclear medicine, and the operating/surgical areas—is controlled by department employees with the assistance of security. Policies and procedures concerning these areas are contained in the security program.

Another means of controlling access is by providing guidelines for patient visitation to the hospital. Patient visitation regulations establish and govern visiting hours for the hospital. Intensive care units and Women's Center patient areas are addressed separately.

4. Vehicular access and traffic control to emergency service areas: The physical layout of the hospital and its various campuses provides vehicular access to these service areas. This access is maintained by regular security patrols 24 hours a day. Security officers assigned to the respective campuses have the primary responsibility for maintaining this access on a daily basis and in any emergency situation. The high priority of getting emergency vehicles into this area is coordinated through communication between ED personnel and the security officer on duty. When requested, the officer on duty can provide immediate traffic control, to include the resources of the environmental services department, the engineering department, and the police department.

5. Lost and Found: The security department operates the hospital Lost and Found 24 hours a day. Officers on duty can accept property that has been found or initiate incident reports concerning that has been reported lost. All found property is turned over to the director of security for storage.

V. TRAINING

As with all employees, security officers attend a formal orientation program instructed by the education department. The director of security attends and instructs all new hire employees at these orientation classes. The director disseminates information concerning routine and emergency security reporting procedures, crime prevention, and parking policies.

The education department has annual refresher training for all employees, including security officers.

Emergency procedures are reinforced to security officers during their field training officer program. Emergency procedures are published in all hospital phone directories for further reinforcement and easy reference. The hospital *Safety and Emergency Preparedness Manual* outlines tasks to be performed in the various departments in case of an emergency including security.

Additional emergency policies and procedures—including those for civil disturbances, hostage incidents, patient abduction, news media relations, and workplace violence—are contained in the security program.

Officers are tested in a variety of subject areas considered to be the basic tasks performed by security. The field training officer (FTO) program is facilitated by an experienced security officer or supervisor. Each officer is given a list of tasks which he or she is responsible for researching. Each task must be performed correctly in the identified manner before the officer can be signed off on that task. This list, with the signature of the officer/supervisor, becomes part of the officer's permanent training file.

The director of security assists in preparing department-specific policies and procedures related to security for various departments throughout the hospital when requested. The director also provides employees with security-related training, upon request.

Coursework in other subject areas is conducted on a regular basis with all officers, based on the need as it arises. This may include refresher courses on areas already instructed. Coursework is delivered by several different methods. If the subject is academic in nature, lectures with audiovisual aids are used, followed by testing to ensure understanding.

Other types of coursework require the student to demonstrate proficiency in the skill before he or she passes the subject or coursework.

_____

Director of Security

_____

Coordinator of Adminstrative Services

Appendix 4-C

(*Hospital Name*) Quality Assessment of Security Services for 1998

CONCLUSIONS

A. Based on an assessment of security for 1997, four recommendations were made: to improve documentation, the chain of command, training of new employees, and identifying officer competencies followed by training.

   1. After the implementation of a formal incident-reporting procedure, over 400 security incident reports were completed during 1998.
   2. A formal security management plan was written and distributed to all three campuses for dissemination to all security personnel as well as hospital department directors and nurse managers.
   3. The director of security sought a more active role with a physical presence in new employee orientation. This request was granted. The director now briefs all new employees on incident reporting, parking, sensitive areas, and current criminal activity within and around the hospital campuses.
   4. Competencies were identified that are required by security officers. Officers were trained in the use of pepperfoam and handcuffing techniques. Officers also received in-service training in state law, the use of force, hospital safety and emergency preparedness policies, and patient confidentiality.

RECOMMENDATIONS

   1. Initiate training for security officers in methods to deal with verbally and physically abusive individuals to increase their confidence in potentially volatile situations. Implement nonviolent crisis intervention training.
   2. Hold refresher sessions in 1999 on the use of force, pepperfoam, and handcuffing techniques.
   3. Increase crime prevention presence throughout the hospital system by dissemination of information and lectures.
      -Continue presence in new employee orientation/security training, targeting 100 percent of all new employees.
      -Reduce by 5 percent incidents of crime at the hospital.

-Reduce by 20 percent incidents of unlocked doors on evening/night shift.

ACTIONS

1. The director of security has initiated nonviolent crisis intervention training for security officers and all hospital employees. By the end of the first quarter of 1998, 28 persons will have been trained.
2. Refresher sessions for officers in the use of force, pepperfoam, and handcuffing are planned for the third and fourth quarters of 1998.
3. Guest lectures and the acquisition and dissemination of crime prevention information have already occurred as of the first quarter of 1998.

EVALUATION (through first quarter, 1998)

1. The initial response from the students in the nonviolent crisis intervention training has been positive, especially as it addresses handling physically abusive individuals. One department is scheduling special classes for all its employees.
2. At the end of the first quarter, annual refresher training in the skills identified above has yet to occur; however the fourth quarter is targeted.
3. As of the end of the first quarter, all employees in new hire orientation have received security training.

Appendix 4-D

Security Department Performance Improvement Project

PROBLEM

Security officers are called away from their interior and exterior building patrols to open doors for employees. Environmental Services is the organization that requests this service most often. Each office cleaned while it is not open for business has to be opened by security.

DISCUSSION

Suggestions were solicited from all security personnel as to how this service could be performed in a manner that would free the officer to accomplish uninterrupted patrols of hospital properties. The focus of the project was Environmental Services, since these employees were the primary users of this service from security.

There had been negative experiences in the past with issuing keys to Environmental Services employees. Office staff complained of unauthorized access after business hours, and there were other allegations.

DESIGN

It was suggested by one security officer that Environmental Services employees check out keys from the security officer on duty for the work area that they needed access to. If any problems arose in that area as a result of a complaint from office staff, security would simply check the log and see who checked the key out that day for that work area.

Log books were placed in the security office. Environmental Services personnel signed out keys at the beginning of their shifts and turned them in at the end. The same procedure was implemented on a smaller scale at other campuses. No change occurred at the Women's Center.

After consultation with administration and the Environmental Services department director, the new procedure was implemented.

MEASUREMENT

The director of security used the monthly shift activity report as the means to assess the success of the new procedure. Report data from previous months was compared with data from the month of July, to determine if fewer doors were being opened by security.

GOAL/OBJECTIVE

Reduce door openings by security officers.

RESULTS

Door openings on all campuses combined averaged 395 per month for the three months before implementation of the new process. In the first month the new process was implemented, this number was reduced by 155 door openings, or 57 percent. In the one campus in which the procedure was partially implemented, door openings were reduced by 26 percent from the previous month. The campus where the procedure was implemented on a larger scale experienced a 54 percent reduction from the previous month. The Women's Center experienced no change of any significance as the procedure was not implemented.

ASSESSMENT

It is apparent that implementation of the new process reduced the number of door openings in proportion to the extent to which it was implemented on the respective hospital campus: the more extensive the implementation, the more significant the reduction of door openings by security officers.

Chapter 5

Security Recordkeeping

CHAPTER OBJECTIVES

1. Understand the importance of accurate recordkeeping.
2. Appreciate how task analysis can increase productivity, reduce costs, and provide more efficient security.
3. Learn how to conduct a productivity study.
4. Learn how long to keep security documents.

INTRODUCTION

How important is proper recordkeeping and documentation? Consider the following three scenarios. What do they have in common?

Mid-Sized Hospital in an Urban Area

A security director receives a call from the risk manager and is informed that the risk manager has received a letter of complaint from a plaintiff's attorney. The letter states that the attorney's client was visiting a patient at the facility 11 months ago. During the visit, for no apparent reason, he was confronted by security, taken to the security office, questioned by security and police, then escorted off the property. The attorney informs the facility that it must agree to a pay a settlement to the plaintiff or he will sue the facility for damages for slander and false imprisonment. The risk manager asks the director to bring the report on the incident to her office so they can review it. Unfortunately, the security director can not locate any report about the incident. He is able to retrieve, through the payroll department, the names of the officers believed to have been on duty on the day in question. Unfortunately, the officers no longer work at the facility, and no one knows their whereabouts. If you were the risk manager, what would you think about the professionalism of the security director and the department?

Smaller Facility in a Suburban Setting

The facility is facing serious budget cuts, and each director has been asked to meet with the finance committee to justify the next year's budget for his or her department. The committee asks the security director to justify the number of full-time equivalents (FTEs) in the department. The director knows that the officers are always very busy and that current staffing levels are not only justified, they are actually too low. He says this to the committee, but he has no documentation to back up his statements. If you were on the committee, how would you vote on the security department's budget?

Large Facility Connected to a Medical School and University

The security director is conducting an officer's yearly evaluation. He has graded the officer "below average" on quantity of work. When the officer asks the director to explain the below-average rating, the director says that the officer "just doesn't look as busy as the other officers." The officer asks for a list of the criteria used in the performance rating. The director admits that no quantitative measures are used in the review, only the opinions of the director and the officer's immediate supervisor. The officer appeals his review to the vice president of human resources. If you were the vice president, what would you think?

Security directors encounter situations like these every day. They are learning that if they do not have good recordkeeping procedures and quantifiable methods for making decisions, those decisions may be questioned and in many cases overturned. The decisions the directors make are probably the correct ones, but without supporting documentation, they can not defend their actions.

They need to establish a "paper trail" that will support their actions. Security incident reports, shift reports, task analysis reports, reports to the safety committee, annual officer evaluations and job descriptions, and reports of investigations are just a few of the countless documents the director needs to evaluate and effectively manage the department. This chapter discusses various ways the director can increase the efficiency of the security department and quantify its needs for resources.

TASK ANALYSIS

When a consultant is called upon to review and analyze a security department, one of the most common concerns is that the security director believes the department is understaffed. In many cases, the director is correct, but he or she has no evidence to prove the point. However, in just as many cases the problem is not the number of employees assigned to the department but how they are used. Just as the facility conducts a security audit to determine its risks, the security department can conduct a task analysis to determine the most efficient and cost-effective method of staffing. What tasks do the security officers do? How long do the tasks take? How often are they performed? What competency level is required to do each task? How many hours are spent per week, month, and year performing a particular task? These are some of the questions that must be answered to efficiently manage a security function.

A task analysis looks at each part of a job—how it is performed and what type of training is needed to perform it. Each part of a job is a "mini-job" unto itself. For example, if you decide to wash your car, that is the job. The tasks for this job are getting the bucket ready, parking the car near the hose, washing the exterior, washing the interior, rinsing, drying, and waxing. In addition, each task can be divided further into subtasks.

For example, if the task is getting the bucket ready, the subtasks are deciding what kind of detergent to use, gathering the cloths and sponges, getting the bucket, and filling it with water. Every task in the job can be broken down into its subtasks. For the audit, you would also note the average time it takes to satisfactorily complete each task.

SAMPLE TASK ANALYSIS

A security officer is on patrol inside the facility. A visitor stops the officer and asks how to get to the admitting department. The officer escorts the visitor to the admitting department, then returns to his patrol. Similar requests are made of the officer four more times during the patrol. He completes seven patrol rounds; without any interruptions, he could have completed eight internal patrol rounds of the facility during his shift. (Facilities should be broken into patrol zones, each of which takes an average of 30–60 minutes to patrol.)

On the day we are examining, the officer is scheduled to work eight hours. There is always down time in calculating actual work time versus scheduled work time. Most management engineers assume that a person is actually working between 85 percent and 90 percent of a work shift. This is the target range for productivity. Down time includes personal time (making a phone call, using the restroom); fatigue (people do not work as quickly near the end of a shift because they are tired); and delay (waiting for an elevator, being stuck in traffic). On the day in question, the officer has 480 minutes (8 hours × 60 minutes) of scheduled work time. We expect him to work anywhere from 408 to 432 minutes.

The next assumption for our discussion is that we have timed—over a two-week period several times during the year—each task the officer performs. We know that the average time to stop a patrol, help someone locate a department in the facility, and return to the patrol is six minutes. On our review day, the officer helped five people locate areas of the facility and completed seven one-hour patrol rounds. Thus, the actual work completed by the officer was 30 minutes of assisting visitors and seven hours of patrol, for a total of 450 minutes and a productivity rate of 94 percent.

Productivity Rates

An officer's productivity rate can vary greatly even from one day to another, but the director is looking at department averages. The director may calculate—after reviewing all officers in the department on random days throughout the year—that the department's average productivity rate is 88 percent (within the average range of 85 percent to 90 percent). If one officer consistently performs at 78 percent, the director may want to counsel the officer to help him or her reach the average. Likewise, if the time standards are correct and one officer consistently achieves over 100 percent productivity, an inquiry should be made to make sure that the *quality* of the work performed is consistent with the department's expectations.

It should be expected that the different shifts will have a different mix of performed work time. For example, third shift should be able to make more external vehicular patrols than first shift, because there will be less traffic. And first shift will probably have more assistance calls for service because more people are at the facility during that shift. Reviewing and posting monthly productivity reports for the shifts can be a way of setting up friendly competition between shifts, but again, the director must emphasize that it is the quality of the work that matters.

CODING AND LOGGING TASKS

How can the security director keep track of the various tasks and times? Most facilities assign code numbers for tasks; for example, assisting a visitor may be Code 2. Each time that task is completed, the officer radios in to the dispatcher, who then records the task on a shift log sheet (Exhibit 5–1). At the end of a 24-hour period, these numbers are entered onto the daily log (Exhibit 5–2).

These log sheets can be used to document the work performed by the security department as a whole and how much time is spent on each task. For example, a department of 10 full-time officers should perform between 17,680 and 18,720 hours of work per year. Using the reporting system described above, the director can track tasks and productivity rates and produce the report shown in Table 5–1.

This method also demonstrates to upper management that all members of the security department are aware of the importance of performing their jobs within an acceptable range of productivity.

Kinds of Tasks

The security task analysis also helps to determine the type of training, education, and experience needed to perform a task. For example, some security departments are also responsible for courier service. The officers deliver mail, packages, and medical equipment throughout the central facility and to outside facilities. If this kind of service is of sufficient volume that a security officer is performing the task over half of a shift, should a security officer be doing it, or should the security department hire a part-time courier? Perhaps a closer look is necessary.

If the deliveries are within a set time frame—for example, 8:00 a.m. to 12:00 p.m. each day—it would make sense to reduce the security officer force by ½ FTE and hire a part-time courier at a lesser wage. However, if the deliveries are throughout the shift, it would be impossible to offset any security staffing by hiring a courier, because the courier would have to

Table 5–1 Security Department Task Report

Function	Times	Hours
Patrol, internal	12,800	6,400
Patrol, external	13,500	6,750
Assist visitor/employee	6,000	600
Escort staff	2,100	210
Incidents	2,081	3,021
Safety checks	365	365
Fire drills	12	12
Other services	2200	733
TOTAL		18,091 (91% productivity rating)

Exhibit 5–1 Shift Log

1-Incident	-	13-	-
2-Visitor/Employee assistance -		14-Special detail	-
3-Jump start	-	15-Patrol round	-
4-Tire inflate	-	16-Challenges	-
5-	-	17-Camera scan	-
6-Supply/delivery run	-	18-Gate problem	-
7-Escorts	-	19-Tickets	-
8-Codes	-	20-Traffic/Valet hours-	
9-Auto unlock			
10-Door unlock	-	21-Post hours	-
11-Door lock	-		
12-Misc. assistance	-		

Unit #	Duties	Weapon #	Unit #	Duties	Weapon #

Time	Unit	List all misc. activity - Assistance calls - incidents	Tally

be available during the entire shift. The next option would be for the facility to hire a courier service that can respond and make deliveries on short notice. This type of service may be more costly in terms of cost per delivery, but the facility must consider the possibility that a security officer would be away from the facility, making a delivery, when an emergency arises. To reach a balance of service (deliveries) and security (officers always present) the facility could contract with the courier service only for off-property deliveries.

Exhibit 5–2 Daily Log

	FIRST	SECOND	THIRD	TOTAL
Larceny (misd.)				
Larceny (felony)				
Damage to property				
Breaking/Entering				
Suspicious person/activity				
Trespass				
Disturbance				
Missing patient				
Assault				
Domestics				
Visitor restriction				
Auto accident				
Personal injury				
Alarm activated/reset				
Maintenance report				
Special report				
Items found				
Unsecured area				
Other				
Visitor/employee assistance				
jump start				
tire inflate				
food run				
supply/delivery run				
escorts				
codes				
auto unlock				
door unlock				
door lock				
misc. assistance				
ambulance run				
special detail				
patrol round				
challenges				
camera scan				
gate problem				
tickets				
traffic/valet hours				
post hours				

Date: _____   Day: _____

The key point to remember in this discussion is to look at a job as a series of individual tasks and subtasks. What is needed to do the task, by whom is it best performed, and what is the most productive and cost-effective manner?

Measuring Performance

By analyzing the components of a job, the director can also establish standards to measure the performance of the job. For example, the job description for a security officer may list as job functions patrolling the facility, assisting visitors, writing reports, etc. What do these functions mean? Without measurable tasks within a job, it is very difficult, if not impossible, to measure performance. However, if standards are set—for example, officers should conduct eight patrol rounds per shift, and a patrol round consists of patrolling a designated area and making contact with at least one staff member per department during the patrol—then there is something to measure.

In reviewing all jobs in the department, the security director should note any factors that might cause the task itself or the productivity rate to vary. If the facility is under construction in a certain area and security is charged with interim life safety, the director should note that the patrol function in that area will take longer than normal. As the facility changes, it is necessary from time to time to alter, add, and delete functions. One consultant tells the story of accompanying a security officer on a patrol of a facility. Several times, the officer went to an empty storage room and noted that the area was secure. When the consultant asked why it was necessary to repeatedly patrol an empty storage room, the officer explained that it used to be the pharmacy storage area, and the shift orders still instructed the officers to patrol the area at least four times per shift. This kind of inefficiency dramatically distracts from the professionalism of a security department. The security director must make sure that the activities of the department meet the facility's *current* needs.

WHAT KIND OF REPORTS ARE NEEDED?

In many facilities, the security department's incident report is used for any and all incidents, statements, investigative reports, and so on. That approach may seem to work for a small security department that reports few incidents, but even in a small department that is a short-sighted view. Having specific reports for different kinds of events can accomplish several things. First, by asking for certain information, a report form can help ensure that the officer gathers the pertinent facts. Thus, for example, if a standard incident report is used to document an auto accident, the officer may forget to ask for the owner's insurance information or the vehicle identification number, because there is not a line on the report for that information. The following are the basic report forms that a security department should use.

- *Incident Report Form:* Used for basic reporting of an incident. It should ask for all basic information and have an area for the officer's narrative of the event. The form should have an area to enter a case number (Exhibit 5–3).
- *Supplement Report Form:* This form is used to supplement the initial security incident report. It is a valuable tool for investigators to document their activities on a particular case.

• *Statement Form:* This form is used to take statements from all concerned parties—victim, witness, and suspect. The form should include a statement for the person to sign certifying that the statement is true and was freely given without promise or inducement (Exhibit 5–4).

Many departments color-code incident reports, supplement forms, and statement forms to enable someone to find them quickly in a case file.

• *Trespass Warning Form:* Standardized form that an officer can attach to an incident report stating that a suspect was given a trespass warning and describing the nature of the warning.

Exhibit 5–3 Security Incident Report

Report No. _____   Shift _____

Report Date _____

Occurence Date _____

Confidential

S / M / T / W / T / F / S

Time of incident _____

Location of incident _____

____ Larceny (Misd.)	____ Missing patient	____ Alarm activated/reset
____ Larceny (Felony)	____ Patient restraint	____ Maintenance report
____ Damage to property	____ Assault	____ Special report
____ Breaking/entering	____ Domestics	____ Items found
____ Suspicious person/activity	____ Visitor restriction	____ Other (specify): ____
____ Trespass	____ Auto accident	_____
____ Disturbance	____ Personal injury	_____

NAME: DOB: RACE: SEX: W / S / V

DEPT. (if employee): _____   PHONE:

ADDRESS: APT. #:   CITY   STATE: ZIP:

DRIVER'S LICENSE: CAR MAKE: MODEL: YEAR: TAG:

HT: WT: HAIR: EYES: GLASSES: ATTITUDE: G / F/ P

DRESS:

OTHER DISTINGUISHING FEATURES:

NAME: DOB: RACE: SEX: W / S / V

DEPT. (if employee): _____   PHONE:

ADDRESS: APT. #:   CITY   STATE: ZIP:

DRIVER'S LICENSE: CAR MAKE: MODEL: YEAR: TAG:

HT: WT: HAIR: EYES: GLASSES: ATTITUDE: G / F/ P

DRESS:

OTHER DISTINGUISHING FEATURES:

continues

NAME: _____ DOB: _____ RACE: _____ SEX: _____ W / S / V

DEPT. (if employee): _____ PHONE: _____

ADDRESS: _____ APT. #: _____ CITY _____ STATE: ____ ZIP: _____

DRIVER'S LICENSE: _____ CAR MAKE: _____ MODEL: ____ YEAR: ____ TAG: _____

HT: _____ WT: _____ HAIR: _____ EYES: _____ GLASSES: _____ ATTITUDE: G / F/ P

DRESS: _____

OTHER DISTINGUISHING FEATURES: _____

PLACE OF INTERVIEW: _____ TIME INTERVIEW BEGAN: _____ TIME ENDED: _____

_____ Evidence Seized   _____ Articles Recovered   _____ Articles Stolen/Missing

ITEM(S)   DEPT.   APPROX. VALUE _____

_____

_____

_____

_____

_____

OFFICER'S STATEMENT: _____

_____

_____

_____

_____

_____

_____

_____

_____

_____

_____

_____

_____

_____

_____

_____

_____

ACTION TAKEN:

_____ Released   _____ Arrested   _____ Medical help

_____ Trespass warning given and released   _____ Placed in police custody   _____ Terminated

_____ Ejected from property   _____ Parents called

STATUS: _____ COURT DATE/TIME: _____ FINE/SENTENCE: _____

REPORTING OFFICER: _____ OFFICERS INVOLVED: _____

INVESTIGATING/ARRESTING POLICE OFFICER: _____ CPD REPORT NO: _____

- *Auto Accident Report:* This form is used to document vehicle accidents that occur on the property. The report should include an area for the officer to sketch the accident scene (Exhibit 5–5).
- *Safety Hazard Report:* Used to document an existing safety hazard. The form should specify that, if possible, a photograph should accompany the report. The routing of the report should include the facility's safety officer.
- *Personal Injury Report:* This report is used to report all personal injury cases, both employee and nonemployee. It should prompt the officer to note such details as whether the victim wears glasses, what kind of shoes the victim was wearing, and what the weather was like on the day in question. The facility's risk manager should be able to help design the form.

Exhibit 5–4 Statement Form

Case Type: _____ Case Number _____ Page _____ of ____

Statement of: _____ Age _____ DOB _____

Address: _____ Phone _____

Connection with case: W / S / V   Were taken: _____

Date: _____   Time:_____

_____
_____
_____
_____
_____
_____
_____
_____
_____
_____
_____
_____
_____
_____
_____
_____

I certify by my signature that the above statement is true to the best of my knowledge. No threats, promises, or inducements have been made to me with regard to this statement.

Witness: _____   Signed: _____

_____   Address:_____

Date: _____ Time: _____

Exhibit 5–5 Auto Accident Form

```
                                              ┌─────────────────────────────┐
                                              │ Case #:                     │
                                              └─────────────────────────────┘
                                                       Supplemental (  )
Date of Accident: _____         S  M  T  W  T  F  S        Time: _____
Date of Report: _____         Time: _____  No. of Vehicles: _____
Location of Accident: _____

      VEHICLE 1 ( ), HIT & RUN ( )            VEHICLE 2 ( ) PEDESTRIAN ( ) OTHER ( )
```

VEHICLE 1 ( ), HIT & RUN ( )	VEHICLE 2 ( ) PEDESTRIAN ( ) OTHER ( )
Driver: _____	Driver: _____
Address: _____	Address: _____
City: _____ State: __ Zip: __	City: _____ State: __ Zip: __
Phone W: _____ H: _____	Phone W: _____ H: _____
License #: _____ State: _____	License #: _____ State: _____
Exp. Date: _____ DOB: _____	Exp. Date: _____ DOB: _____
Restriction Code: _____	Restriction Code: _____
Owner: _____	Owner: _____
Address: _____	Address: _____
City: _____ State: __ Zip: __	City: _____ State: __ Zip: __
Phone W: _____ H: _____	Phone W: _____ H: _____
VIN#: _____	VIN#: _____
Plate: _____ State: _____ Year: __	Plate: _____ State: _____ Year: __
Veh. Year _____ Make _____	Veh. Year _____ Make _____
Model _____ Veh. Type Code _____	Model _____ Veh. Type Code _____
Vehicle Drivable . . . . yes ( ) no ( )	Vehicle Drivable . . . . yes ( ) no ( )
Insurance Co. _____	Insurance Co. _____
Policy #	Policy #

Other Property Damaged: _____

Owner Name: _____ Address: _____

Ambulance Requested . . . . Yes ( ) no ( )   If yes, Ambulance arrived at _____ hrs

Injured taken to: _____

Responding Police Department _____ Report # _____

continues

Exhibit 5–5 continued

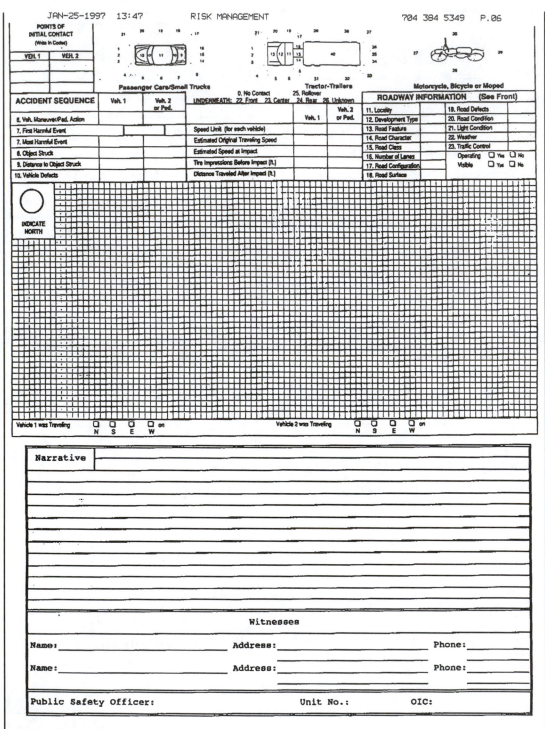

These are the most common forms used by security officers in reporting incidents. For a full review of forms, see *Security and Safety Administration in Health Care Facilities: Forms, Checklists and Guidelines* (Aspen Publishers, Inc., 1997). This publication contains hundreds of sample forms and reports that can be adapted for use.

HOW LONG SHOULD A REPORT BE KEPT?

The length of time a report should be kept depends on the nature and severity of the incident. In most cases, security incident reports should be kept for three to five years. However, the policies and procedures for destroying reports should include communication with corporate counsel. If a lawsuit has been filed against the facility that concerns a security incident, it may be necessary to keep the report and accompanying documents until the lawsuit is litigated, including any appeals.

HOW ARE SECURITY REPORTS TRACKED?

Security reports can be tracked manually or by computer, and you can use various systems for case numbering.

Computer Software

There are numerous software packages on the market to assist the security director in tracking incidents and producing reports. Some of these packages use a modern version of the "clock wind" system, in which an officer patrols a designated area using a handheld bar code reader. The reader reads a bar code for the area, and the location and time are entered into its memory. At the end of the shift, the reader is downloaded into the security computer and a printout of the shift activities is produced. Some systems also have generic report features loaded into the software, so that the officer can simply enter the numerical code for a specific type of incident and the software will generate a report.

Incident and tour software packages have improved greatly, but they still have some drawbacks. For some facilities, cost is an issue: these systems can cost from $4,000 to $10,000. Second, if the computer is producing the reports, an officer may be less likely to remember an incident, which will hurt his or her credibility in court. Third, most of these systems are not easy to customize, and the department's ability to conduct task analyses and productivity studies may be reduced.

Case Numbering Systems

Whether the department uses a computerized system or a manual system to collect data and track incident reports, case numbering is necessary. There are two main methods of numbering cases.

Year and Chronological Numbering

In this method, the year is entered and the case number is sequential. An example of this type of case number would be **99–882** (1999 fiscal year, the 882nd case handled by the department). In using this system, you start the new year when the facility's fiscal year begins. This is extremely important for budgeting. The department must be able to show the number of cases it handled in the fiscal year, because all department budgets are allocated for a fiscal year, not a calendar year.

Full Date and Time Numbering

In this system, the full date and time of the report are used as the case number. For example, **9906221300-01** would indicate that the case was recorded on June 22, 1999, at 1:00 p.m. (1300) and it was the first (01) case recorded at that particular time. If other cases happened to be recorded at the same time, they would be numbered consecutively: −02, −03, etc.

In addition to case numbering, the department must keep a log of the assigned case numbers. Most departments assign case numbers in chronological fashion (i.e., 1–xx . . .), regardless of the case tracking system they use. The important components of a case log are case number, day, date, shift, nature of report, open/date closed.

The first three items are self-explanatory. "Shift" indicates the time frame during which the incident occurred. This knowledge can help an investigator track down witnesses later. "Nature of report" refers to the type of incident—was it a safety hazard, auto accident, theft?

Open/date closed: Is the case open (there is more work to be done on it) or closed (no further work)? Some facilities allow the security director to close cases that cannot be resolved "by exception," meaning that the case is unsolvable because of lack of evidence or possibly that the department has fully investigated the case and identified the perpetrator but does not have sufficient proof. Cases closed by exception should be reviewed periodically to see if there might be new evidence that would allow the department to reopen the case.

KEY POINTS

- Recordkeeping is essential for
  –litigation
  –program qualification
  –staff evaluations
- A task analysis is needed to establish true standards.
- Security should compile monthly, quarterly, and yearly reports that document the performance of the department and of individual officers.

Chapter 6

Security Officer Selection and Training

CHAPTER OBJECTIVES

1. Understand the type of security officer who normally succeeds in a health care setting.
2. Know some of the personality traits of a good officer.
3. Know why training is important.
4. Determine the subjects that all training programs should cover.
5. Determine how much training is needed for various facilities.
6. Learn which organizations have recognized training programs.

INTRODUCTION

What kind of person makes a good health care security officer? What education level and what type of experience are needed? These questions can be answered with two more questions: What do you expect of the officer, and what is the facility's philosophy?

In the past, it was believed that someone who had law enforcement experience was automatically qualified for a security job. Many of the technical skills a law enforcement officer learns are transferable to the health care setting: interviewing, crime scene search, and report writing, to name three. But a health care security officer must master many other skills to be successful.

The main problem law enforcement officers usually have in their transition to private security is *mindset*. They are accustomed to telling people what to do and having them do it or risk arrest. In private security, the officer must ask for compliance, and may have to rely on the powers of persuasion to get it. For some law enforcement officers, that transition is too difficult to make.

The same problem is found among former military personnel. The military relies on strict obedience and clear guidelines. That works for the military but not for private security, especially in a health care setting—there are just too many variables in the equation.

Security in a health care facility is not based on a set of black-and-white rules; in fact, most of the time, the officer operates in a gray area. Perhaps the rules say that visitors are not permitted after 9:00 p.m., but what if a loved one is dying? The rules say that this is a No Parking area, but what if the driver is a chemotherapy patient who is so weak he can hardly walk? The health care security officer encounters these kinds of exceptions to the rules every day.

The ideal prospective candidate should possess some law enforcement/security skills, such as a basic understanding of constitutional and criminal law, investigations, and patrol procedures. However, it is more important that the candidate can demonstrate—either through past employment or formal education—the ability to work with people who are under stress. Excellent communication and interpersonal skills and the desire to help others are far more important for the successful health care security officer than any other attribute. It is not surprising that off-duty firefighters and paramedics adapt well to the health care security environment.

Security officers in a health care facility should base all decisions on what is best for the patient. If they use that as the yardstick, they will be correct most of the time.

What kind of educational background is appropriate for a security officer? A high school diploma is necessary, and more and more hospitals are requiring at least one year of college. Some prefer an associate degree. The dynamics of working in a stressful, socioeconomically varied environment require that the officer possess logic, excellent communication skills, a cool head, and an understanding of the reason he or she is employed: to assist in treating the sick and injured. Technical skills can be taught, but attitude and the willingness to serve others must come from within. Look for these qualities when interviewing applicants.

One of the best tools a security manager can have at his or her disposal in hiring is a well-thought-out job description. It should be objective-based and should cover the main areas of responsibility. Be sure to let prospective applicants read the job description. Then ask them to tell you how they would accomplish the tasks outlined. Listen for the candidate who uses too many "command"-type words—"I would INSTRUCT, ADVISE, TELL . . ." Why not ASK? See Appendix 6–A for a sample job description.

WHY TRAIN?

The two main causes of security officer turnover are low pay and boredom. Even in a busy facility, the duties of a security officer can become repetitious. Certainly there are days when an incident or incidents get the adrenaline flowing and make the job exciting. However, the purpose of security is to be proactive and preventive, so, ironically, the better job people are doing, the more bored they may be.

The pay structure for security has increased in the past several years. As municipalities reduce their budgets for police departments, it has become the job of corporate America to establish its own security programs. In the past, pay was low because officers were not trained and not expected to do much, and contract companies stressed low costs to secure contracts. Most companies that contract with a security guard and patrol service still have no idea what they are purchasing. Security is not the purchasers' forte and their only concept may be that of the night watchman. Demanding more of security, requiring a higher level of education from applicants, and establishing a quality in-house training program will justify higher wages.

BENEFITS OF A TRAINING PROGRAM

Reducing turnover and increasing wages are not the only benefits of establishing a quality training program. In our litigious society, "negligent security" is one of the fastest-growing areas for lawsuits. In most years, more lawsuits are filed against hospitals for inadequate or negligent security than for malpractice. Attorneys, and the general public, no longer view health care entities as off-limits when it comes to filing security-related lawsuits. Hospitals, especially, are viewed as large, multicorporate entities with very deep pockets.

One large retirement center and nursing home learned a hard lesson about inadequate security. The company did have a security department; however, it required only a high school diploma to become an officer. No previous experience was required and the company did not have ANY training program. An incident occurred in which one of the residents was assaulted and robbed. The resident's husband, who also received injuries, call the "emergency security phone number," as he had been instructed when he and his wife moved to the facility. It took the security officer 10 minutes to respond (he was on the other side of a 200-acre campus, patrolling on foot, because the company would not provide security with a vehicle). When he got there, he did not know what to do. To compound the problem, the wife went into cardiac arrest. The officer had not received any first aid or CPR training, despite the fact that security was supposed to be the first responder for medical emergencies on the property. Luckily (and no thanks to the security officer), both residents survived. In the ensuing lawsuit against the facility for inadequate and negligent security, the plaintiff's attorney cited 37 times that the words "safe" and "secure" had been used in the company's promotional material. It didn't take a jury long to decide that the company had breached its contract by not providing a safe and secure property, and that the security program was, in the words of one juror "a sham." The jury returned a multimillion dollar verdict against the company.

There are a number of important benefits of training.

- Training can increase morale by giving the officers a chance to work together. Too often a security department can become fragmented by shift rivalry. It then becomes three separate departments, rather than one group working toward a common goal.
- Training can make the job more interesting and increase the personal growth of the individual officer. Officers learn skills that they can use while working in security and that they can apply if they decide to go into public police work. One facility established such a high-quality program and produced such superior security officers that the local police department established a solid working relationship with the security department. They included the department on their radio frequency, held joint briefings, and helped to design specialized training programs.
- Training can upgrade the expectations of the department. Rather than being the stereotypical night watchman, the department can establish itself as a partner in rendering quality patient care. Medical staff are very education- and training-oriented, because that is required in their field. The medical staff want to be assured that everyone else who is helping to care for patients, even indirectly, is also appropriately educated and trained. Having a quality training program and letting the medical staff know about the qualifications and training of the security officer can help eliminate the "us versus them" divisions that exist in some health care facilities.
- Training can also help prepare a facility for a crisis. For example, in the case of a bomb threat, security should be able to take the lead and facilitate the search, call analysis, and liaison with law enforcement. Likewise, in the prevention of infant abductions, security should be the department that keeps abreast of cases, outcomes, methods, and training

for the staff. Security should be a resource for policy formulation regarding how to deal with violence in the workplace, how to deal with verbal aggression, and other topics. Security must also be part of any and all disaster training, in the facility and at the local or state level.

In addition to security officer training, the Joint Commission on Accreditation of Healthcare Organizations requires training for employees on security-related topics if they work in a "sensitive area." The sensitive areas are determined by a yearly security audit.

HOW MUCH TRAINING IS ENOUGH?

There is no set answer to this question. To determine the amount of training that is needed, start by reviewing the security department mission statement and the duties required of the officers. If they are required to patrol the property, they should be trained in proper foot and, if applicable, vehicle patrol. If they are expected to assist in restraining patients, they should be trained in restraints. In other words, the amount of training must be relative to the tasks to be performed. For basic training, it is safe to say that a minimum of 40 hours of training on core topics should be required. In some states, security officers must complete a state-required training program. If so, the facility should make sure all regulatory requirements are met and, in addition, topics related to health care security are included in the officer's training.

If a lawsuit results from an officer's actions, training procedures and records are sure to be reviewed. Attorneys for both sides will review the topics in the training program, the qualifications of the instructors, and the method of testing. Most facilities fail miserably on keeping records of training. They usually pass a class roster around during the inservice and use the roster for their training record. But attorneys want to see evidence that (1) the officer attended the entire class and (2) he or she learned the material. Pre- and posttests are absolutely necessary to document inservice training. In addition, officers should be retested periodically to make sure they have retained the information. If an officer fails the posttest or fails to correctly answer questions on key topics (for example, use of force), he or she should be retested after a review of the subject.

Training methods are another topic for discussion. Many facilities use videotapes in their training programs. Training tapes can provide a good overview of a subject in a relatively short time. They can be used to train officers individually as they are hired or in a group session. Make sure that the tapes are up to date and are specific to health care security where necessary. For example, most videotapes used to teach an officer basic reporting skills probably cover the same material: that a report should be concise, accurate, timely, etc. However, a videotape on health care security may also include a special section on patient confidentiality.

In addition to videotapes, training should include lectures and the opportunity for questions and answers. Learning in a group enables the student to test his or her understanding of the material against the understanding of others in the class. The instructor, by using structured questions to the class, can make sure that the key points of the subject are understood.

Hands-on training should be used whenever possible, and must be used for some subjects, such as handcuffing, baton use, CPR, verbal de-escalation, and patient restraints. In these areas, practice is the key to success. The security officer should receive periodic follow-up training in all of these areas.

TRAINING RESOURCES

A number of excellent training tapes can be found on the market.

Communicorp,[1] long recognized as a leader in health care security officer videotape training, is an excellent resource. The company offers tapes covering a wide range of generic security training topics, as well as the following health care security topics:

The Joint Commission and the Role of Security	Disaster Response
Assault Prevention in the Hospital	Hospital Parking Lot Security
Basic Hospital Investigations	Courteous Enforcement
Linen Losses and the Security Officer	New to the Hospital
Emergency Department Control	Securing the Pharmacy
Fire Response Control	Focus on Responsibility
Loss Prevention and Materials Management	Orientation to Hospital Safety
Physical Aggression in the Hospital	Calming the Aggressor
Hospital Security and the Joint Commission	Quality Security
Infant Abduction Prevention	Appropriate Use of Force

Another excellent resource is **Professional Security Television Network (PSTN)**[2] in Carrolton, Texas. PSTN offers a video training academy for security officers through which it maintains training records for officers and awards them a certificate of completion. The company offers a specialized Academy in Healthcare Security. In addition to a large inventory of generic security training videos, PSTN offers a wide range of security management tapes and the following tapes specific to health care security:

Interacting with Disturbed Persons	High-Rise Building Security
Disaster Management	Access Control
Bloodborne Pathogens	Loss Prevention
Controlling Aggressive Individuals	Fire Apparatus
Emergency Department Security	Drug Diversion
Parking Lot Security	Crowd Control at the Healthcare Facility
Use of Patient Restraints	Violence in the Emergency Department
Disaster Management for Healthcare	A Mock OSHA Inspection

The **International Association for Healthcare Security and Safety (IAHSS)**[3] offers several training programs. Its 40-hour Basic Security Officer Training Program provides adequate generic training for the security officer, with an emphasis on health care security. As this book goes to press, IAHSS is in the process of developing an Advanced Security Officer Training Course. The following subjects are covered in the training program:

Basic Training Certification Program

Introduction to Healthcare Security	Pharmacy
Security as a Service Organization	Emergency and Mental Health Units
Public/Community/Customer Relations	Support Units/Auxiliary Services
Employee/Labor Relations	Healthcare Vulnerabilities/Risks
Patrol and Post Procedures/Techniques	Access Control Concepts/Systems
Security Interactions with Patients/ Visitors/Employees	Physical Control Measures
	Basic Safety Concepts
Self-Protection/Defense	Fire Prevention
Professional Conduct and Self-Development	Fire Control/Response
Crisis Intervention	Bomb Threats/Procedures
Interview/Investigation	Disaster Control/Response
Report Preparation/Writing	Civil Disasters
Report Utilization	Criminal and Civil Law
Judicial Process/Courtroom Procedure/Testimony	Narcotics and Dangerous Drugs
Nursing Units	Public Safety Interactions/
Business Office	Liaisons

IAHSS also offers a Supervisor's Training Program and a Safety Training Program. Each of these programs is 20 hours, and they cover the following topics:

Supervisor's Training Program

Introduction to Supervision	Effective Communications/Management Skills
Contemporary Issues in Healthcare	Self-Improvement
Supervisory Responsibilities	Civil Liability and the Supervisor
Employee Relations and Employee Appraisals	Safety
	Budgeting and Cost Control
Authority and Control	Principles of Customer Relations
Leadership	Professionalism and Ethics
Handling Complaints and Grievances	

Safety Training Program

Regulatory Agencies	Special Healthcare Settings
Healthcare Safety Programs	Radiation Safety
Accidents and Injuries	Construction/Renovation Safety
Fire Safety	Hazard Surveillance
Emergency Preparedness	Hazardous Materials and Emergency Response
Infection Control	
Equipment Management/ Personal Protection	Hazardous Materials/Waste Management

Another excellent training program, although not specific to health care, is offered by the **International Foundation for Protection Officers (IFPO)**.[4] The program offers training for the security officer, who earns the designation of Certified Protection Officer, and for the supervisor, who earns the designation Certified Security Supervisor.

Many facilities use a combination of IAHSS Basic, Safety, and Advanced programs, along with several tapes from Communicorp's basic orientation training and a monthly tape from PSTN for continuing education. In addition, the facility should make sure that security officers receive annual CPR training. In most cases, security will be the first responder to all emergencies outside the facility.

KEY POINTS

- Ongoing training can provide the facility with a more professional officer and improve morale.
- The amount of training needed depends partly on the expectations the facility places on its security officers.
- The Joint Commission requires security orientation and ongoing training for employees in sensitive areas.
- The following companies/organizations offer training programs: Communicorp, PSTN, IAHSS, and IFPO.

REFERENCES

1. Communicorp, Inc., 160 North Wacker Drive, Chicago, IL 60606, (800) 367-9274.
2. Professional Security Television Network, 1303 Marsh Lane, Carrolton, TX 75006, (800) 942-7786.
3. International Association for Healthcare Security and Safety, P.O. Box 637, Lombard, IL 60148, (708) 953-0990.
4. International Foundation for Protection Officers, 3106 Tamiami Trail North, #269, Naples, FL 34103, (941) 430-0534.

Appendix 6–A

Sample Job Description—Security Officer

JOB TITLE: Security Officer

DEPARTMENT: Security services

CLASSIFICATION:

JOB SUMMARY

Performs general security work in the protection of persons and property and the enforcement of all applicable policies, rules, and regulations of _____ and applicable federal, state, and local laws to prevent losses due to accidents and incidents.

JOB RELATIONSHIPS

- Responsible to: Director of security services
- Assignments received from: Shift coordinator or security officer II
- Nature of supervision received: General supervision from the assistant security director. Immediate supervision from the shift coordinator. With the exception of hiring and termination, which must come from the director. Director is responsible for hiring and promoting the security officer.
- Positions supervised and nature of supervision given: None
- Interaction with: All other departments, both medical and nonmedical, within the hospital, as well as patients, visitors, and occasionally other persons outside the hospital

MAJOR JOB FUNCTIONS

The following list summarizes the major functions of this individual's job. He or she may perform other duties, both major and minor, that are not mentioned below. Specific functions may change from time to time.

- Provides for the safety and security of all persons (patients, visitors, and staff) and for property of the facility.
- Enforces all federal, state, and local laws as well as all hospital policies and procedures.
- Maintains professional competency by staying up-to-date on the changing trends of security procedures and practices.
- Understands and demonstrates the proper guidelines for the use of force.
- Complies with organization and department policies and procedures.

JOB QUALIFICATIONS

The following qualifications are the minimum requirements necessary to perform this job adequately. However, any equivalent combination of experience, education, and training that provides the necessary knowledge, skills, and abilities would be acceptable, subject to any legal or regulatory requirements. Must be certified in cardiopulmonary resuscitation (CPR) to be released from probation.

Education:	One year of college training from an accredited college in law enforcement, security, or a related field or completion of basic law enforcement training and six months of college training. Successful completion of the following or will complete within six months:

- International Association for Healthcare Security and Safety basic certification
- International Association for Healthcare Security and Safety basic safety certification program
- Professional Security Television Network basic certification program, and the hospital's basic security training program

Work experience:	Six months' prior experience as a noncontract security officer or law enforcement officer, one year preferred.
Knowledge, skills, and abilities:	Some knowledge of security and law enforcement practices. Ability to produce a concise, accurate, well-written report. Ability to solve problems on an independent basis. Possession of a valid driver's license. Ability to work independently or as part of a team.
Special conditions:	Be able to work outside in all types of weather. Be able to stand and walk for long periods of time. Cognizant that the possibility of physical confrontation increases the likelihood of injury. May be required to do light to heavy lifting. Requires walking up and down stairs during routine patrols. May require running up and down stairs and climbing ladders in emergency situations. Requires stooping, kneeling, crouching, twisting, bending, and reaching overhead. Must possess manual dexterity. Must be able to listen and hear machinery sound changes, whistles, cries for help, screams, alarms, and traffic

noises. Must be able to distinguish basic colors and have excellent depth perception and side vision. Free of night blindness. May be required to rotate and work long, irregular shifts. May be exposed to infectious diseases and hazardous materials.

Chapter 7

The Service Side of Security

James P. Finn

CHAPTER OBJECTIVES

1. Know the difference between "essential" and "ancillary" service functions.
2. Understand the usual service activities performed by health care security departments.

INTRODUCTION

The health care facility security department provides two kinds of services: *essential* services and *ancillary* services. Essential services are those that every security department in the health care profession typically provides; ancillary services are those that may be provided by the security department or by another entity within the organization.

ESSENTIAL SERVICES

Essential services include the following:
Escorts
Patrols
Door locks/unlocks
Key control
Patient restraints
Visitor control
Emergency response
Parking control
Alarm monitoring
Money escorts

Escorts

"Escorts" refers to physically escorting employees, visitors, or patients to their vehicles or other destinations. The primary reason for this service is personal safety. Escorts are an important part of the security function and should always be treated as a number one priority for a security department. Departmental policies and procedures must be developed, and the program should be advertised so staff and visitors understand that the service is available and, more important, how to access it. Typically, escort programs are available 24 hours a day, but users should be encouraged to call in advance so officers can plan to break away from their patrols or other assignments to provide the escort. The security officer providing the escort, either by vehicle or on foot, should accompany the person, check inside the vehicle, and stay there until the person has started the car and driven away. The beginning and end of the escort should be radioed back to the security command point and recorded on the security log.

Patrols

Patrols have always been the primary responsibility of security. Patrol patterns and sequences vary depending on the size of the facility and the department, but two aspects remain constant: both internal and external patrols are performed. Patrols are the backbone of a well-designed security department. By patrolling the facility, officers can ascertain where vulnerabilities exist, maintain good working relationships with other staff, and note opportunities for improvement in security. Every officer should understand the importance of patrols in relation to the mission of the health care security department.

Patrol rounds should be staggered to avoid establishing a pattern that could be easily figured out by someone who wants to commit a crime at the facility. Another excellent idea is to code patrol areas and change the codes often. If you use two-way communications to report each area patrolled, anyone who has a radio scanner can easily determine where your security officers are at any given time. By using codes and changing them often, it is less likely that a perpetrator will know where security personnel are.

Internal Patrols

The purpose of the internal patrol is to make visual contact with all internal components of the facility. It is important for security staff to visit every area, from the penthouse to the sub-basement, looking for, reporting, and correcting potential safety and security problems. One of the main reasons security patrols were instituted years ago was to look for fires that may occur in vacant or sparsely inhabited parts of a building. The role has expanded to include securing areas to prevent theft or crimes of opportunity. Internal patrols are also used to build rapport with other staff. One of security's best weapons in preventing crime is to have the support of all staff members in the facility, so that they will call and report any unusual situation or behavior. Patrols are typically a continuous effort: whenever security officers are not busy with other assignments, they should be patrolling the building.

External Patrols

The first external patrol on a shift (especially on the evening and night shifts) should be a foot patrol, to ensure that all external entrances and exits are secure. Subsequent patrols should be made of all parking areas, looking for suspicious activities or customer service opportunities. The officer should also check for burnt out lighting and for overgrown landscaping that may need pruning to increase security in a given area.

Door Locks/Unlocks

Door locking and unlocking should always be handled by the security department. In addition to the personal safety aspect, this policy will ensure that a record is kept of when and for whom access was granted. Such an audit trail can be essential for a later investigation. Many facilities maintain a grand master key system, and security is usually able to access or secure any area in the facility.

Key Control

Key control is one of the most important functions of the security department. Depending on the size of the facility, there may be hundreds of keys in use at any given time, and any key that is not secure is a potential disaster. It is very important that key inventories be maintained and key use tracked. All keys should be maintained in a locked cabinet, preferably in an area where there is constant supervision. All keys issued should be recorded on a log sheet that identifies the key number, time of issue, person the key was issued to, and the time it was returned. Procedures should be in place for periodically auditing the key cabinet, either at shift change or when personnel from the area are relieved by someone else. At each change, an inventory and verification of keys should be made.

The biggest problem with signing out keys is getting them back. It is not uncommon for staff members to sign out a set of keys and, hours later, punch out and go home, forgetting they have the keys in their pocket. Meanwhile, the security department also changes shifts, a key inventory is completed, and a set of keys is missing. (If an inventory had been taken an hour before the end of shift, this discrepancy would have been found and the individual who signed out the keys could have been contacted and reminded to bring them back.) The main concern with keys leaving the facility is that they could be duplicated and used to commit a crime at a later date. For this reason, all keys should be stamped with "Do Not Duplicate," and arrangements made with engineering personnel or a locksmith to duplicate keys only at the request of the security manager. This procedure will allow the security department to maintain a master list of how many keys have been made for any given area and to whom they were issued.

Patient Restraints

One of the most despised duties of the security department is patient restraint. Because of its 24-hour staffing and the perceived physical strength of officers, security is invariably called upon to help restrain combative patients. It is important for security staff to receive as much training as possible, and it is equally important that other staff receive this training as well. Most injuries that occur to security officers happen during a patient restraint, and the number one cause of injury is that the people involved in the restraint had no clue as to who was supposed to do what. The facility should provide group training sessions with all personnel who will be involved with patient restraints—typically security, emergency departments, psychiatric departments, and patient care technicians. Also, if everyone understands that the patient's nurse is the responsible party and should direct the activities of the restraint, there is less likelihood of injury.

Visitor Control

The issue of visitor control is constantly changing. At one time, the most difficult thing to do at a hospital was to visit a loved one. Everyone was stopped in the lobby at a "police sergeant-type" desk, a visitor's pass was required to get on the unit, and each patient was allowed only two visitors at a time. Now most facilities have a "hotel-type" visitor access policy, in which anyone, at just about any time, is allowed to visit. No passes are required, and patient rooms can fill up with people as long as they do not cause any trouble. You can imagine what this kind of visitor access does to the integrity of security programs.

Security officers and other hospital staff must be alert to the potential problems associated with this influx of the general public. It is not uncommon that some of these visitors get tired of sitting in the patient's room and decide to venture out and see what else is happening in the facility; many times, it is these persons who are involved in crimes of opportunity. In the process of wandering through the hospital, they find an unguarded purse or an unlocked office area and succumb to temptation.

After-hours access by the public to the facility should be controlled by using one entry portal. In most instances, the emergency department is a prime location for this access point because of its around-the-clock staffing. Employees should also be required to use only one access point. The more entry/exit points a facility has, the more opportunities exist for theft.

Sometime a patient or staff member may ask security to ensure that a certain person is not allowed access to them while they are in the facility. The security department should have a procedure for handling this kind of visitor restriction. Consult the facility's legal counsel, especially for policies that deal with patients or their guardians. Visitor restrictions for hospital employees are typically easier to handle, because facilities have a clear right to keep employees from being interrupted at work. The extent to which this policy is developed is up to the facility; **at minimum, the procedures should include the following items:**

- The person requesting the restriction must contact the security department in person to provide the name of the individual who will be restricted, a physical description, and the reason for the request.
- The staff member must sign a liability release form that gives the security department the authority to ask the restricted person to leave the premises and, if that person refuses, authorizes the security department to have the individual arrested for trespassing.
- The form should state that the requester will appear in court on behalf of the security department if necessary.

Always verify the identity of the person requesting the visitor restriction.

Emergency Response

Next to the need for physical security as a deterrent, emergency response is probably the biggest reason security departments have survived the trend to downsize or even eliminate them completely from the health care setting. In this section we will discuss emergency situations that occur outside the realm of organized responses to fires, disasters, and hazardous spills. (Those areas are covered in Chapters 23 and 28.)

In the early days in the profession of health care security, emergency response usually meant dealing with unruly patients and visitors. Over time, security departments have had to develop strategies to respond to more aggressive behavior and even violence. It is not uncommon for security departments to handle numerous calls for emergency response every day, from the intoxicated, uncooperative patient in the emergency department to the distraught family member or the mentally ill patient on a psychiatric ward. The need for trained security personnel to respond quickly and professionally is greater than ever, and the security department should develop protocols to handle all possible emergency situations.

Parking Control

Just as it is important to control access to the facility, it is important to have control over parking areas. Today's health care facilities are mini-municipalities, with a large number of perplexing parking issues. They are constantly challenged to provide parking for employees, inpatients and outpatients, physicians, construction personnel, and vendors. Most facilities do not have enough parking to accommodate all the requests, and it is usually the job of the security department to develop a systematic approach to how, when, and why certain parking areas are reserved for specific groups.

Begin with a site drawing of the campus, then prioritize and assign the available parking spaces in the way that best supports the facility's mission. Typically, facilities will need to address the following areas:

Parking for Physicians and Other Employees

In most cases, local ordinances specify the number of parking spaces needed—usually a minimum of one space for every physician on staff and one space for every employee (using the worst-case shift demand). Facilities typically have reserved designated parking areas for physicians. The security department may also elect to designate an area near the entrance for second shift employees. This strategically allows security to place employees so they can be easily observed while second shift employees leave work in darkness and third shift employees arrive. The natural order of things will allow third shift employees to have the next closest parking because they will occupy space vacated by first shift employees. The end result is second and third shift staff parking in one general area, which allows security officers to efficiently monitor these areas during shift change.

Visitor Parking

Local ordinances may require that one visitor parking space be provided for each patient room. Generally, visitor parking areas are established according to projected flow patterns. The majority of visitor parking is located near the main entrance to the facility and is removed from employee and physician parking areas. Separate parking facilities are made available for areas such as the Emergency Department or Outpatient areas that would typically need access during hours when the main entrance would be secured.

Handicapped Parking

Local ordinances usually require 1 handicapped space per 100 parking spaces, and a certain percentage of them must be wheelchair-accessible spaces. However, these requirements may not be adequate for a health care facility, which may designate additional handicapped parking as it sees fit. Parking for handicapped employees should be in a different area than parking for handicapped visitors and patients.

Parking designation and control are issues that require a lot of attention. Many organizations worry only about having enough space, when they might be making an effort to use the space they have to better advantage.

Alarm Monitoring

Because most security departments operate on a 24-hour basis, they are usually responsible for monitoring all the various alarms in a facility. Security also monitors certain equipment, described below, 24 hours a day. Changes in business practices or an effort to maximize human resources may mean that security also installs and monitors the burglar alarm systems, not only in the main facility but in all buildings that the corporation owns, rents, or leases. This can add up to big savings: hardware can be purchased directly from a supplier and installed and monitored by the facility, eliminating all installation and monitoring fees. In addition to burglar alarms, many security departments also monitor various ancillary alarms located throughout the building, such as fire alarms, generator alarms, pump alarms, and refrigerator alarms associated with the laboratory (blood bank). It is imperative that policies and protocols be developed with step-by-step processes to follow for each and every alarm, including who gets notified when an alarm is activated.

Money Escorts

A tremendous amount of money changes hands every day in a health care facility, and all security professionals know that whenever large amounts of money are being transported, there is a serious threat of something going wrong. First, the security department must have a good understanding of all money transactions that take place within the organization and must complete a risk assessment for each type of transport. The department must be familiar with all locations that are transporting money to other locations using public access. (Off-site facilities may transport their money to the hospital's business office at the end of the day. Business office staff may go out and collect parking lot money or pay telephone money.) If it is determined that some of the activities involve a high risk, security should meet with the department heads and other people involved and decide whether there is a way to make the activity less risky or whether a security officer is needed to physically escort these money transports.

If security escorts are used, officers will need policies and procedures to follow, including how often escorts will be needed and when, how much money will be transported at any given time, whether the escort will be armed or unarmed, how the money will be concealed, and the path of travel. It is best to travel through areas that are under camera surveillance; this allows for another set of eyes supervising the escort and provides a video record should an incident occur. Officers should be trained on what to look for and how to react to a robbery attempt. It is always better to give up the money than take the chance of someone getting injured, or worse.

ANCILLARY SERVICES

Ancillary services that may be provided by the security department include the following:

Auto unlocks
Battery jump starts
Tire inflates
Tire changes
Vendor identification
Staffing information areas
Courier services
Switchboard/PBX operation
Patient valuables
Lost and Found
Morgue responsibilities

Auto Unlocks

Many institutions no longer provide auto unlocking services because of the associated liability, but quite a few security departments still offer this service. Unlocking a locked car used to be a very easy task; however, in recent years, auto manufacturers have added safety features that make it more difficult. Many vehicles have electronic locks, which increase the likelihood of damage to the locking mechanism, and factory-installed alarm systems are apt to go off if the vehicle is not unlocked quickly.

If the facility decides to add or continue this service, officers must receive the proper amount of training and be tested on their competence before they are allowed to perform auto unlocks. The officer must be sure to verify that the person who is making the request is in fact the owner of the vehicle and must obtain a signed liability waiver from the vehicle's owner before proceeding. Offering this service is good public relations, but remember that even a signed release does not always mean that the facility will be clear of liability if the car is damaged.

Battery Jump Starts

Most health care facilities perform courtesy jump starts on their campus. This is very good customer relations, but it is not without risk and liability. It is extremely important that security staff wear protective equipment and understand the proper way to connect and disconnect the jumper cables. Numerous problems can cause the battery to explode, and improper jump starts can severely damage a vehicle's electrical system. As with auto unlocks, a liability waiver should be obtained from the owner of the vehicle before the jump start is initiated.

Tire Inflates

During external patrol rounds, security officers may come upon vehicles with flat or very low tires. Some security departments inflate tires using a portable air tank. The motivation to provide this service is a desire to get enough air in the tire so the person can make it to a repair shop, rather than having security become involved in changing the tire.

Tire Changes

Tire changes are probably one of the most controversial services provided by security because of safety and liability issues. Some departments refuse to change flat tires for anyone, opting instead to offer to inflate the tire so the person can get to a repair shop or call a wrecker service to change the tire for them. If a facility chooses to extend this service, it is important that officers receive sufficient training and are given the proper tools to perform the task to minimize the chance of injury or damage. It is a good idea to obtain a liability waiver from the owner before beginning.

Vendor Identification

From a security perspective, it is important to identify as many individuals as possible, and vendors are no different. Policies and procedures should be developed to identify all vendors allowed on site. Even though this seems overwhelming, enlisting the help of the Purchasing and Engineering Departments can accomplish this goal. During business hours, all vendors coming to the facility to visit nursing units or department managers should report first to the Purchasing Department so that their presence in the facility is known and the appointment is verified. Engineering departments should take responsibility for assuring that all construction and subcontractors are properly signed in and identified. The security department should be used for nonbusiness hours sign in and identification for vendors. Even though it is an almost impossible task to identify every vendor in a facility at a given time, a well-formed plan gives security departments the edge when it is necessary to verify a person's authority to be on the premises.

Staffing Information Areas

Security personnel are probably the most knowledgeable employees in the facility when it comes to knowing where everything is located, so they are ideally suited to staff information areas. This arrangement can be a great asset to the department as well: it makes for good customer relations and allows security to have outposts at strategic locations throughout the facility, typically in the main lobby, in the emergency department, and at the entrance to the parking facility. There is no better security tool than a trained security professional with good observation skills. Having a constant security presence in these locations can make a big difference when it comes to prevention.

Courier Services

As 24-hour service departments with staffing that is essentially continuously mobile, it is not surprising that many security departments have added a courier function, especially after hours and on a STAT basis. It is important that procedures are in place to handle calls for courier services: all calls should be recorded on the security log, noting the time the call was received, when the officer was dispatched, and when the service was completed. A bonded courier company should be on call to handle emergency orders if circumstances prevent the security officer from making a pickup or if the pickup would require the officer to be away from his or her primary duties too long. The final decision to send a security officer away from the campus should always be made by someone in authority—a security supervisor, nursing shift manager, or administrator on call. Coverage for emergency situations must be maintained if at all possible.

Switchboard/PBX Operation

As part of the trend to increase operational efficiencies, many security departments have inherited switchboard operations, especially during the late night and holiday shifts. This makes sense. Security departments are traditionally the hub of all communications throughout an organization and are normally the first point of contact for emergencies and other calls for assistance. In addition, most security officers have an excellent understanding of the need for positive, effective communications and are well equipped to establish priorities.

Before adding the switchboard function to the security department, it is important to know how much traffic the switchboard has and when most calls are received. Knowing how much traffic the switchboard receives, as well as the peak times for traffic, will help to determine whether or not using security monitoring personnel to double as the main facility switchboard is a viable option. The main objective is to determine if adding the switchboard function to security monitoring personnel will be detrimental or not to existing security monitoring functions. What usually happens is a compromise, in which a full-time operator handles the switchboard when it is busy (during the day) and the security monitoring person takes over when traffic is light (during the night shift, from 11:30 p.m. to 6:30 a.m., and on some holidays).

If the organization chooses to operate the switchboard from the security office, other factors need to be considered. Many switchboard areas house the master fire alarm reporting system, emergency call lines to initiate response to heart attacks, and backup and emergency paging systems. If the facility is considering moving the switchboard function, it will have to duplicate some of these systems or tie slave monitoring equipment to them. This can be very costly.

Patient Valuables

Security staff are often called to take possession of jewelry or large sums of cash from a patient. Every health care facility should have written policies and procedures for handling patient valuables. The crux of the policy should be that every effort is made to tell potential patients to leave their valuables at home. But this does not always happen, so organizations need to protect patients, and themselves. Most thefts are crimes of opportunity, and a patient with cash or jewelry is a temptation to be avoided.

The initial patient registration form should ask whether the patient has any jewelry or cash. Patients should be encouraged to send valuables home with their spouse or significant other. If they choose to keep the items with them or have no one to give them to, the facility should offer to secure their property. Valuables collection must be a systematic procedure, with built-in checks and balances. All items should be inventoried in front of the patient and placed in a tamper-proof envelope. The patient's name, the date, and a list of the contents should be written on the envelope. The person collecting the valuables and the patient sign the envelope.

If the patient is admitted to the emergency department (ED) and is unconscious, emergency care will no doubt take precedence over valuables collection; however, this is where patient valuables are most likely to be reported missing, so it is imperative that the ED establish strict policies for valuables collection. If the patient is unconscious, two employees (or an employee and a friend or family member of the patient) should collect and inventory the patient's valuables. The patient's name is written on the envelope, and it is signed by the two people.

Once the valuables have been collected, the envelope is delivered to the location where it will be secured—usually the business office or security office, where there is a safe or strongbox. It is most important to maintain the chain of custody throughout this process. The envelope delivery is entered into a log, including the name of the person who delivered it and the person who received it, the date and time, the contents, patient's name, and receipt number. The receipt should be given to the patient or placed on the patient's chart.

When the patient is discharged, the process is reversed: the receipt is verified against the logbook and the contents of the envelope are verified by the patient or designee, who signs the receipt. The outgoing side of the log is completed: date, time, person receiving the property, property released, and name of the employee who released the property. These steps can be time-consuming, but it is very important that the chain of custody and inventory of items be maintained for legal purposes.

Lost and Found

There will be times when patients, visitors, and employees will lose or forget articles while in the facility. Because it is known that this will occur, a well-organized system must be established to handle items turned in as lost and found. Items turned in must be logged, investigated, and secured until a potential claim is received. There must also be procedures established for how long an item will remain in lost and found (typically 90 days) and what will happen to an item stored beyond the established time frame. Some organizations return found items to the person who turned them in, if that person requests it. If items in lost and found can be traced to a given person, and that person is no longer a patient or employee of the facility, a certified letter should be sent to the owner informing them that the item(s) is in the facility's possession and that they have X number of days to contact the facility to claim the item(s). Once a claim is made, it is very important to verify the identity of the person claiming the item(s), if known, or have a reasonable surety that the items in question do in fact belong to the individual making the claim.

Morgue Responsibilities

More and more security departments are becoming involved with the process of receiving and releasing bodies. This is a large responsibility, and includes collecting valuables, maintaining the integrity of evidence, dealing with distraught family members, and notifying pathologists, the coroner, and funeral homes.

Policies and procedures should be in place for each of the different ways the organization may receive bodies: from the nursing units, ED, birthing center, or operating room. If the facility has a contract with the county or other municipality, it will also receive DOAs. It is a good idea to check with the local coroner and medical examiner, as well as the chief pathologist, to determine the protocols for handling each situation without disturbing evidence or complicating an investigative autopsy.

Policies and procedures should also be in place for collecting, securing, and releasing valuables. The usual guidelines for collecting and securing valuables apply, but it must be ascertained who is the legal next of kin and thus has the authority to retrieve any possessions obtained from the body. The organization's legal department and risk manager should be involved in developing policies for this situation.

KEY POINTS

- There are two kinds of security service:
  - Essential (those that most security departments perform)
  - Ancillary (those that security may perform for the facility)
- Essential services may include, but are not limited to, escorts, patrols, door locks/unlock, key control, patient restraints, visitor control, emergency response, parking control, alarm monitoring, money escorts.
- Ancillary services may include, but are not limited to, auto unlocks, battery jump starts, tire inflates and changes, vendor identification, staffing information areas, courier services, pay phone collection, switchboard/PBX operation, patient valuables, Lost and Found, morgue responsibilities.

Chapter 8

Security Awareness Programs

CHAPTER OBJECTIVES

1. Understand why security awareness programs are important.
2. Review some of the most common security awareness programs

INTRODUCTION

Health care facilities offer a unique set of challenges when it comes to security. Most are large complexes, covering many acres or city blocks. They have numerous entrances/exits and are "open" 24 hours a day. They are a place to heal the sick and injured; a place where human stress is at a very high level. These facilities have a population that is largely unable to defend itself from attack, and goods—from drugs to blankets—that attract the criminal element. It is impossible to hire enough police officers to guarantee public safety. The same holds true for private security in a health care setting. **How can we increase the level of security in a cost-effective manner? The answer lies in increasing the awareness of everyone in the facility, and the following are some of the ways this can be achieved.**

COST AWARENESS

The climate in health care today is one of cost containment, but what good does it do to trim expenses if theft is occurring? Let everyone know the impact that even minor theft can have on the facility. Make sure employees know how much it costs to replace items and that the cost of theft directly affects how much money is available for patient care and employee pay and benefits. Use the facility newspaper; hold a contest to see who can guess the cost of various items.

SECURITY NEWSLETTER

A newsletter can be an extremely effective security awareness tool if it is done correctly. Have the security department publish a newsletter giving information on the kinds of incidents that have occurred and on crime prevention tips. Shift-specific information is particularly effective. A newsletter is also an excellent place to showcase new security equipment

95

and programs, and to introduce new security officers to the staff. Appendix 8–A contains the text from a sample newsletter.

SECURITY FAIR

Hold a security fair. Invite vendors that specialize in home security and personal security devices, local law enforcement crime prevention departments, and so on. An excellent time to hold the fair is just before vacation season. Contact travel agencies and ask them to participate. Most will give away road maps, luggage tags, and hotel safety tips. The idea is to increase everyone's general sense of security awareness. The employees will appreciate the "freebies" and the information.

SECURITY SEMINARS

Sponsor free employee crime prevention/security seminars on topics that are not necessarily related to a health care facility, such as rape prevention, crime prevention for the elderly, child abuse prevention, and home protection. The idea is to offer topics that are of interest to employees. The concepts they learn at these seminars will carry over to the workplace. They will become more aware of the potential for crime and will be more likely to report suspicious activity.

SECURITY ALERT MEMBER PROGRAM

The Security Alert Member (SAM) program is highly effective. In every health care facility there are several departments whose employees move throughout the facility daily. Environmental services, materials management, and diet and nutrition are some of those departments. Train those employees to be alert for suspicious activity. Teach them the who, what, when, where, and how method of reporting, as well as how to report their observations to security. You can roll out the program by having several employees in those key areas wear buttons to attract attention. The first button, "SAM IS COMING," is worn for several weeks. The next button is "SAM IS HERE," and the last one is " I'M SAM." The curiosity of other staff members will increase communication and awareness.

HOSPITAL WATCH

This program, patterned after the highly successful Community Watch programs, is a great complement to the SAM program. The idea, again, is to increase awareness by involving the facility staff. Figure 8–1 is an example of a Hospital Watch pamphlet.

SECURITY LIAISON PROGRAM

This program aims to increase communication between security officers and other staff members. In many facilities, an "us versus them" feeling exists. This program helps to bridge that gap by assigning each security officer to a department in the facility. It is best if each shift has its own officer as well. The officers' goal is to learn as much as possible about

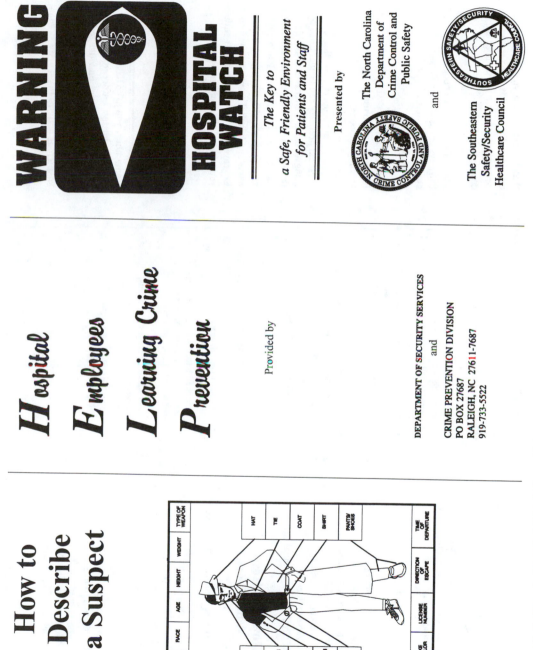

WARNING

HOSPITAL WATCH

The Key to a Safe, Friendly Environment for Patients and Staff

Presented by

The North Carolina Department of Crime Control and Public Safety

and

The Southeastern Safety/Security Healthcare Council

H ospital
E mployees
L earning *Crime*
P revention

Provided by

DEPARTMENT OF SECURITY SERVICES

and

CRIME PREVENTION DIVISION
PO BOX 27687
RALEIGH, NC 27611-7687
919-733-5522

How to Describe a Suspect

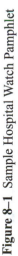

Figure 8–1 Sample Hospital Watch Pamphlet

What Is Hospital Watch?

Hospital Watch is a crime prevention program originating in North Carolina. This program coordinates the efforts of law enforcement, hospital security, and hospital staff to create a safer atmosphere in and around hospitals.

Crime Risk Triangle

Crime follows the path of least resistance. There are three basic elements necessary for a crime to occur: a criminal with the *DESIRE* and *ABILITY* to commit a crime, and a victim who provides an *OPPORTUNITY* for a criminal to act.

How Does Hospital Watch Work?

Hospital Watch breaks the crime risk triangle. Hospital Watch works most effectively by reducing the *OPPORTUNITY* for crime to occur. By learning and practicing basic crime prevention steps, you can significantly reduce the likelihood of becoming a victim. Target-hardening—or making hospitals more secure—forces the would-be criminal to increase his *ABILITY* or go out of business. We can do little to control the *DESIRE* of an individual to commit a crime.

It Is Important that Everyone Know Their Role!

The Security Liaison Officer

- Maintain a good working relationship with law enforcement, hospital security, and hospital staff.

- Keep floor captains informed about crimes in and around their areas. Supply quarterly community safety reports by mail.

- Survey areas upon request for suggestions/recommendations to improve security.

- Identify and check out suspicious activity reported in area. Report findings to floor captains.

The Floor/Department Captain

- Attend two meetings a year.

- Report all information received from members of Hospital Watch to the security liaison officer.

- Coordinate supplies: signs, decals, literature.

- Constantly enlist the support of other employees.

The Member

Watch for suspicious vehicles parked on or near the grounds. Be prepared to write down a license tag number and description.

Watch for suspicious people in the hallways or the office. Report anyone who is soliciting, trying doors, etc. to security.

Keep the suspect description sheet handy. Learn to use it. Practice describing someone.

Engrave your property. Medical and personal property can be identified by using an electric engraver available through the security liaison officer (or purchased on your own). Photograph your property with the department's name and hospital name engraved on it. Engrave your personal property with your driver's license number.

Remember, you are ONLY the eyes and ears for law enforcement. You are not expected, nor encouraged, to physically intervene in a situation. Simply use the phone to report any suspicious activity to security as soon as possible.

Figure 8–1 continued

the departments and their employees. They should conduct a security survey of their department and attend department meetings. The officers should file a monthly report to the director of security, describing what they have accomplished in their assigned departments. The officers' job is to bridge the communications gap and help the department learn sound crime prevention methods.

Once the department employees get to know the officers, they will feel more comfortable calling them with problems, suggestions, and information. This program also ensures that most of the facility is surveyed frequently for security problems.

CRIME PREVENTION THROUGH ENVIRONMENTAL DESIGN

While not a new concept, these programs have gained favor rapidly in the past few years. Some of the key components are to use the design of the buildings, lighting, landscaping, and so on to deter crime. For example, the facility should take advantage of any natural barriers—hedges, treelines, rivers, etc.—to help protect the core of the facility by establishing observable boundaries. On the other hand, the facility should be aware that overplanting can increase the possibility of crime. If the foliage blocks lighting or closed-circuit television (CCTV) surveillance, the opportunity for a crime may increase. Many facilities have increased the lighting in the parking lots/decks far above industry norms. This can be one of the most cost-effective crime deterrents. Building architecture is important—small changes in building plans can increase security; for example, the use of glass-walled elevators in a parking deck rather than regular walls.

The key to these programs is to decide (1) what needs to be protected and (2) why it should be protected. List the areas in descending order of importance and determine whether possible defensive options exist that can be used to better advantage. See Appendix 8–B for information on crime prevention through environmental design.

Appendix 8–A

Security and Public Safety Newsletter

SECURITY NEWS AND VIEWS

Each quarter the Security Department will be sending you a newsletter informing you of the happenings on your shift. The newsletter will also have tips to help you stay safe.

Third Shift Activity Summary

	April–June
Misd. larceny	19
Felony larceny	24
Damage to property	2
Breaking/entering	8
Suspicious person	6
Trespass	4
Disturbances	6
Missing patients	3
Patient restraints	13
Assaults	2
Domestic disturbance	3
Visitor restriction	1
Auto accident	3
Personal injury	3
Alarm activations	18
Maintenance report	6
Special report	0
Found items	5
Misc.	22
TOTAL	148

Monthly Security Tips

Spring and summer mean VACATION TIME for most of us. Unfortunately, criminals never take a vacation. Here are some tips to help you have a safe and secure vacation:

1. If you are going to be away for an extended period of time, consider hiring a housesitter.
2. Put your lights and TV on a timer.
3. Leave window coverings as they normally would be.
4. DO NOT stop deliveries! Have a neighbor pick them up for you, as well as any circulars that accumulate by the front door.
5. Make arrangements to have the lawn cut while you are away.
6. Turn the telephone ringer down.
7. Store lawn furniture, garden tools, hanging baskets, etc., in a secure area.
8. Ask neighbors to look out for your residence while you are away.
9. Leave the phone number with a neighbor of someone to contact in case of an emergency.

Taking these few precautions will make your residence look occupied, and that is the key to residential security while you are away.

Vacationing in a New City?

Your vacation may take you to a new city, with new shopping, museums, sports, and nighttime entertainment. But before you get involved in these activities . . .

1. Buy a city map and ask about local traffic laws or regulations that you aren't familiar with.
2. Designate someone to point out streets or landmarks needed for directions so the driver can concentrate on the road.
3. There may be areas of the city you should avoid. (Crime, heavy traffic, construction, etc.) Check with local police, hotel personnel, taxi drivers, and friends about problem areas.
4. Convert as much cash as possible into travelers checks.
5. To foil pickpockets, carry valuables such as wallets, keys and passport in your <u>front</u> pants or skirt pocket.

Hotel and Motel Safety

Your hotel or motel may be your "home away from home" but it is not as secure. Hotel staff will enter your room to clean, room service may bring meals, and so on. You are in a different environment. Follow these tips to ensure your safety:

1. Be sure to lock your door and windows when you're in your room, as well as when you leave.
2. Know who is knocking before you open the door.
3. Keep your jewelry, cash, and valuables locked in the hotel safe, not lying around your room.

4. Inventory your belongings nightly.
5. Locate the fire exits, and count the doors between your room and the closest exit.
6. Do not smoke in bed.
7. Do not let young children swim without adult supervision.
8. Always take your room key with you. When you check out, return it to the front desk.
9. Remove bags from your luggage rack or inside the car. Lock them in the trunk, or leave them inside.
10. When you are packing to depart, be sure you haven't left anything.

Appendix 8–B

Crime Prevention through Environmental Design

Reducing the Odds: Prevent the Next Crime

To protect your property, a thoughtful and thorough approach to crime prevention is a must. This commonsense approach is suitably called crime prevention through environmental design (CPTED).

CPTED suggests that the form and arrangement of buildings and open space can either encourage or discourage crime. CPTED attempts to reduce crime and the fear of crime by reducing criminal opportunity and fostering positive social interaction among the users of a space. The emphasis is on prevention rather than apprehension and punishment.

The three elements of CPTED are territoriality, surveillance, and access control. Together, these elements can strengthen total premises security and personal safety.

TERRITORIALITY

Territoriality is a person's innate desire to protect or defend his own space. The extent to which people will defend territory depends on their personal investment in or responsibility for that property. For example, homeowners are likely to risk their lives to defend their homes against an intruder who is threatening a spouse or child.

Criminals seek out places that do not exhibit a great deal of territorial control. Places that are unwatched or uncared for make excellent locations for selling drugs, committing robberies, and painting graffiti. The following are several economical, commonsense steps you can take to protect your business:

- Clearly define your property through the use of natural or manmade borders.
- Improve the interior and exterior appearance of your environment.
- Personalize the environment by showing ownership.
- Make special provisions for areas that attract undesirables.
- Initiate Business and Community Watch programs in your neighborhood.

SURVEILLANCE

To defend your property against crime, you must be able to see illegal acts taking place. Surveillance puts the offender under the threat of being observed, identified, and apprehended.

The following tip will help you maximize visibility in your business setting:

- Improve indoor and outdoor lighting. Illuminate all entrances and parking areas.
- Clear windows of all clutter.
- Place employees or trusted members where they can supervise a specific area or activity.
- Control landscaping. Trim shrubbery no higher than two feet. Remove any tree limbs that are six feet or less from the ground.
- Install electronic devices where they will be seen by anyone who enters your building.
- Place restrooms in high-traffic areas.
- Train members, neighbors, and employees in crime reporting. Encourage their participation.
- Involve the entire community in your surveillance efforts.

ACCESS CONTROL

By controlling access, you can funnel people onto your property at specific points where they can be easily observed. Access control denies or restricts access to a crime target, and it also increases the perceived risks of offenders by controlling or restricting their movement. The following are methods of access control:

- Reduce the number of entrances and exits.
- Have a trusted member or employee greet everyone who enters your business.
- Have guests sign in. Give them a visitor badge to display as identification.
- Use a buddy system for people leaving after hours.
- Fence or rope off problem areas.
- Use door and window locks effectively.

CONCLUSION

Encourage your coworkers, employees, members, and neighbors to establish a safe and secure environment by implementing the three basic elements of CPTED:

1. Territoriality: A space has both a clear definition and a specific purpose. The community in which the space is located has ownership.
2. Surveillance: Maximize visibility in the space to maintain a safe environment.
3. Access Control: Monitor those who use the property by assisting legitimate users in their activities and discouraging trespassers.

Problem	On the site	In/around the Neighborhood	Communitywide
Graffiti vandalism	Educate the private property owner or manager about steps to reduce the vulnerability of the property to graffiti vandalism.	Improve opportunities for surveillance:	Increase access control:

Problem

Graffiti vandalism

On the site

Educate the private property owner or manager about steps to reduce the vulnerability of the property to graffiti vandalism.

Increase access control:

- Install fencing or other barriers to the property.
- Install shrubbery along the base of the wall or structure to inhibit easy approach by vandals.

Improve opportunities for surveillance:

- Focus increased lighting on exterior wall of property.

Define territory:

- Recover damaged surface with community or prevention-oriented mural designed by residents or the property owner and residents.

In/around the Neighborhood

Improve opportunities for surveillance:

- Add street lighting along perimeter of facility.
- Dedicate targeted patrols.
- Organize a block watch.

Communitywide

Increase access control:

- Control access to graffiti paints and other implements.
- Provide for increased penalties for property defacement by gang-related graffiti.
- Require property owners to remove graffiti within a specified time period.
- Outline the support local government will provide for property owners in graffiti removal.
- Specify the type of graffiti-resistant coating that must be used on exterior surfaces of buildings.

Improve opportunities for surveillance:

- Establish city agency–supported citizen patrol to provide law enforcement with information on graffiti-plagued properties.

Define territory:

- Educate property owner about cost-effectiveness of graffiti-resistant coating material and other prevention strategies.
- Educate school-aged youth about graffiti vandalism as a serious crime with consequence for the offender and the community.

Crime Environment	Crime Environment	CPTED Strategies	CPTED Design Directive
Parking lot Larceny from auto Robbery from person Assault Auto theft Vandalism	1. Layout of parking lot area conflicts with traffic and pedestrian flow.	1. Improve design of parking lot	1. Main entrance should be marked with double yellow lines and reflector. Need directional sign to Park and Ride area more clearly marked. Add three-way stop to main entry. Traffic island at main entry should be moved to form an all-way or three-way stop. Place crosswalk at bottom of Park and Ride lot.
	2. Lack of lighting	2. Improve lighting in parking lot	2. Have lighting evaluated.
	3. Poor location for bus stop.	3. Relocate bus stop.	3. Bus stop should be moved to northwest corner of main entrance above the Park and Ride lot.

Chapter 9

Security Equipment

CHAPTER OBJECTIVES

1. Discuss the standard issue items for a security officer.
2. Debate the argument for arming or not arming the security staff.
3. Know how to properly select a security vehicle.

INTRODUCTION

Security equipment can be anything from a flashlight to sophisticated electronic equipment. The security director can, through the use of various kinds of uniforms and equipment, set the tone and image for the department. The image the department displays should be congruent with the facility's and the department's mission statements.

UNIFORMS

There are several choices for the security uniform. Some health care facilities use plainclothes security officers, who are identified only by a facility name badge. The problem with this approach is that security officers are often called upon to defuse disturbances, so it is necessary that they quickly gain control of a situation. If they are not easily identified as security, their task may be more difficult. Security should be easily recognized by all staff, visitors, and patients who come unto the property. In most facilities, only security administrators—the director, assistant director, etc.—wear plain business attire.

The military- or police-style uniform is the traditional look for security. Wearing this kind of uniform helps the officer control disturbances and provides a deterrent to crime. The uniform is versatile—it can be worn indoors or outdoors in all climates. If an officer is required to conduct patrols both inside and out, or foot patrols in areas such as boiler and mechanical rooms, this kind of uniform will handle the wear and tear. If the military-style uniform seems too regimental, it can be softened by hospital logo accessories and by wearing a baseball-type cap. To distinguish supervisors from officers, most facilities have them wear a different color shirt, usually white for supervisors, blue for officers.

How many uniforms does an officer need and who should supply them? There is no set answer to these questions. The number of uniforms needed varies. Some facilities require security officers to do light maintenance work, or to patrol dirty areas or outside in extremely inclement weather. These factors can reduce the life of a uniform. Areas that have wide temperature swings usually require officers to have both cold and hot weather uniforms. Most facilities issue (or require an officer to purchase) three shirts and two pairs of pants for full-time employment.

Many facilities furnish uniforms to the officers and charge the officer a small weekly uniform expense. Others require the officers to purchase their own uniforms. For a newly hired officer, the cost of several uniforms may be too much, so the department may arrange for the officer to purchase the uniforms through a payroll deduction plan: the uniform company bills the facility for the uniforms, and the facility deducts a set amount from the officer's pay until the uniforms are paid for. The officer is required to sign a statement acknowledging the uniform debt to the facility and agreeing that if the uniforms are not paid for at the time of termination, the balance will be deducted from his or her final paycheck. This way the officer is spared a large cash outlay, and the facility makes sure the officer has enough uniforms to maintain a professional image. Most facilities will replace a uniform item if it is worn out or damaged in the line of duty. Some facilities that require officers to purchase their own uniforms agree to provide new uniforms after one year of service.

The other style of uniform seen in health care facilities is the blazer with contrasting slacks. Usually the slacks are gray and the blazer blue. Most facilities that use this uniform identify the officer by means of a breast patch. This can be a very professional look, but it is normally not a serviceable uniform. It makes working outdoors in weather extremes difficult and the style defeats two main purposes of a uniform: the officer is not as easy to recognize as one in a military-style uniform and the image may be too "soft" to deter an offender.

Some facilities use a combination of styles: field officers wear the military-style uniform, supervisors wear the slacks and blazer with breast patch, and security administrators wear normal business attire. This combination can work well, especially for large departments that have several layers of personnel.

Regardless of the uniform style chosen, one of the keys to the image of the department is a professional-looking officer. Not only must the uniform be clean, pressed, and properly fitting, the officer must adhere to strict personal grooming standards. The appearance of each officer reflects on the director and the facility.

OFFICER EQUIPMENT

The officer should carry and use only equipment that is issued and/or authorized by the director of security. There can be no exceptions to this policy. Too many times an officer has injured someone in an altercation and it is later found that the officer used an unauthorized weapon. The most likely culprit is a metal flashlight. Unfortunately, many facilities do not issue flashlights to officers, which means the officers purchase their own flashlights. The cost of providing officers with flashlights is very minor compared with the cost to settle a lawsuit if an officer strikes someone with a metal flashlight.

The type of equipment issued to an officer varies according to the level and type of services expected of the officer. If the officer will be called upon to assist with patients, he or she must be issued rubber gloves. If the officer is expected to make minor maintenance repairs or checks, appropriate equipment should be issued. The best way to avoid unauthorized equipment is to issue everything an officer needs. The following are the main pieces of equipment issued to security officers.

Notebook and Pen

Often overlooked, this can be an officer's most-used equipment. The best size is the 3-inch by 4-inch flip pad that many facilities can make in their own print shops. These notepads can hold the radio codes for the department, emergency codes for the facility, and key questions to ask on the scene of a crime. Some even contain foldout maps of the facility grounds. Officers should always use black ink to facilitate clear copies of reports.

Handcuffs

Make sure they work properly and are not rusted or bent. In addition, do not issue the handcuffs until the officer has been trained in how to properly apply and double lock them. Some people think that an officer should not handcuff a suspect because it places him or her under arrest, and if the person is later released the facility is liable for false arrest. The use or nonuse of handcuffs is irrelevant: if a person is restricted in his or her freedom to move or leave an area, that is the basis for a false arrest, not the use of handcuffs. One facility never allowed its officers to carry any restraining devices. When a consultant asked them how they restrained someone when it was necessary, they replied, "We get as many people as we can, throw the suspect to the ground, pile on, and hold him until the police arrive." Handcuffs should be used as a defensive device only, to keep someone from injuring him- or herself or others. They should never be used in an offensive manner, for example, striking someone with them or applying them too tightly.

Baton

Like handcuffs, batons should be issued and used only for defense. The officer must be thoroughly trained in the use of the baton before it is issued and must understand that he or she must *never* strike someone in the head area with the baton. Several baton types are available: the straight baton, the handled PR-24, and the metal expandable flex baton. The expandable baton is easier to carry, but officers should receive extra training in its use because of its increased potential for inflicting injury.

Protective Spray

Again, training is the key. Officers should not be issued protective spray until they have been trained in its use. Most states require the officer to receive training from a state or manufacturer-certified trainer. As part of the training, many states require the officer to be sprayed with the product.

Most facilities that use protective spray use pepper foam with a 10 percent oleoresin capsicum pepper formula concentration. The foam is not as easily picked up by interior air handlers and spread throughout the facility. If officers are issued the spray/foam, they should also be issued and carry the reversal spray and towelettes. The officer should only leave a suspect under the influence of the spray/foam until restraining devices are fastened. The suspect should be taken to the emergency department, if possible, and checked to make sure he or she has recovered from the spray/foam. See Appendix 9–A for a suggested policy and procedure for the use of pepper spray.

Firearms

To arm or not to arm officers is a decision each facility must make. The International Association for Healthcare Security and Safety (IAHSS) adopted the following position in October 1992:

> The decision whether or not a healthcare facility's security officers carry a weapon, or the type of weapon, is best determined by the individual facility based upon a needs assessment. If the decision is made that security officers are to carry a weapon, the officer must be thoroughly trained in the use of the weapon prior to being issued. All policies and procedures regarding weapon usage should be reviewed by corporate attorneys representing individual institutions.

What would constitute a needs assessment? Several factors must be reviewed. First, the crime rate in and around the facility. A higher crime rate, especially one with violent crime, may dictate that the officers must be armed. Second, what is the local law enforcement response time? In some rural facilities, law enforcement response time may be so long that the security officers are essentially on their own. The level of professionalism of the officer must also be considered. The officer must be intelligent, trainable, and mentally and emotionally stable. Some facilities will not consider an officer eligible to be armed until he or she successfully completes a probationary period. The type of tasks the officer is asked to perform should also be reviewed. If officers are asked to patrol parking lots and off-campus buildings alone, it may be necessary for them to be armed.

One might think that the sight of an armed officer in a health care setting could make staff, visitors, and patients feel uneasy; however, if the officers are well trained and professional, the opposite will occur. Patients, visitors, and staff will feel safer knowing that an officer has all the tools necessary to protect them. In addition, the presence of a firearm can be a deterrent to crime and make the officer look more professional than the so-called Rent-a-Cop guard.

If the facility decides to arm the officers, they must also carry handcuffs, baton, and protective spray/foam. In addition, the officer's training must have included verbal noncrisis intervention. The facility must make sure that it can show that the officer had other means of protection available before the final resort to a firearm.

The type of firearm is also debatable. Many facilities allow security officers to carry the same weapon used by local law enforcement. It is this author's opinion that a .38 or .357 revolver is a better choice. First, a revolver requires less training and is easier to use for the less-experienced officer. The revolver is also less offensive looking than an automatic pistol. The security officer should never remove the revolver from its holster or fire the weapon in an offensive manner, as law enforcement officers may be required to do. The more clearly security officers can show that their actions were purely defensive, the fewer problems they will have if a shooting situation occurs.

The holster used by the officers is also important, especially when carrying the weapon in or around the emergency department. The holster must be a department-issued safety holster with a hammer strap. It must hold the firearm steady and close to the body. A holster that requires the weapon to be pushed down and then pulled forward is generally considered the best type.

Appendix 9–B is a sample policy and procedure outlining an approval process and suggested training program for firearms. Of course, the facility should determine what the local and/or state requirements are for the issuance and use of firearms by security personnel.

Security Vehicles

Many factors bear on the decision of what type of, if any, security vehicle to use. Again, the expectations for the security department and the tasks officers are called upon to perform will influence the decision. Other factors to consider are climate, types of parking facilities, and volume of calls for service. If the facility is in an area that experiences heavy snowfall and security is expected to pick up staff from home and bring them to the facility in inclement weather, a four-wheel-drive is a must. If security also serves as a courier for the facility, a van or pickup truck with a cover may be better.

The kind of patrols performed by security will also dictate the type of vehicle. If the patrol area is small and includes parking decks, a rear-wheel vehicle normally gives better service—the constant turning of the vehicle in a small lot or parking deck will make the tires wear out much faster on a front-wheel-drive vehicle because of the engine weight. If the patrol area is extremely large, a front-wheel-drive may give better gas mileage. The size of the vehicle is important. If security is expected to escort employees to their vehicles, a full-size vehicle or mini-van would probably be the best choice.

Some facilities have found that electric golf carts or bicycles work well to patrol a small, flat campus. The problem with the golf cart, of course, is the down time when the battery is being recharged. And a bike patrol may not always be possible because of weather conditions. However, if the facility is located in a moderate climate, the bike patrol is a good idea. Not only can the officers maneuver through parking lots easily and quickly, but riding a bike helps them stay physically fit.

Regardless of the type of vehicle used, a preventive maintenance program must be in place and shift-by-shift inspections of the vehicle should be performed. The facility should also establish a policy concerning investigation and, if necessary, discipline if an officer is involved in an accident. Appendix 9–C is a sample policy for patrol vehicles and Appendix 9–D is a checklist for inspecting a vehicle.

KEY POINTS

- The term "equipment" can mean many things; however, the following are the items usually associated with security in a health care facility:
  - –uniforms (there are at least three options)
  - –notebook and pen (essential items)
  - –handcuffs (hands-on training is necessary)
  - –baton (hands-on training is necessary)
  - –protective spray (hands-on training is necessary; foam is preferred over spray)
  - –firearms (arming security officers is an individual facility decision)
  - –vehicles (auto, truck, van, golf cart, bike can all be used in special circumstances)

Appendix 9–A

Pepper Spray—Policy and Procedure

	Issued By:	Policy #:
	Prepared By:	Revision #:
	Approved By:	Effective Date:
Subject:		Page of

PURPOSE

To provide guidelines on use of defensive sprays.

POLICY

The thrust of our security program is geared at prevention. The patrolling security officer will not be equipped with firearms. An armed security force contributes to the enforcement philosophy, and one hasty decision by an individual could cause untold ramifications to everyone.

PROCEDURE

1. Security officers can be equipped with defensive sprays designed to subdue aggressive individuals. Security personnel will carry defensive sprays in holsters on the equipment belt with the safety on. Officers will not patrol with spray carried in hand.
2. All officers will complete a training program conducted by either the local police department or other metro area police department before they are allowed to carry the spray. The training may require the officer to be sprayed with the defensive spray.

3. Experiencing the spray will help the officer not to panic should he or she be sprayed during use or by someone carrying the spray.
4. Defensive sprays are to be used only as a last resort to protect patients, visitors, or employees from physical harm. After use of the spray, officers shall remain with the subject for 45 minutes and visually observe the subject until he or she has recovered from its effects.
5. Any officer who uses the defensive spray for whatever reason during the course of his or her duties will be suspended until the manager of safety and security or the director of material and environmental services conducts an investigation of the incident.
6. Should the investigation find that the officer acted reasonably, the individual will be allowed to return to work for the next regularly scheduled shift. If the investigation reveals that the officer's use of the spray was unwarranted, the employee shall be subject to immediate termination.
7. Termination will be made only after the director of human resources and performance improvement has reviewed the findings and agrees with the recommendation.

Appendix 9–B

Firearms—Policy and Procedures

POLICY

Public safety/security officers are authorized to carry firearms in the performance of their duties after having met the following criteria, completed the required training, and been approved by the State Private Protective Services Board.

PROCEDURE

Basic Qualifications

1. The officer has been employed with the department for a minimum of six months and has successfully completed and been removed from probation.
2. The officer has successfully completed the public/safety security basic training program and demonstrated competence in all areas.
3. The officer must meet the state requirements for an armed security officer.
4. The officer must submit to a yearly drug screening.

Approval Process

After meeting the basic qualifications, the officer must request in writing to the director to become an armed officer. The request will be reviewed by the preliminary review board. If the request is approved by the preliminary board, the officer will appear before an oral board. The officer will complete a written exam and appear before the oral board. The oral review board will question the officer on background, training, legal issues, and deadly force and will ask the officer to respond to various scenarios.

In the event an officer fails to successfully complete any portion of the approval process, the officer may submit another request after six months.

Training Program

After successfully completing the approval process, the officer must successfully

1. Complete the public safety/security firearms training program.
2. Pass a written examination with a minimum score of 80%.
3. Demonstrate proficiency on an approved day course or fire with a minimum of 80%.
4. Demonstrate proficiency on an approved night course or fire with a minimum of 80%.
5. Demonstrate proficiency on a simulated realistic shooting situation with a minimum score of 80%.
6. Demonstrate proficiency in the safe handling of a firearm.
7. Demonstrate knowledge of the state laws governing the use of firearms by a security officer.
8. Demonstrate knowledge of the department's public safety/security policies and procedures governing the use of a firearm by its security officers.

Standard Operating Procedure: Firearms

The following policies and procedures will govern the use of firearms by security officers:

1. Firearms will only be carried by an approved, trained, and registered officer.
2. An officer will, at all times when on duty have his or her firearm registration permit displayed on the outermost garment.
3. Firearms other than department-issued firearms will not be used in the performance of a public safety/security officer's duty.
4. Only ammunition that is issued by the department will be carried or used.
5. The firearm of the uniformed officer will always be worn on the utility belt. Uniformed officers will not carry concealed weapons.
6. Public safety/security officers will not carry backup weapons.
7. Firearms owned by the facility will not be used for target practice, even on one's own land, except for authorized and supervised training at an approved range, under the supervision of the firearms instructor.
8. No department firearms will be signed out for personal practice. Practice sessions can be scheduled with the firearms instructor at the officer's expense.
9. No alterations or repairs will be performed on any firearms by an officer.
10. Public safety/security officers are responsible for cleaning and maintaining departmental firearms. Damages or repairs that are needed should be reported to the firearms instructor.
11. If a firearm is drawn for any reason except authorized training, a full written report of the circumstances will be made immediately by the officer in charge (OIC) on duty. Included in this report will be a written statement by the officer involved. A follow-up investigation will be conducted by the director of the security department. The officer will be suspended during the investigation.
12. If a firearm is discharged for any reason except authorized training, a full written report of the circumstances will be made immediately by the OIC on duty. Included in this re-

port will be a written statement by the officer involved. The director and firearms instructor will be notified immediately. A follow-up investigation will be conducted by the director. The officer will be suspended during the investigation.

13. Deadly force may not be used for the protection of property.
14. Officers are not to fire at, above, or in any direction to prevent a suspect from fleeing. Warning shots are not justifiable and will not be tolerated under any circumstances.
15. Officers will never point a firearm at any person without justifiable cause or protection of life. Pointing a firearm at a person or threatening use of an unholstered or holstered firearm could result in a conviction for assault.
16. A firearm can be used only to protect the officer's life or the life of another person from the imminent use of deadly force.
17. Any time an officer enters an area where firearms are not permitted, the officer will unload the firearm and secure it.
18. Any time an officer exchanges a firearm with another officer, the firearm will be unloaded and the cylinder will be open. The barrel of the firearm will be pointed in a safe direction. This procedure will be conducted out of the view of the public and other staff.
19. All armed officers will comply with the department handcuff and baton policy at all times when on duty.
20. Failure to comply with any of the department policies and procedures, or to maintain the degree of proficiency outlined regarding firearms, will result in disciplinary action including suspension of approval to carry firearm, suspension form duty, and/or termination.

Appendix 9–C

Procedures for Patrol Vehicles

PROCEDURE

I. **Patrol Vehicle Accidents**

A. When a department vehicle is involved in <u>any</u> accident, a report will be completed by the officer in charge (OIC). Also, the appropriate law enforcement agency will be contacted at the time of the accident for a report. The accident will be reviewed by the OIC, assistant director, and director.

B. If the accident is determined to be the result of the driver's negligence, the driver will personally be held responsible for the first $50 in repairs and will receive a written warning.

C. If the same driver is involved in another accident, he or she will be responsible for the entire deductible amount of the department's insurance policy and will receive a three-day suspension without pay.

D. If there is any further accident or abuse of a department vehicle, the driver will be responsible for all repairs and will be terminated.

II. **Security Department Vehicles Are Not Emergency Response Vehicles**

A. No 10-33 traffic (emergency).

B. All traffic laws must be obeyed.

C. The overhead lights (bar-lights) are to be used for visibility purposes only.

D. Vehicle traffic stops are to be made on health care facility property only. Do not make vehicle stops on public property.

E. Vehicle must be operated in a safe manner. Any deliberate abuse or misuse will not be tolerated.

F. Failure to obey the above will result in disciplinary actions as follows:

1. First offense—written warning
2. Second offense—written warning
3. Third offense—written warning
              3-day suspension
4. Fourth offense—Termination

III. Vehicle Inspection

A. A vehicle inspection form must be completed by the driver prior to the start of his or her shift.

B. Any damage that is noted by the driver must be reported to his or her supervisor before the vehicle is moved.

Department vehicles are highly visible pieces of equipment and must be used and maintained in the appropriate manner.

Appendix 9–D

Vehicle Checklist

Date: _____

Shift: _____

Vehicle number: _____

Gas Level: _____ Oil Level: _____ Mileage: _____

		NOTE ANY PROBLEMS IN THIS SPACE	FIXED BY	DATE
E	Front			
X	Right side			
T	Rear			
E R	Left side			
I	Roof			
O R	Tires			
I	Condition			
N	Tickets			
T	Gate openers			
E R	Radio			
I	Air tank			
O R	Slim jim			
	Jumper cables			
L	Interior			
I G	Parking			
H	Turn signals			
T S	Flashers			
Y	Brakes			
S	Reverse			
T E	Spotlight			
M	Bar lights			

Vehicle acceptable? _____ Yes _____ No   Officer: _____

123

Chapter 10

Electronics in Health Care Security

William P. Gibbons III

CHAPTER OBJECTIVES

1. Know the basic components of an electronic security system.
2. Understand when and how the various components can/should be used.

INTRODUCTION

The use of electronics to achieve a higher level of security has become commonplace in the health care setting. As budgets are trimmed, the security director is faced with the task of offering the same, if not a higher, level of protection as when funds were more plentiful. In most cases, the only way to achieve this goal is through the use of electronics.

Although electronic security equipment has become more affordable, it still is a considerable investment; however, the security director should remember that the electronic equipment does not receive benefits, does not take days off, and does not expect salary increases every year. Will electronics ever totally replace qualified security officers? No. Should a proper mix of security personnel and electronics be used in a fully supported, high-quality program? Yes.

Many factors should be considered when using electronics. Security directors should ask themselves, What do I hope to achieve with this equipment? What is the threat level for personal safety in the area? When do the threats occur? Do I need historical documentation of events? How can I determine the budget for purchasing the equipment? What equipment is available that will do the best job at the lowest cost, for both purchasing and maintenance?

In the electronic security market, there are many different types of cameras, card access systems, alarms, and radios, and countless companies selling and installing equipment. How does the security director know where to turn? The best source is personal referrals from your peers. If this source is not available, the next best guide is the *American Society of Industrial Security Buyer's Guide* (Phillips Business Information, Potomac, MD: Mark Kimmel Group Publisher, 1997). This guide, while it does not recommend any of the companies listed, is an

125

excellent resource. **The key components of an electronic security system are closed-circuit television, access control, tour management systems, intrusion alarms, intercom alarms, panic alarms, and radios.**

CLOSED-CIRCUIT TELEVISION (CCTV)

The basic CCTV system includes cameras, monitors, and VCRs.

Cameras

Some important factors must be considered when designing an electronic security system. First look at lighting. Good lighting can provide two advantages: (1) it allows better personal viewing of employees and guests in parking lots and other outside areas at night, and (2) it boosts the performance of the CCTV system. If lighting is a problem at the facility, it will also be a problem for electronics. System design is a very important aspect of the operation of any electronic security system. Choosing the right camera for the lighting conditions and the right zoom or fixed lens is at the heart of the system. With the correct camera and lens selection, security officers will be able to use a well-designed CCTV system to cover a large area rather than employing more officers.

Black and White versus Color

In most cases, perimeter cameras should be black and white rather than color. Black and white is more effective at night because less light is required to give full video pictures. Outside color cameras require more light and do not perform well at night.

High-Resolution versus Standard Resolution

High-resolution cameras have sharper edges and more detail in the pictures than standard resolution cameras and therefore work well for parking lots and other perimeter applications. Standard resolution cameras do not have well-defined pictures, but they are less expensive than the high-resolution series. High-resolution and standard resolution cameras are available in 24VAC, 12VDC, or 115VAC versions. These cameras can be outfitted with motorized zoom lenses as well as fixed lenses.

Lens

Most CCTV cameras come with a 16mm lens, which gives the camera a field of vision similar to the human eye. If a smaller lens is used—4mm or 8mm—the image will be a wider view, but it will seem farther away. Conversely, if a larger lens is used—25mm—the image will appear closer and larger, but the field of vision will be narrower.

Overt versus Covert

Should the cameras be overt (plainly visible) or covert (hidden)? The answer lies in the purpose of the camera. For example, a camera used in a parking lot/deck probably would be overt, to let the public and the criminal element know that you have CCTV and are watching their activities. If the camera is to be used as an investigative tool, then perhaps it should be covert. Cameras can be disguised as smoke detectors, clocks, wall switches, laptop computers, and so on. Both overt and covert cameras can be used to videotape activities or can route the video to the head-in (control) equipment.

Monitors

Video monitors are an important part of the CCTV security system. They are available in different sizes. Nine-inch monitors are usually used with individual cameras or multiple cameras tied to a switcher (switchers are discussed under Video Management); 12-inch monitors are usually used with multiplexers or quad-splitters (also discussed under Video Management). Larger monitors—such as 17-inch and 20-inch versions—can be used with multiplexers, quad-splitters, and matrix switchers. Color monitors can also be used with color equipment and are available in various sizes. Monitor size depends on the specific application and the number of cameras in a given system. Regular television sets cannot be used in CCTV systems.

The monitoring station must be designed with ergonomics in mind, because an officer may be sitting there for 8–12 hours at a time. Monitors must be arranged so the officer can watch as many screens as possible at one time.

The control, or head-in, system should be designed for ease of operation. Individual monitors for each camera usually do not work well, because the pictures are spread out and are very difficult to watch. Multiplexed or quad pictures on one monitor are much easier to view. Multiplexers are high-tech video compression devices that can produce 16 individual video pictures on a single video monitor. Quad units are also compression devices, except their capability is limited to compressing only four cameras on a single monitor. Videotape can be used to record all pictures at one time for archiving video information.

Video Management

Video management is an important part of any CCTV system, and ease of operation and efficiency will pay off during an emergency. Selecting the right equipment for a given situation will make security personnel more valuable.

In the past few years, a number of pieces of equipment that manage video quite well have arrived on the market. Quad-splitters (or quads) can be used for a four-camera system that is either black and white or color. These devices will compress video and show all four cameras either individually or all four on a single monitor. A number of manufacturers build and sell quads, which are available in many different sizes and shapes to meet any requirements.

Multiplexers are available in a 16-camera or 9-camera design. These devices compress video and reproduce all cameras onto one monitor or can show just one camera at a time. Both can be purchased in black and white or in color versions, and either simplex or duplex. With a simplex multiplexer, you can record all cameras, but if recorded video needs to be played back, the system cannot view and record live cameras at the same time. The system is either playing back or recording, not both. With a duplex multiplexer, you can record and play back simultaneously. Duplex units are generally more expensive but usually more efficient. Two video recorders must be used for simultaneous recording and playback of video.

Switchers are used to switch video from one camera to another. The switched-on camera is the only video shown on the monitor (see Figure 10–1). Switchers are not used much anymore because quad-splitters and multiplexers offer better performance.

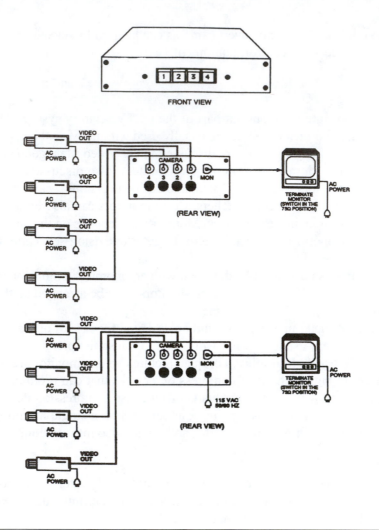

Figure 10–1

Microprocessor-controlled systems offer the best video management tool. They are available in different camera and monitor configurations to fit any application. These systems can control pan, tilt, and zoom cameras, and can select cameras for display on monitors. Microprocessor-based systems can also respond to alarms from doors and switch the appropriate camera to the alarm area. One person can control many cameras—pan and tilt as well as fixed cameras, black and white or color.

Another type of control is hardwired, which means that a multiconductor copper wire must be pulled between pan, tilt, and zoom cameras and the control point or security station. Hardwired controls are used to control camera pan and tilt functions and the zoom lens. Many hardwired controls are in use today and will continue to be used where economic controls are needed.

VCRs

VCRs are another important part of the security control system. The time-lapse machine is usually used because a single T-120 videotape can be used and can record many hours of video—from 6 to 960 hours. VCRs can be used with multiplexers, and all cameras (up to 16) can be recorded. The recorded video can be played back through the multiplexer as a single-camera full-screen picture or all 16 cameras on the screen at the same time. It is a good idea to number the tapes and rotate them so you do not use the same tape all the time. The time-lapse VCR should be serviced at least every 12 months—a new head, new belts, and alignment are required. Figures 10–2 and 10–3 show how VCRs are installed.

Accessories

Once the control and video management equipment are selected, it is time to select camera accessories. Pan and tilt units will be required to move the cameras and lenses up and down and back and forth. These units are manufactured in standard voltages; the one most often used is 24VAC, which is safe for technicians to work with outside without fear of electrocution. Pan and tilt units are available in various load ratings. Housings are used to protect the camera and lens from harsh weather and other conditions. Housings can be bought with heaters and blowers if the camera and lens will be used in extreme cold or heat. Sunshields are also available to decrease the heat buildup from the sun during the summer months. After

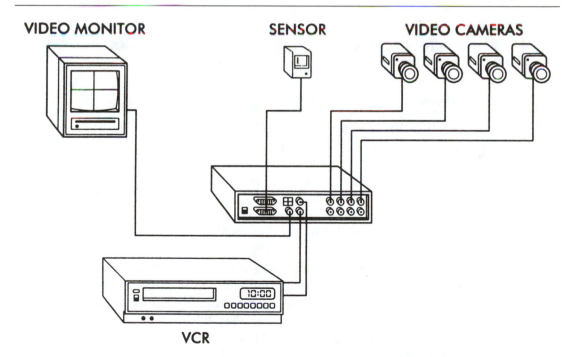

Figure 10–2

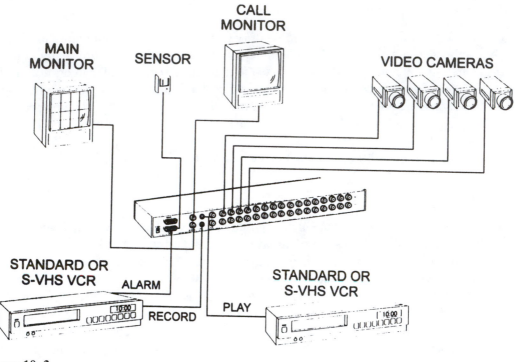

Figure 10–3

---

you select a location for the camera, you can choose the appropriate camera mount for the pan and tilt size and the weight load.

Transmission Methods

Coaxial (coax) cable is the most commonly used transmission method in CCTV systems. Coax cable is inexpensive and can be installed up to 1,000 feet using RG59 cable (if it is pulled farther than 1,000 feet, you will need amplification). The cable is susceptible to lightning and noise, so it must be routed away from lighting power lines and building services. Check your local electrical code before installing the cable. It is rated at only 300 volts, so it is not legal to pull it through the same conduit with power wires. In some cases, plenum cable must be used in ceilings. Cable is pulled from the camera to the control and video management equipment.

Fiber optic cable is the best choice for transmission. It can be run extreme lengths without any video loss. Fiber optic cable can be pulled in ceilings, but plenum-rated cable may still need to be used. Interface modules must be used at both ends of fiber cable to convert to useful signals. Fiber optic cable is much more expensive than coaxial cable, but if long lengths are required and lightning is a problem, it is worth the extra cost.

Telephone line transmission should be used only when there is no other option. At its very best, telephone line transmission will provide poor video quality. If telephone lines are the only path available, try to obtain dedicated lines, that is, two uncut wires from camera to monitor. Interfaces will be required on phone lines, as with fiber optic cable.

Microwave transmission is very expensive, and when it is used on long paths (three to six miles) it is not dependable because of weather and natural barriers such as trees. This transmission method should not be used unless there is no other choice.

ACCESS CONTROL

Once the CCTV system is in place, it is time to consider access to the facility. Keys are normally used to secure doors, but there is a major drawback to keys: they can be duplicated. If a master key is lost and duplicated, security is also lost, and the whole building will have to be re-keyed. Cipher locks and keypads are two other methods for controlling access. Cipher locks have mechanical pushbuttons that, when pushed in the right order, will unlock the door. Keypads operate in the same manner, except that they use electronic technology. The disadvantage of the cipher lock and the keypad is that many people will have to know the number. Also, there is no audit trail to track who opened the door.

Card Access

Card access control is an alternative. With card access, it is possible to know who unlocked the door and when. **Some of the common technologies used in access cards are bar code, magnetic strip, Wiegand, and proximity.**

Bar code systems use cards that have bar codes printed on the back. The code is usually covered by a material that makes it difficult to copy but still allows the reader to read it using photoelectric technology. The bar code is arranged so that the reader may read three of the nine numbers. For example, the first three numbers denote the particular facility, and the remaining numbers can be used for individual information. This type of card technology produces a high level of security.

Magnetic cards have a magnetic strip on which information is stored, similar to tape used in recording devices. These cards can be altered or forged and are not a good choice for high security.

Wiegand cards have 20 to 40 bits of unique information embedded in them. By having this limited data capability, this system has limited application. It can be used only where small amounts of data are needed.

Proximity cards are very popular and very difficult to duplicate. The card is available in two types: active and passive. Active cards are not as widely used—they are thicker and somewhat larger because they contain a small battery that gives the card a large sensitivity area. Passive cards, on the other hand, are widely used. These cards are the same size as a credit card and are easily carried in pockets and wallets. The read distance (about one to four inches) is shorter than that of the active card, but the passive card can be left in the cardholder's pocket or wallet and still read. The reader sets up a radio frequency (RF) when the card is placed in the RF field. If the card is valid in the database, the door will open.

Door Hardware

Whichever card access system is selected will require door hardware. Strikes in door frames are easily installed. The knob set stays in place, and the strike plate in the frame is changed out with a strike. The strike plate is the small piece of metal in the door frame that the lock bolt slides into. The strike itself is installed in place of the strike plate, and, when electrical impulses are applied, it allows the strike to move in such a manner as to allow the bolt to go back into the lock set. The strike is wired to the card access hardware. Another way to secure the door is with a magnetic lock. The lock is wired to the card access hardware in the same manner. Using magnetic locks requires crash bars on doors in order to disconnect power from the magnetic locks.

TOUR MANAGEMENT SYSTEMS

How can you make sure that the security officer is actually checking key locations? The answer lies in a tour management system.

Once the card access system and locking hardware are in place, security officers can use one of two tour systems: a mechanical clock or an electronic system. The mechanical clock system, which has been used for many years, requires the officer to use a key to imprint the time and location on a paper chart in the clock. The newer electronic systems use magnetic strips at each check station. A data acquisition unit reads and records the strip location. When the officer returns to his or her post, the data acquisition unit is placed in a cradle that downloads the recorded information to a computer hard drive. Reports can be generated from the downloaded information.

INTRUSION ALARMS

If outlying buildings must be secured and cameras and access systems are not used, an intrusion detection system should be considered. Internally, intrusion alarms can be used to add another level of security to sensitive areas.

There are many different kinds of alarm systems, but they all can be reduced to a simple process. The sensors receive a signal (a door opened, a window broken); they transmit the signal over an electrical circuit to the control unit, and an alarm is sounded or transmitted. The alarm may be a loud horn, a telephone call to the police, etc.

Basic alarm systems are not expensive and can be designed to sense door intrusion, glass breaking, changes in room temperature, or motion. Alarm systems can be interfaced with other electronic security equipment such as a CCTV system.

INTERCOM/AUDIO ALARMS

These alarms have their best application in parking decks. In many ways, they work like a normal station-to-station intercom: if someone needs nonemergency help, he or she can push the button on the intercom and talk directly with the monitoring station, which is usually security. But these alarms also can be set to "open" at a predetermined decibel level. When this occurs, an alarm sounds at the monitoring station and security can have direct audio communication with the area. These systems also can be interfaced with the camera system: if an alarm notification is received, the central processor can interface with the CCTV system and that level of the parking deck will be immediately brought up on the video monitors and videotaped.

PANIC ALARMS

In areas where there is a likelihood of personal attack or robbery—such as the business office, pharmacy, psychiatric units, and emergency department—panic alarms should be considered. These are simply contact switches that cause an alarm to sound at the monitoring location. One tip on installing these alarms: if they are installed under a desk, make sure the alarm button is recessed so people do not hit it by accident with their knees.

Certain staff members can also carry a personal panic alarm. These look like small garage door openers, but they are actually radio transmitters that are received at a control unit. They are ideal for use in a psychiatric unit. The control unit can be installed at the nurse's station. If a staff member has a problem, he or she can push the personal alarm, which does not make any noise in their hand but sounds at the nurse's station.

RADIOS

The radio is the single most important piece of equipment for the individual security officer. Using the radio, officers can receive assignments, call in their location, and, if necessary, call for assistance. Cellular phones are used widely but are expensive because of the cost of air time, so radios should be used whenever possible. A number of companies manufacture two-way radio equipment and cellular phones.

UHF and VHF equipment operate at different frequencies. The UHF type is more popular, because licenses are easier to obtain and the radios work well inside buildings. It is almost impossible to get a clear VHF frequency from the Federal Communications Commission because of high demand. Both kinds of equipment can be used with earphones, so the security officer can walk around the facility without disturbing others.

The security industry is constantly changing, and new and improved products appear on the market often. Before buying any electronic security products, do as much research as you can to determine what products will best fulfill your particular security requirements.

KEY POINTS

- Health care facilities are turning to electronics to offset the loss of personnel from budget cutting.
- The most common electronic equipment used in security is:
  –CCTV (cameras and camera accessories, monitors, VCRs, switchers)
  –access control equipment
  –tour management systems
  –intrusion alarms
  –intercom alarms
  –panic alarms
  –radios

Chapter 11

Maternity Center Security

John B. Rabun, Jr.

CHAPTER OBJECTIVES

1. Understand the scope of the problem of infant abduction by people outside a family.
2. Learn a profile of the typical infant abductor.
3. Use recommended guidelines to help prevent and respond to an infant abduction.
4. Know about the possible legal liability associated with an infant abduction.
5. Realize that infant security measures must exist in other areas of the health care facility, not just in the birthing center.
6. Know how to educate the parents of infants concerning infant abductions.
7. Learn how to conduct a self-survey of a facility concerning infant abductions.

The text in this chapter is primarily taken from "For Healthcare Professionals: Guidelines on Prevention of and Responses to Infant Abductions" by John Rabun, vice president and chief operating officer of the National Center for Missing and Exploited Children (NCMEC). The material in this chapter and in the appendix is available from the NCMEC and is reprinted with permission of the NCMEC, copyright 1989, 1991, 1992, 1993, 1996, and 1998. All rights reserved. National Center for Missing and Exploited Children® is a registered service mark of the National Center for Missing and Exploited Children.

This "Self Assessment for Healthcare Facilities" is from *For Healthcare Professionals: Guidelines on Prevention of and Response to Infant Abductions* by John B. Rabun, Jr. It is reprinted with permission of the National Center for Missing and Exploited Children (NCMEC). Copyright © NCMEC 1989, 1991, 1992, 1993, 1996, and 1998. All rights reserved. National Center for Missing and Exploited Children® is a registered service mark of the National Center for Missing and Exploited Children.

Contributing to particular sections were Ian Chambers, marketing manager for the commercial/industrial division of the Sensormatic Electronics Corporation; Jim Crumbley, director of protective services, Scottish Rite Children's Hospital; Connie Blackburn Furrh, RN, corporate risk manager and safety officer for project development at Renaissance Healthcare, Inc.; and Janet Lincoln, RNC, MSN, former director of maternal-child health, Hoag Memorial Hospital-Presbyterian.

The Recovery section at the end of the chapter was written by David H. Sells, Jr., and is not part of "For Healthcare Professionals: Guidelines on Prevention of and Responses to Infant Abductions."

INTRODUCTION

> On Father's Day a young mother sat in her room in a secure and well-managed private health care facility in North Carolina feeding her newborn infant. A woman in a nurse's uniform came into the room and told the mother that she was taking the infant to have him weighed and tested. The mother handed her infant over. Within minutes, the infant was out of the health care facility, abducted by the woman impersonating a nurse. Happily, thanks to a speedy response by law enforcement and effective media coverage, the child was recovered two days later, unharmed. When questioned, the abductor, convicted for kidnapping, said simply, "I wanted an infant for myself."

While not a crime of epidemic proportions, the abduction of infants from health care facilities by people who are not family members has clearly become a subject of concern for parents, nurses who care for mothers and newborns, health care security and risk management administrators, law enforcement officials, and the National Center for Missing and Exploited Children (NCMEC). With the goal of preventing crimes against children, NCMEC—in cooperation with the Federal Bureau of Investigation (FBI), the International Association for Healthcare Security and Safety, and the University of Pennsylvania School of Nursing—has studied infant abductions from health care facilities, homes, and other sites and considers most of them preventable.

Based on a study of cases from 1983 through 1997 (see Exhibit 11–1 and Table 11–1), it is estimated that there are between 12 and 18 infant abductions by nonfamily members per year nationwide. Because a number of cases may not be reported to NCMEC or other organizations, this estimate may be conservative. (As a point of comparison, there are approximately 4.2 million births yearly in the United States at more than 3,500 birthing facilities.) Ninety-seven of the cases studied were abductions from health care facility premises, and 57 were infant abductions from the home, following most of the same patterns as the health care facility abductions but with the addition of violence committed against the mother. Seventeen additional infants were abducted from other places such as malls, offices, and parking lots. Of the facilities in which infants have been abducted, 12 percent of the abductions occurred in facilities with no more than 200 beds, 42 percent of the abductions occurred in facilities with between 201 and 400 beds, 16 percent of the abductions occurred in facilities with between 401 and 600 beds, and 30 percent of the abductions occurred in facilities with more than 600 beds. Of all the infants abducted from health care facilities, 94 percent were located and safely returned, usually within a few days to two weeks. Anecdotal evidence would suggest that there may be numerous abduction attempts at birthing facilities each year.

The typical health care facility abduction involves an unknown abductor impersonating a nurse, health care facility employee, volunteer, or relative to gain access to an infant. The obstetrics unit is open and inviting. Patients do not stay long, so they have little time to get to know staff members. In addition, obstetrics units can be filled with medical and nursing staff, visitors, students, volunteers, and participants in classes in parenting and newborn care. With so many faces on these units, intruders are not likely to be noticed. Because there is generally easier access to a mother's room than to the newborn nursery and newborn infants today usu-

Exhibit 11–1 Infant Abductions, 1983–1997

Abductions at health care facilities	97	Located = 92
		Still missing = 5
From mother's room	55 (57%)	
From nursery	14 (14%)	
From pediatrics	16 (17%)	
Outside hospital but still on health care facility grounds	12 (12%)	
With violence to mother	3 (3%)	
Abductions at homes	57	Located = 52
		Still missing = 5
With violence to mother	16 (28%)	
Abductions at other places	17	Located = 16
		Still missing = 1
With violence to mother	3 (18%)	

Note: To date, there has been no use of violence (or attempts) against the mothers or health care staff *within* the health care facility; however, there is clear evidence of increasing violence by abductors when the abductions move outside of the health care setting.

ally stay with their mothers rather than in nurseries, most abductors con the mother into handing over the infant.

TYPICAL OFFENDER

The offender is typically an overweight female somewhere between the ages of 12 and 50 who has no prior criminal record. If she has a criminal record, it is usually for crimes such as shoplifting, passing bad checks, and forgery. She is likely to be gainfully employed. While she appears "normal," the woman most likely is compulsive, suffers from low self-esteem, has faked one or more pregnancies, and relies on manipulation and lying as coping mechanisms in her interpersonal relationships. Sometimes she wishes either to "replace" an infant she has lost or to experience a "vicarious birthing" of a child she is for some reason unable to conceive or carry to term. The infant may be used in an attempt to maintain or save a relationship with her husband, boyfriend, or companion (hereinafter referred to as "significant other"). On occasion, an abductor may be involved in a fertility program at or near the facility from which she attempts to abduct an infant. Of the 164 cases where the abductor's race is known, 68 are white, 65 are black, and 31 are Hispanic. The skin color of the infant almost always matches that of the abductor or her significant other.

Approximately half of the infants are seven days old or younger when taken. The abducted infant is perceived by the abductor as "her newborn baby." Data do not reveal a strong gender preference in the abduction of these infants.

Although the crime may be precipitated by impulse and opportunity, the abductor has usually laid careful plans for finding another person's infant to take and call her own. In addition, prior to the abduction, the offender will often exhibit nesting instincts by announcing her pregnancy and by purchasing items for an infant in the same way an expectant mother pre-

Table 11-1 Infant Abductions in the United States, 1983–1997, by State

State	Number of Reported Infant Abductions
Alabama	3
Arizona	3
Arkansas	2
California	27
Colorado	5
Connecticut	2
Delaware	1
District of Columbia	5
Florida	11
Georgia	6
Illinois	6
Indiana	1
Iowa	1
Kansas	1
Kentucky	1
Maine	1
Maryland	8
Massachusetts	1
Michigan	3
Mississippi	2
Missouri	4
New Jersey	3
New Mexico	4
New York	9
North Carolina	4
Ohio	4
Oklahoma	3
Oregon	2
Pennsylvania	5
Puerto Rico	2
Rhode Island	1
South Carolina	4
South Dakota	1
Tennessee	4
Texas	22
Virginia	3
Washington	3
West Virginia	1
Wisconsin	2

pares for the birth of her child. The positive attention she receives from family and friends validates her actions. Unfortunately, this nesting activity feeds the need for the woman to produce an infant at the expected time of arrival.

Many of these abductors have a significant other at the time of the abduction, and a high percentage of them have already given birth to at least one child. When women are married, cohabitating, or involved in a relationship at the time they abduct an infant, their significant other—sometimes a considerably older or younger person—is not known to be involved in the planning or execution of the abduction but may be an unwitting partner to the crime. The significant other is often very gullible, wanting to believe that his companion indeed gave birth to or adopted the infant now in her possession. The significant other may vehemently resist law enforcement officials' attempts to retrieve the child.

The vast majority of these women take on the "role" of a nurse and represent themselves as such to the mother and anyone else in the room with the mother. Once the abductor assumes this role, she asks to take the infant for testing, weighing, photographing, and so on. Obviously, arriving at the decision to ask the mother if the abductor can take the infant for a "test" or "photograph" takes forethought on the part of the abductor.

The pretense of being someone else is most often seen in abductors who use interpersonal coping skills such as manipulation, conning, and lying. These women demonstrate that they are capable of providing good care to the infant once the abduction occurs. The infants who have been recovered seem to have suffered no ill effects. The offenders, in fact, consider the babies to be "their own." There is no indication that these are "copycat" crimes, and most offenders can be found in the same general community where the abduction occurred.

These crimes are not always committed by the stereotypical "stranger." In most of these cases, the offenders made themselves known and achieved some degree of familiarity with health care facility personnel and procedures as well as the infant's parents. The abductor, a person who is compulsively driven to obtain an infant, often visits the nursery and maternity unit for several days before the abduction, repeatedly asking detailed questions about procedures and the layout of the maternity unit. In the case cited at the beginning of this chapter, the offender had taken the infant from a room with which she was highly familiar: her daughter had given birth there just four months earlier. Moreover, these women usually impersonate nurses or other health care personnel, wearing uniforms or other staff attire. They have also impersonated lab technicians; social workers; home health nurses; Women's, Infants', and Children's Program staffers; photographers; and other professionals who may normally work in a health care facility. They often visit more than one health care facility in the community to assess security measures and infant populations.

The abductor may also follow the mother home. Although to date there has been no use of violence against mothers within the health care facility, 28 percent of the abductions from homes involved some form of violent act against the mother, including homicide (see Exhibit 11–1). In the last few years, in-home abductions have become more common.

The abductor may not target a specific infant for abduction. When an opportunity arises, she may immediately snatch an available victim, often be visible in the hallway for as little as four seconds with the infant in her arms, and escape via a fire exit stairwell. Since the abductor is compelled to show off her new infant to others, use of the media to publicize the abduction is critical in encouraging citizens to report situations they find peculiar. Most often, infants are recovered as a direct result of the leads generated by media coverage of the abduction when the abductor is not portrayed in the media as a "hardened criminal."

In 1995, for the first time in more than a decade, the incidence of infant abductions from health care facilities decreased. Infant abductions in health care facilities in the United States declined by 82 percent overall. There has been a slight increase, however, in the last two years. Thus, the overall decline is now 64 percent. This reduction seems directly attributable to five years of proactive education programs. The primary seminar, Safeguard Their Tomorrows, is sponsored by the Association of Women's Health, Obstetric, and Neonatal Nurses; the National Association of Neonatal Nurses; and NCMEC and is underwritten by Mead Johnson Nutritionals and Sensormatic Electronics Corporation. Education has greatly increased the awareness of nursing and security staffs in health care facilities nationwide. In the last eight years, I have provided direct educational training to more than 45,000 health care professionals and informal on-site assessments of maternity units for approximately 675 health care facilities in Canada, the United Kingdom, and the United States. In addition, NCMEC has distributed more than 187,000 copies of its award-winning publication *For Healthcare Professionals: Guidelines on Prevention of and Response to Infant Abductions* (formerly titled *For Healthcare Professionals: Guidelines on Preventing Infant Abductions* and *For Health Care Facility Professionals: Guidelines on Preventing Abduction of Infants from the Hospital*).

Susie was married, was in an abusive relationship with her spouse, participated in two support groups for battered women, and had three children who were removed from her care by Child Protective Services. Susie began "announcing" to people in January that she was pregnant and started to visit a local children's health care facility where she informed the staff that her infant was going to be born with a heart problem. She frequently showed staff members a sonogram of her infant despite the fact that she was not pregnant.

In November the women in her support groups asked about the impending birth of Susie's child. Since Susie did not appear to be pregnant, the women accused her of faking the pregnancy. Apparently feeling pressured to "give birth to her baby," Susie went to the children's health care facility, arrived on a floor where a code blue was in progress, disconnected an infant from a cardiac monitor, put the infant under her sweater, and walked out of the health care facility.

Susie's sister-in-law, learning of the abduction through the media and suspecting that Susie's "baby" was the child who was abducted from the health care facility, called the police. Upon investigating, the police found the child, an altered birth certificate for the child, and a roll of film that contained pictures of a pregnant-looking Susie. Although Susie did not harm the infant, she had placed raisins in the infant's navel to make it look as if the child were a newborn.

INTRODUCTION TO GUIDELINES FOR HEALTH CARE PROFESSIONALS

The guidelines highlighted in bold print in the following sections are essential. Quality management and team review processes should address each item at least quarterly. All other guidelines listed are highly recommended. Appendix 11–A, a self-survey, summarizes the guidelines.

Safeguarding newborn infants requires a comprehensive program of health care policy; education of and teamwork by nursing personnel, parents, physicians, security officers, and risk management personnel; and coordination of various elements of physical and electronic security. Collectively, all three actions foil the efforts of potential abductors. Without question, the first two elements can and should be immediately implemented at all health care facilities.

A multidisciplinary approach to the development of specific health care policies and plans for responding to critical incidents is needed to effectively combat this infrequent and highly visible crime. Nurse managers and supervisors may be well suited to take a lead role in this approach because of the holistic philosophy of nursing, the large amount of time nurses spend with parents and infants, the educational component of nursing care, and the ability of nurse managers and supervisors to incorporate teaching infant safety to parents and other staff members. Additionally, obstetric, nursery, and pediatric nurses have close working relationships that would help them implement effective policies and improve processes. In the health care facility, nurses are "surrogate parents" and the front line of defense in preventing abductions and documenting any incidents that occur.

Electronic security measures are simply modern tools used to back up health care facility policy and nursing practices. Not only do these devices discourage or deter potential abductors; they may also enhance the ability of nursing, security, and risk management personnel to work as a team. Closed-circuit television (CCTV), access control, and infant bracelet alarms are useful devices for deterring abduction. First, these systems are reliable when properly installed. They are constantly vigilant, unaffected by distractions, lunch breaks, and shift changes; however, these systems are not infallible and need to be checked. Second, and more important, they document and deter (not simply prevent) an abduction. They may also help resolve and document "false alarms" of systems for supervisory follow-up. Third, CCTV cameras and alarm panels, coupled with security signage, serve as a visual deterrent to the potential abductor. These devices clearly increase the potential for immediately locating the abductor and recovering the newborn. But they in no way diminish the parents' responsibilities to their newborn infants.

In the fall of 1995, at approximately 10:00 a.m., a woman claiming she was a university student conducting research entered the room of a patient who had recently given birth to an infant. The woman stayed with the patient all day, leading staff to believe that she was related to or a friend of the new mother. When the mother went to the bathroom around 5:00 p.m., the "researcher" removed the infant from the bassinet and exited the room. The image of the abductor "arm carrying" the infant from the room, as well as a nurse approaching the abductor and telling her to return to the room, was captured by videocameras.

Upon returning to the victim mother's room, the abductor located a tote bag, placed the infant inside, and exited the room cradling the tote bag in her arms. This image was also captured by the strategically placed videocameras.

These taped images of the abductor were immediately provided to the local media. When aired on television stations that day, viewers called with information that was instrumental in identifying the abductor. As a result, law enforcement officials were at the home of a member of the abductor's family when she arrived with the infant later that day.

Personnel should be alert to unusual behavior. Health care security, nursing, and risk management administrators should remind all personnel that the protection of infants is a responsibility of everyone in the facility, not just security personnel. One of the most effective means of thwarting, and later identifying, a potential abductor is using phrases such as "May I help you?" while carefully observing behaviors and noting a physical description. All personnel should be alert to unusual behavior, including

- repeated visiting "just to see" or "hold" the infants
- close questioning about facility procedures and layout ("When is feeding time?" "When are the babies taken to the mothers?" "Where are the emergency exits?" "Where do the stairwells lead?" "How late are visitors allowed on the floor?" "Do babies stay with their mothers at all times?")
- taking uniforms or other items used to identify health care facility staff members
- physically carrying an infant in the health care facility corridor instead of using the bassinet to transport the child, or leaving the health care facility with an infant while on foot rather than in a wheelchair
- carrying large packages (e.g., gym bags) off the maternity unit, particularly if the person carrying the bag is "cradling" or "talking" to it

Be aware that a disturbance in another area of the health care facility may create a diversion that facilitates an infant abduction (e.g., fire in a closet near the nursery or loud, threatening argument in the waiting area).

GENERAL GUIDELINES

Persons exhibiting the behaviors described above should be reported immediately (to the nurse manager or supervisor, security, and administration), positively identified, kept under close observation, and interviewed by the nursing supervisor and facility security personnel. Report and interview records on the incident should be preserved.

As part of contingency planning, the backbone of prevention, every health care facility must develop a written prevention plan for infant abductions. In the plan for critical incidents, each facility should designate a staff person who will be responsible for alerting other birthing facilities in the area when there is an attempted abduction or when someone is identified who demonstrates the behaviors described above but has not yet attempted to abduct an infant.

Each facility should develop a concise, uniform reporting form to facilitate the timely recording and dissemination of this information. (Exhibit 11–2 shows a sample form.) Care should be taken that this alert does not provide material for a libel or slander suit against the facility by the identified person.

Personnel should notify the police, then NCMEC at 1-800-THE-LOST (1-800-843-5678), of all attempted abductions.

PROACTIVE MEASURES

Facilities must develop written plans discussing ways to prevent abductions.

Exhibit 11–2 Sample Notification Form

TO: Area Birthing Facilities

RE: Unusual/Suspicious Activity

FROM: City Hospital Birthing Facility Staff

Following is a description of an unusual/suspicious incident that occurred at our facility. Please inform us if you experience any incidents of this nature.

Occurrence date(s) _____   Time(s) _____

Description of subject

   Name/alias(es) _____

   Sex _____

   Approximate age _____

   Race _____

   Height _____

   Weight _____

   Hair _____

   Eyes _____

   Clothing _____

   Unusual characteristics _____

Synopsis of incident _____

For additional information, contact _____ at ( ) _____.

Facilities notified:

National Center for Missing and Exploited Children notified?
If not, please call 1-800-THE-LOST (1-800-843-5678).

Immediately after the birth of the infant, identically numbered identification bands should be attached to both the infant (two bands) and mother (one band). One band should also be attached to the mother's significant other or infant's father when appropriate. If the fourth band is not used by the father or mother's significant other, that fact must be documented. That band may be stapled to the chart or cut and placed in the "sharps box."

Prior to the removal of a newborn from the birthing room (within two hours of the birth), the following tasks should be completed:

- The infant should be footprinted.
- A color photograph of the infant should be taken.
- A full physical assessment of the infant should be performed and recorded.

The footprints, photograph, physical assessment, and documentation of the placement of the identification bands, including their number, must be noted in the infant's medical chart.

Footprints of each infant should be taken at birth, admissions, and readmissions to pediatrics. The infant's full foot should be sparingly inked, and a complete impression should be made using light pressure. Ridge detail on the ball of the foot should be visible in the impression.

Occasionally, footprints of the newborn are unreadable. Footprints are an excellent form of identification if an abducted infant is recovered many months later. Health care facilities should take good, readable footprints of the infant. They should consult their local FBI office or law enforcement agency for appropriate techniques, paper stock, and various inked and inkless products.

Like footprints, cord blood taken at the time of delivery is an excellent form of identification. (Currently, DNA testing is expensive, and it takes a minimum of six weeks to issue the results.) Health care facilities should store a sample of cord blood for identification purposes until the day after the infant is discharged from the health care facility.

Another form of identification successfully employed by some health care facilities is antibody profiling. Because a mother and her infant share the same antibody profile for the first year of the infant's life, a "biological barcode" can be created from one drop of blood from the infant and one drop of blood from the mother to look for a "match" in cases where there is a question concerning the infant's identity.

Facilities must take clear, high-quality color photographs of all infants (at birth and up to six months of age upon admissions), including a close-up of the face (taken "straight on").

When completing the physical assessment of the infant, personnel should make sure to identify any marks or abnormalities such as skin tags, moles, and birthmarks. While the footprint, photograph, and assessment must be placed in the infant's medical records, parents may wish to keep a copy of this information for their own records.

Facilities must require all personnel to wear up-to-date, conspicuous color photo identification badges. Personnel, including physicians, in direct contact with the infants should wear a form of unique identification used *only* **by them and known to the parents (e.g., a distinctive and prominent color or marking to designate personnel authorized to have direct contact with infants).** Forms of identification should be worn above the waist on attire that will not be removed or hidden in any way. Paraphernalia (pins, advertisements) should not cover name or position on identification badges. Identification systems should include provisions for all personnel in direct contact with infants, including students and temporary staff. For example, unique temporary badges that are controlled and assigned each shift could be used. Facilities need to modify the identification process to accommodate people with various disabilities.

The guidelines for parents (listed in "What Parents Need to Know" below) must be distributed to parents in childbirth classes, on preadmission tours, upon admission, at postpartum instruction, and upon discharge. (Also consider posting this information on patients' bathroom doors.) **This same information needs to be distributed to all new and current staff members and physicians and their staff members who work with newborns and child patients.**

Staff, at all levels, must receive instruction on protecting infants from abduction, including, but not limited to, information on the offender profile and unusual behavior, prevention procedures, and critical incident responses.

To safeguard the infant while being transported within the health care facility, the following measures should be taken:

- Only an authorized staff member (or person with an authorized identification band for that infant) should be allowed to transport a child.
- An infant should never be left in the hallway without direct supervision.
- Infants should be taken to mothers one at a time. Health care facility personnel should never group babies while transporting them to the mother's room, nursery, or any other location.
- Babies should be pushed in a bassinet, not carried.

Require anyone transporting the infant outside of the mother's room (including the mother, father, or any other person designated by the mother) to wear an identifying wristband. Wristbands should be readily recognizable and have the same numbers for all people associated with one infant.

Infants must always be in direct line-of-sight supervision by a responsible staff member, the mother, or other family member or close friend designated by the mother. This procedure should even be followed when the infant is with the mother and she needs to go to sleep or the bathroom or is sedated. If the mother is asleep when the infant is returned to the room, staff should be careful to fully awaken her before leaving the room.

The mother's or infant's full name should not be posted where it will be visible to visitors. If necessary, use surnames only. Do not publish the mother's or infant's full name on bassinet cards, rooms, or status boards. Charts, patient index cards, and other medical information should not be visible to anyone other than medical personnel. Be aware that identifying information in the bassinet (such as identification cards with the infant's photograph and the family's name, address, and/or telephone number) may put the infant and family at risk after discharge. Keep this information confidential and out of sight.

A new mother, with the help of the infant's maternal grandmother, was settling in on her first day back home after delivering an infant at the local health care facility. A sign on the house's front window and balloons tied in front of the home announced the arrival of a new infant.

On that day a young woman who appeared to be pregnant knocked at the family's front door. Claiming to be lost, she asked to use the telephone. While in the home the young woman asked to use the bathroom. Upon exiting the bathroom, with a gun in one hand and a knife in the other, she demanded that the two women hand over the infant. When they refused to hand over the infant, the intruder shot and stabbed both women, fled with the infant, and discarded the gun along the side of a road.

While the infant was located unharmed three days later and her grandmother recovered from the injuries sustained during the abduction, the infant's mother died.

During the investigation, police found that the abductor had visited the health care facility where the infant was born several days prior to the abduction. Investigators determined that the abductor—while looking through the health care facility's nursery window—obtained a significant amount of personal information about the victim family from an information card located in the infant's bassinet.

Facilities should establish a policy controlling access to the nursing unit (nursery, maternity, neonatal intensive care, pediatrics) to maximize safety. At the front lobby or entrance to the maternity unit, facility personnel should ask visitors which mother they are visiting and for how long. If no name is known or given, personnel should decline admission and alert health care facility security, the nurse manager or supervisor, facility administration, or the police. Especially after regular visiting hours, there should be a system to positively identify visitors (preferably with a photo identification).

The person taking the infant home from the health care facility should be required to show an identifying wristband. The bands on the wrist and ankle of the infant should match the bands worn by the mother and father or significant other. It is important to follow the health care facility's protocol for Joint Commission on Accreditation of Healthcare Organizations (Joint Commission) Sentinel Event reporting.

If the facility's public relations department still releases birth announcements to the news media, no home address or other unique information should be divulged that would put the infant and family at risk after discharge. Also, while giving yard signs away may be considered good marketing, posting these signs increases the risk of abduction.

In mid-1996 some health care facilities began posting birth announcements on their Web sites. These on-line birth announcements often included photographs of the infant and his or her parent(s). These birth announcements should never include the family's home address and should not provide the full name (use S. and D. Smith or Sam and Darlene S., for instance). Additionally, **the facility should not post this information on its Web page until after both mother and infant have been discharged from the facility and after the parents have signed a consent form**. Ideally, there should also be some kind of password assigned so that the parents control who may access the announcement.

When providing home visitation services, personnel entering patients' homes need to wear a unique form of identification used only by them, strictly controlled by the facility, and known to the parents. Facilities should consider utilizing a system where the mother is called before the visit to inform her of the date and time of the visit, name of the visitor, and visitor's requirement to wear a photo identification badge. (See discussion of identification badges above.) For additional information on this topic, see "Outpatient Areas" below.

It was feeding time on the maternity floor of a health care facility in Maryland. While in her room feeding her newborn infant, the mother was approached by a woman dressed in a health care facility lab coat and uniform. The woman informed the mother that her son needed to be taken for routine tests and would be returned to her in a few minutes. The mother relinquished her infant to "the nurse," who left the room. Minutes later an oncology department staff member saw "the nurse" carrying the infant on a different floor. This staff person suspected that something was wrong and called the nursery to check on the situation. Health care facility security was notified by the nursery staff and as the abductor exited the building with the infant in her arms, she was stopped by security staff, who had surrounded the facility. Due to the actions of an alert nurse and the responsiveness of the security personnel, this abductor never left the health care facility grounds and the infant was quickly reunited with his mother.

PHYSICAL SAFEGUARDS

Every health care facility must develop a written assessment of the potential for an infant abduction. This assessment should be performed by a qualified professional (e.g., certified protection professional, certified health care protection administrator, risk manager) who identifies and classifies vulnerabilities within the health care facility. The application of safeguards (guidelines, systems, and hardware) should depend upon the risk potential determined and reflect current professional literature on infant abduction. This process should be ongoing; targets, risks, and methods change, particularly when there is new construction.

Alarms, preferably with time-delay locks, should be installed on all stairwell and exit doors on the perimeter of the maternity, nursery, neonatal intensive care, and pediatrics units. There should be a policy of responding to alarms. Responsible staff should silence and reset an activated alarm only after direct observation of the stairwell or exit and the person using it. The alarm system should never be disabled.

Optimally, video recording should be tied to alarm activity. If the alarm is activated, the situation should be properly documented, a report on the incident should be submitted to the proper authority within that facility, and security should review the tape.

All nursery doors must have self-closing hardware and remain locked at all times.

If there is a lounge or locker room where staff members change clothes and leave clothing, all doors to that room should have self-closing hardware and be under strict access control (locked) at all times.

A needs assessment for an electronic asset surveillance (EAS) detection system should be documented. Such a system would utilize an EAS infant bracelet that is always activated and tied to video recording of the incident and alarm activation. If a health care facility installs an infant EAS system, the system should always be operational. Staff should never get in the habit of turning the system on only when they suspect a problem. Such habits present major liability risks.

Facilities should install a security camera system (using time-lapse loop tape, as banks do) or digital recording technology to monitor activity in the halls of the maternity and pediatrics floors. Cameras should be placed in strategic spots to cover the nursery, hallway, stairwells, and elevators and adjusted at an angle that is likely to capture an abductor's full face. Facilities should retain videotapes for a minimum of seven days before reusing.

One camera should be positioned to capture the faces of all persons entering the main entrance of the maternity unit. This video should be at or near real-time recording and on at all times. There should be signs alerting the public that the area is being electronically monitored. Someone must be responsible for the management of videotapes and recording equipment.

Because the lighting conditions in health care facilities are usually both good and stable, it is better to use color cameras and accessory equipment. Color film makes identification easier.

It is important to have an audit trail on videotape with as much information as possible to aid in investigations. (The abductor is likely acquainted with the facility and has probably evaluated the situation prior to acting.) Ideally, a facility would have one dedicated videocassette recorder per camera running real-time recordings continuously. It may be preferable to use video multiplexers and time-lapse videocassette recorders to change the tapes every 12 hours. The closer to real-time recording, the more information is on tape per camera.

Facilities should consider integrating the video system with alarms from devices such as electronic asset protection panels, magnetic contacts on emergency exit doors, and motion detectors in stairwells. This can result in automated responses by the system.

Moveable cameras, referred to as "pan and tilt domes," with high-resolution imagers and zoom lenses provide much more detailed images than fixed cameras. If they are programmable, high-speed domes can "pattern" and respond to alarms even if the domes are aimed in the opposite direction. Since many of the areas in the health care facility, particularly corridors, look similar, it is important to select programmable, on-screen titling that varies with the pan and tilt position. Thus, when a tape is being presented for evidentiary purposes, there is no question which camera it was and where it was pointing; the information is overlaid on the video pictures.

In stairwells that contain videocameras and are not commonly traveled, these cameras should be equipped with video motion detectors that are integrated with the system as outlined above.

PLAN FOR RESPONDING TO CRITICAL INCIDENTS

General

Every facility must develop a written critical-incident-response plan so that staff can act quickly if there is an infant abduction. All these protocols and critical-incident-response plans must be written out and communicated to all staff members within the maternity unit. Records must be maintained to verify attendance at staff training concerning these plans. Other departments (including communications/switchboard, environmental services, accounting, and public relations) should also have written plans to follow in the event of an abduction.

When formulating the critical-incident-response plan, facilities need to consider several items.

- openness and visibility of facility
- entrance and exit doors
- alarm systems
- staffing patterns, including number of staff members who are visible on the unit

The plan must discuss how incidents will be handled at different times of day. For example, if the incident occurs at shift change, the plan must include a provision for holding staff on the shift scheduled to leave until excused by law enforcement (or designated health care facility authority).

Using a code word (e.g., code pink, code stork) to alert health care facility personnel that there is a missing infant is appropriate as part of the health care facility's critical-incident-response plan. It is the responsibility of health care facility staff to secure the facility and search for the infant. In this process, care should be taken to avoid adding descriptive phrases to the code such as "missing infant."

The plan must include a provision to designate a staff person (usually the security director) to act as the liaison with law enforcement.

As noted above, it is important to follow the health care facility's protocol for Joint Commission Sentinel Event reporting.

Personnel should call NCMEC at 1-800-THE-LOST (1-800-843-5678). It is in an excellent position to advise, provide technical assistance, network with other agencies and organizations, assist in obtaining media coverage of the abduction, and coordinate dissemination of the child's photograph as mandated by federal law (42 USC 5771 and 42 USC 5780).

A media or crisis communication plan should be developed to brief the media on the incident (with the approval of law enforcement), enlist their aid in publicizing the abduction, ensure accuracy of the description of the infant and abductor, coordinate photo dissemination, and provide appropriate access to victim parents while protecting their privacy.

In 1995, the NCMEC received a telephone call from a law enforcement contact who indicated that he had received sketchy information about a possible infant abduction that had occurred four days earlier in a major metropolitan area located within a 50-mile radius of Washington, DC. NCMEC staff members proceeded to contact law enforcement officers in that community to obtain further information and offer assistance.

NCMEC provided technical assistance and distributed posters of the composite sketch of the abductor. Unfortunately, no photographs of the infant were available. Media coverage of the incident was limited to local television stations and the newspaper in the city where the abduction occurred. Investigators did not elect to expand the media coverage to other media markets surrounding their city.

Nine days after the abduction, a staff person at a Washington, DC youth shelter called NCMEC's toll-free hotline regarding a young woman with an infant. The shelter staff member reported that the young woman was not properly caring for the infant and was being evasive about their identity. The staff member asked whether the infant could be a missing child. NCMEC staff members instructed the shelter staff member to call the investigators in charge of the case. The information provided by the shelter staff member led to the recovery of the infant and the arrest of the abductor that same afternoon.

The suspect told law enforcement officials during an interview that she had no intention of ever returning the child and that she had planned to change the identity of the infant, obtain false documentation for herself and the child, and take the infant to a large metropolitan area to "hide."

Had NCMEC staff members not been aware of this abduction, it is likely that this child might not have been recovered.

Nurses in Maternity Units

Nurses who suspect that there has been an infant abduction should immediately search the entire unit. Time is critical. They must count all infants and question the mother of the infant thought to be missing as to other possible locations of the child within the facility.

If an infant abduction is suspected, nurses should immediately call facility security and/or other designated authority per their facility's critical-incident-response plan. Where a facility has no security staff, nurses should immediately call the local police department and make a report. Then they should call the local FBI office.

Nurses should protect the crime scene (area where the abduction occurred) in order to preserve the subsequent collection of any forensic evidence by law enforcement officials. This duty should be relinquished to security officers and subsequently to law enforcement officials upon their arrival.

Staff members should move the parents of the abducted child (but not their belongings) to a private room off the maternity floor. The nurse assigned to the mother and infant should continue to accompany the parents at all times, protecting them from stressful contact with the media and other interference. Staff members should secure all records and charts of the mother and infant, check for adequate documentation, and notify lab and place stat hold on infant's cord blood for follow-up testing. Facilities should consider designating a room for other family members to wait in so that family members have easy access to any updates in the case and parents have some privacy.

The nurse manager or supervisor should brief all staff of the unit. In turn, nurses should then explain the situation to each mother while the mother and her infant are together. Mothers should never hear this news from the media or law enforcement. The nurse manager or supervisor should also be available to relay messages between law enforcement officials and parents.

A staff person (preferably the nurse assigned to the mother and infant) should be assigned to be the single liaison between the parents and facility after the discharge of the mother from the facility.

Nurse managers or supervisors should be sensitive to the fact that the nursing staff may suffer post-traumatic stress disorder (PTSD) as a result of the abduction and make arrangements to hold a group discussion session as soon as possible. All personnel affected by the abduction should be required to attend this session. Such a session will allow facility personnel a chance to express their emotions and deal with the stress resulting from the abduction. Care should be taken not to discuss case details before any criminal or civil trials are concluded. Certain staff members may require further assistance to psychologically integrate this incident and return to their duties on the unit. Facilities should make every effort to assist these staff members with this process. Facilities should consider inviting the investigators of the law enforcement agencies handling the case to this session.

NCMEC is an important resource for assessing and handling PTSD among staff. Individual health care facilities are often so overcome by the enormity of the abduction itself that it is hard to see past the moment to recognize the signs and symptoms of PTSD in their staff. It seems unimaginable to realize that staff suffering from PTSD have to continue working, encourage laboring mothers in bringing forth new life, and allay their patients' fears of this crime. This is their job, but whose job is it to soothe away the nurses' fears and ease their crushed spirits so that they may do their jobs? This time of healing should be strongly encouraged. If facilities do nothing, they may lose some wonderful professionals. Help from NCMEC is a telephone call away. Nurse managers should call 1-800-THE-LOST (1-800-843-5678) for assistance with this healing process.

Security Personnel

If security personnel suspect that there has been an infant abduction, they should call the local police department and make a report. Then they should call the local FBI office or the FBI's Child Abduction and Serial Killer Unit at (540) 720-4700. Then personnel should immediately and simultaneously activate a search of the entire health care facility, interior and exterior. Time is critical.

Personnel should assume control of the crime scene (area where the abduction occurred) until law enforcement arrives. Facility officers should establish a security perimeter around the facility and assist the nursing staff in establishing and maintaining security within the unit (i.e., access control to the unit).

Security officers should ask the police to dispatch an officer to the scene using only the standard crime code number over the police radio without describing the incident. This will help ensure that media and citizens listening to police scanners will not be alerted of the incident before appropriate law enforcement procedures are initiated.

In order to safeguard against "panicking" the abductor into abandoning or harming the infant, security officers should follow the facility's media plan, which should mandate that all information about the abduction is cleared by facility *and* law enforcement authorities involved before being released to staff members and the media. Most often, infants are recovered as a direct result of the leads generated by media coverage of the abduction when the abductor is not portrayed as a "hardened criminal."

Consider limiting official spokespersons to one facility staff person, preferably from public relations, and one law enforcement representative. These persons should be on call throughout the crisis. Security personnel need to brief the facility spokesperson, who can then inform and involve local media by requesting their assistance in accurately reporting the facts of the case and soliciting the support of the public. Personnel should be as forthright as possible without invading the privacy of the family. The family should be apprised of the media plan and their cooperation sought in working through the official spokespersons.

Security personnel should call NCMEC at 1-800-THE-LOST (1-800-843-5678) for technical assistance in handling ongoing crisis management.

Newborn nurseries, pediatrics units, emergency departments, and outpatient clinics for postpartum and pediatric care at other local health care facilities should be notified about the incident and provided a full description of the infant and the suspected or alleged abductor. As part of her plan, the abductor may take the infant to another facility, a private physician, or a public agency in an attempt to have the infant "checked out," obtain a birth certificate for "my child who was delivered at home," or secure public assistance.

In 1994, an infant was abducted from the nursery of Health care facility A, located in a large metropolitan city. The infant was recovered several hours later the same day, and the abductor was arrested.

During the postabduction interview process, law enforcement investigators determined that 10 days prior to the abduction the abductor told her husband that she had given birth to their son at Health care facility B but was unable to bring the infant home immediately because the child required surgery and would be hospitalized for 10 days. Ten days later, when the husband expected the infant to be discharged from Health care facility B, the woman abducted the infant from Health care facility A, took the infant to Health care facility B, called her husband from the lobby of Health care facility B asking him to come pick them up there, and waited in the lobby of Health care facility B for him to arrive.

If authorities at Health care facility A had notified all health care facilities in the city and surrounding area of the abduction, security personnel at Health care facility B might have recognized the abductor as a suspect while she was still sitting in their lobby, and the infant could have been recovered hours earlier.

It was also learned that the abductor had told her husband two years prior to the abduction that she had given birth to a stillborn infant boy at Health care facility B. A check of records at Health care facility B indicated that the abductor had not given birth to a child two years earlier at that facility. Further investigation determined that the abductor had applied to Health care facility A sometime within the year prior to the abduction to become a volunteer. She had specified on her application that she wanted to work in the nursery. It is common for such abductors to misrepresent facts about prior births, or they may visit or try to somehow become "affiliated" with the health care facilities from which they eventually attempt to abduct an infant.

Law Enforcement Officers

Law enforcement officers should treat a case of infant abduction from a health care facility as a serious felony crime requiring immediate response.

Law enforcement officers should enter the child's name and description in the FBI's National Crime Information Center's (NCIC's) Missing Person File. If the abductor is known and has been charged with a felony, officers should cross-reference the infant's description with the suspected abductor in the NCIC Wanted Person File.

Law enforcement officers should call NCMEC at 1-800-THE-LOST (1-800-843-5678). It can provide technical assistance, network with other agencies and organizations, assist in obtaining media coverage of the abduction, and coordinate dissemination of the child's photograph as mandated by federal law (42 USC 5771 and 42 USC 5780).

Parents or law enforcement authorities may request age progression of the infant's photograph as time elapses on the case. An infant's photograph may be "aged" using earlier photographs, computer technology and graphics, data on facial development, and the special skills of medical illustrators (see Figure 11–1).

Law enforcement officers should call the FBI's Child Abduction and Serial Killer Unit at (540) 720-4700 for technical and forensic resource coordination; computerized support for case management; investigative, interview, and interrogation strategies; and information on behavioral characteristics of unknown offenders.

Officers must immediately contact all other birthing facilities in the community and request the retrieval and secure storage of the previous seven days' worth of videotapes or digital disks for review. These videotapes or disks should be treated as photographic evidence.

Officers should consider setting up one dedicated local telephone hotline for sightings and leads or coordinate this function with a local organization.

Polygraphs may be useful with female offenders and their male companions. While polygraphing the infant's father may be useful for eliminating him as a suspect, it should be done early in the investigation. Be aware that polygraphing the infant's mother within 24 hours of the delivery (or while medicated) is not advised.

To deter future crimes and document criminal behavior, the abductor should be charged and every effort should be made to sustain a conviction.

Any release of information concerning an infant abduction should be well planned and agreed upon by the facility and law enforcement authorities. Care should be taken to keep the family fully informed. Consider designating one law enforcement official to handle media inquiries for all investigative data.

Public Relations Officers

As soon as possible after the abduction, public relations officers should contact the local media and request that they come to a designated media room at the health care facility to receive information about the abduction. The media should be provided with the facts as accurately as possible, asked to request the assistance of the public in recovering the infant, and asked to respect the privacy of the family. Public relations professionals should be forthright with the media but release only information approved by the law enforcement authority in

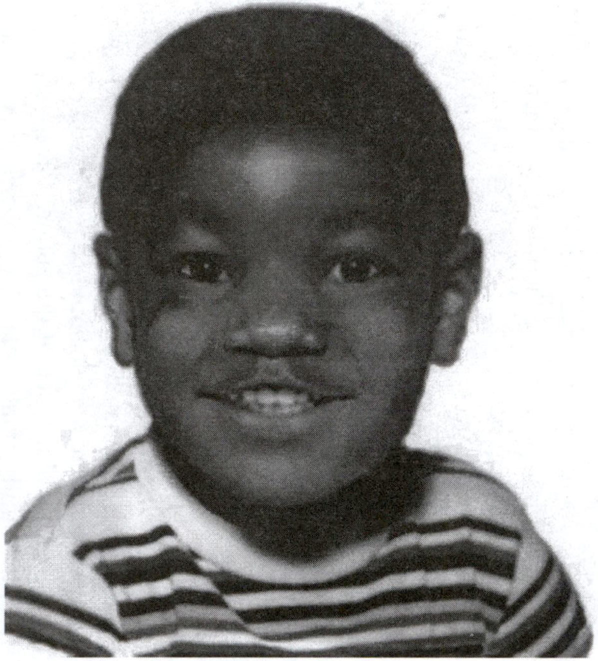

Tavish Sutton

Birth: 02/10/1993

Missing: 03/09/1993

Race: Black

Sex: M

Missing From: Atlanta
                GA
                United States

Age Missing: 0 yrs   Age Now: 5 yrs

Hair: Black

Eyes: Brown

Height: 2'00"

Weight: 8 lbs

The picture shown is a "PHOTO COMPOSITE" of what the child may look like at the age of 4 years. Child was abducted from his hospital room at Grady Memorial Hospital in Atlanta, Georgia, sometime between 6:45 and 7:00 a.m. on Tuesday, March 9, 1993.

Figure 11–1 Photo Composites.

Age Progression by NCMEC 10/13/19

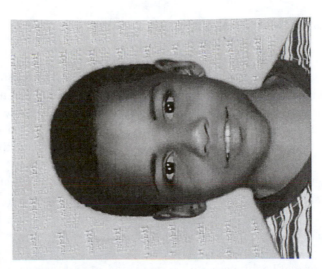

Andre Bryant

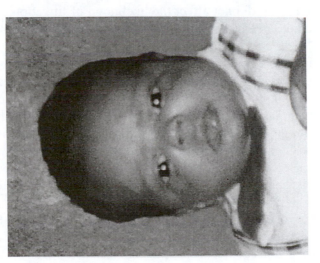

Birth: 02/17/1989

Missing: 03/29/1989

Age Now: 10 yrs

Race: Black

Sex: Male

Hair: Black

Eyes: Brown

Ht: 1'07"

Wt: 10lbs

Missing From:

Brooklyn

NY

United States

Child's photo is shown age-progressed to 10 years. He was last seen with his mother, who was later found deceased. Mother and child had left their residence at about 2 p.m. to go shopping with two black female acquaintances in a burgundy Pontiac Grand Am, possibly with MD tags.

charge of the investigation. Most often, infants are recovered as a direct result of the leads generated by media coverage of the abduction.

Public relations officers should be sure to designate a separate area where friends and family of the parents can gather (away from the press) to receive regular updates on the abduction. Personnel should also designate a separate area for the media to gather and provide them with escorted opportunities to film an obstetrics or nursery area or personnel.

Public relations specialists should prepare switchboard operators with a written response to give outside callers, including anxious parents who are planning to have their babies delivered at that facility.

Personnel should activate the crisis communication plan. It should list steps to be taken, people to be notified, and resources available, such as photo duplication and dissemination.

LIABILITY

Having a solid program of health care policy; education of and teamwork by nursing, parents, security, and risk management; and physical and electronic security helps a health care facility from a legal standpoint if an abduction occurs. In the cases litigated, damages awarded against a health care facility generally have been mitigated when a health care facility is shown to have taken measures to reduce the risk of infant abduction.

CERTAIN FACTORS INCREASE THE LIKELIHOOD OF LITIGATION

- The infant was not recovered within one week of the abduction.
- The abductor impersonated a health care facility employee.
- The abduction occurred during the 1990s.

The location of the abduction did not affect the likelihood of litigation. That is, families sued their health care facilities in equal proportions whether the infant was abducted from the nursery, the mother's room, or a pediatric room.

In cases of infant abduction, a health care facility is potentially liable on several grounds. The first is based on its general duty to take reasonable care to prevent foreseeable harm to its patients. The health care facility could be liable for any physical or psychological harm suffered by the abducted infant. The second area of liability is based on the health care facility's contractual duty to use reasonable care to prevent the occurrence of foreseeable injury to third parties. Thus, the health care facility could be liable to the parents for the costs of any searches and for psychological harm. Another area of liability concerns the need for obstetric and pediatric physicians, especially those in group practice, to have photo identification cards (on-call physicians may not be known by the family or staff).

Today's administrators, risk managers, and security directors must ensure that members of the public trust their facility, that patients are safe, and that staff are prepared if there is an abduction. Though infant abductions do not occur with high frequency in any given area, they do occur. If the potential for infant abduction is ignored, risk managers, nurse managers, and security officers will not be able to properly prepare and perform their job with due diligence.

SECURITY AFTER DISCHARGE

After discharge from the maternity unit, most newborns go home with their families. However, all infants need follow-up care, whether in a special nursery situation immediately after birth or for regular checkups. This section offers advice to health care professionals on helping parents safeguard infants from abduction by someone outside the family whether at home, at a health care facility in either a prolonged or short stay, or at a regular checkup.

Special Nurseries and Pediatric Units

Neonatal intensive care units (NICUs) and pediatric intensive care units (PICUs) normally are in large rooms with multiple bassinets, and parents may not be with their infants at all times. In addition, these units do not often utilize the same level of security that is employed in nurseries for healthy newborns due to monitoring and increased nurse-to-patient staffing ratios.

Because parents often spend time with their infants while in these units, each family member should be positively identified and documented by the nursing staff. Consideration should be given to utilizing multipart patient identification bands for parents and some other form of identification and pass system for family members and visitors approved by the parents.

While there have been no reported cases of infant abductions from NICUs by people outside the family, infant abductions from these units have occurred. These abductions have involved family members of infants who are on "court hold" for such reasons as positive drug screens and custody issues. While these abductions may be reported to local authorities, no national figures have been tabulated.

Problems concerning infant security in such special units are multifaceted. They include

- infant care procedures that result in numerous identification band changes on infants due to reinsertion of intravenous needles, edematous extremities, or weight gain
- designs that divide NICUs and PICUs into small, low-census pods. These areas may be difficult for line-of-sight observation of infants at all times, especially in "rooming-in" situations, and may result in lower staffing patterns.
- security policies and procedures (e.g., allowing parents to carry the infant out of the facility in their arms) that may not be consistent with the maternity department's policies
- large, busy units with multiple caregivers who may not know the parents
- utilization of personnel from registries or traveling nurses who are not required to wear photo or unique identifying badges that are monitored each shift
- lower census and lower staffing patterns that may affect line-of-sight observation
- discharge processes that do not require parents to present an identification band that matches the infant's or do not require verification of identification with an official photo identification card
- a false sense of security (on the part of staff members) that an infant abduction could not occur in NICUs (e.g., probable targets would be "grower" babies, babies ready for discharge, "boarder" babies, or babies who have yet to be placed with a family or picked up by the adoptive family).

While 14 percent of the infants abducted from health care facilities are taken from nurseries, 17 percent of the infants abducted are taken from pediatric units (including children's health care facilities). PICUs present their own security challenges. As in NICUs, parents may not be constantly present. Nurses may not be ever present in the infant's room when family is absent, and infants are not usually placed in a nursery when family members are absent. Thus, pediatric units often are less secure than maternity units and special nurseries.

All items in "Guidelines for Health Care Professionals" above should be considered for NICUs and PICUs. Thus, all facility personnel should wear conspicuous color photo identification. At admission, personnel should footprint and photograph the infant as well as perform and record a full physical assessment of the infant. The footprints, photograph, and physical assessment must be placed in the infant's medical chart. The infant should be footprinted and photographed again later during a long stay (at least monthly) and certainly before discharge.

While transporting infants within the health care facility, personnel must adhere to several guidelines.

- Only an authorized staff member or person with an authorized identification band for an infant should be allowed to transport that child. In cases where the infant needs to be taken for tests in other units of the facility (e.g., X-ray, magnetic resonance imaging), staff should assure parents that the transporter is an employee of the facility and encourage parents to accompany their child. The facility should consider giving pediatric patients priority in testing units to decrease the children's waiting time.
- Infants should be transported one at a time and never left in the hallway without direct supervision.
- Infants should never be carried; they should be pushed in a bassinet.
- Anyone visiting with or transporting the infant—including the mother, father, or any other person designated by the parents—should be required to wear an identifying wristband or produce an official photo identification. As discussed above, all wristbands for people associated with one infant should have the same number. The distribution of identification wristbands needs to be clearly documented, especially to facilitate discharge of the infant. Identification policies should clearly outline steps to be implemented for reapplying matching identification bands when the mother has been discharged from the facility but the infant is still in the facility.
- Infants should always be in line-of-sight supervision by nurses or parents or near the nurses' station. If possible, when not in a special unit, infants should not be placed in rooms next to stairwells and elevators. Children involved with custody or abuse issues should receive greatest priority for this room placement, and security should be notified of their high-risk status.
- An access control policy should be established for the nursing unit to maximize safety. All exterior doors to the unit must have self-closing hardware and be under strict access control (locked). At the front lobby or entrance to the unit, facility personnel should ask visitors which infant they are visiting and their relationship to the child. If no name is known or given, personnel should decline admission and alert health care facility security, the nurse manager or supervisor, facility administration, or the police. There should be a sign-in log for visitors to the unit. It should specify the infant to be visited and require the visitor to show an official photo identification.

In the NICU, infant identification bands applied at birth may be removed due to patient care needs. The removed identification bands should be stapled to the medical record or cut and placed in the sharps box, and this should be noted in the medical record. NICU infants then need to be rebanded with another identification band.

As discharge nears, parents may utilize a rooming-in service to prepare to care for the infant's special needs. It is imperative that security procedures be followed in these situations. For instance, parents in rooming-in situations must always be in line-of-sight supervision of their child.

Upon discharge, staff must check that an identifying wristband appears on the person taking the infant home from the health care facility. Staff must match the bands on the wrist and ankle of the infant with the bands worn by the mother and father or significant other. If parents do not have an identification band that matches the infant's (the one on the infant or stapled in the medical record), require verification of identification with an official photo identification (e.g., driver's license).

Facilities should ensure that infant security policy and procedures are consistent throughout, from the maternity unit to the NICU and PICU. Consistency of policies and procedures will decrease confusion and increase compliance.

Facilities should also implement a policy and procedure that will meet the security needs of an infant who is on "court hold." For example, if the mother is in the well-newborn nursery to visit the infant, she should be under direct supervision and observation.

While infant abductions grab the headlines, more common are family abductions involving custody disputes, child abuse, and Department of Family and Children Services (DFCS) intervention. While this problem is widespread and statistical information is available on the subject, it is likely that family abductions and DFCS intervention are grossly underreported. And, because these cases often involve abuse or neglect issues, the children may be at greater risk than newborn infants taken from maternity units.

Upon admission of a child to a patient room and during the orientation process, nursing staff should ask the parent or guardian if there is any personal circumstance that the facility should be aware of, especially as it relates to a family situation that might place the parent or guardian or child at risk. Special attention should be given to single persons who may be involved in a custody dispute or mothers with a protective order against the infant's father. This line of questioning is best accomplished with a caring attitude. When staff are kind, parents or guardians will often open up about past problems of abuse and even attempted abductions by the noncustodial parent.

Several factors to review when considering how to protect a patient include abduction risk, age of child, probability for violence, and circumstances surrounding the risk. **Protection strategies include**

- "red flagging" the child's name in the system to indicate that no information is to be released
- admitting the child under an assumed name
- placing the child in an isolation room or the intensive care unit
- placing an assumed name on the child's door
- using a wireless CCTV camera with a monitor at the nurses' station so that the child may be closely watched

- increasing the frequency of observation in the patient's area
- posting a description of the potential abductor with security, nursing, and the front desk (reception area)
- posting a security officer at the patient's room, in his or her unit, or on his or her floor

Outpatient Areas

Clinics or postpartum treatment facilities for mothers, pediatric clinics, health maintenance organizations (HMOs), and health care facility waiting rooms should post a sign stating that parents or guardians are not allowed to leave children unattended in the waiting room or relinquish that duty to others. Such facilities should enforce that rule by reminding parents when they violate it. Facilities should post that policy in all the languages spoken by patients in their service area. There should be a policy regarding the identification worn by staff who are authorized to transport and treat the infant, and parents or guardians should be informed of that policy.

Visiting nurses, home health aides, home health care workers, HMO workers, nurses in physicians' offices, and all nursing and medical students should be issued the same photo identification cards. Whenever possible, families should be notified of planned visits to their home and cautioned against allowing anyone to enter their home who does not have the approved form of identification.

The visiting nurses and nursing and medical students should be included under the health care facility's policies and procedures and critical-incident-response plan. All other health care workers need to be included under a critical-incident-response plan from their employer, whether it is a physician, HMO, government agency, or other entity. Care must be taken to encourage physicians in direct contact with infants to fulfill this requirement.

Margaret had been home from the health care facility only a few days after giving birth to her daughter when a woman came to her home announcing that she was a visiting nurse from the health care facility assigned to offer follow-up care for the newborn. The woman was dressed as a home nurse; appeared pregnant; carried medical equipment, including a blood pressure cuff and stethoscope; and had a notebook bearing the name of the health care facility where Margaret had given birth. Two days later the "nurse" visited Margaret a second time. She said that she was being considered for a promotion and asked Margaret to write her a letter of recommendation. While Margaret went into the dining room to get a pen and paper, she heard the "nurse" going out the front door of the house. When Margaret asked where she was going, the "nurse" said that she had forgotten her blood pressure cuff and would be right back. Margaret became suspicious when the "nurse" did not come back. Margaret found that her infant girl was no longer in the bedroom and called the police.

Prior to going to Margaret's house on that second day, the "nurse" informed her husband that it was time for him to take her to the health care facility. He waited in the health care facility lobby while she told him that she was going to be examined. But instead she exited the health care facility and returned to Margaret's home. Upon abducting the child, the "nurse" returned to the health care facility, joined her husband in the lobby, and showed him the infant she had just "given birth to." Suspecting that something was wrong, the husband questioned her, and the couple began to argue. In the meantime, the police began searching for the missing infant and discovered the arguing couple in the parking lot as the abductor attempted to place the child in a car seat in their van. In addition to the car seat, the abductor had purchased formula, infant clothes, and toys.

Homes

Although to date there has been no use of violence against mothers within the health care facility, of the 57 infant abductions from homes between 1983 and 1997 (see Exhibit 11–1), 28 percent involved some form of violent act committed against the mother, including homicide. In-home abductions are becoming more common; therefore, patient education before postpartum discharge is important. Facilities should consider using a signed release form indicating that the parent has received the information (see "What Parents Need to Know" below). There have been several cases where an abductor has made initial contact with a mother and infant in the health care facility setting and then abducted the infant from the home. Therefore, a high degree of diligence should be exercised by the health care facility when releasing information about births. As noted above, it is inappropriate for the health care facility to supply birth announcements to the press that contain a family's complete home address or any other identifying data.

Different techniques are used in abductions inside and outside health care facilities. Since the use of violence is more prevalent in home settings, families should be cautioned to allow only family members and known friends into the home, not merely acquaintances met during the mother's pregnancy or recent health care facility stay.

While pregnant, a mother took her older children to a shopping mall and stopped to observe a woman who was there painting clown faces on children. After a brief conversation the two women exchanged telephone numbers. Although initially the two women did not contact one another, the woman who was painting clown faces located the mother several months later after seeing the birth announcement of her new "friend's" infant in the newspaper. The woman gained entry to the mother's home; shot the mother in the head, killing her; and abducted the infant. The abductor used the moment of the victim mother's death as the time and day of the "birth" of "her" infant. Upon announcing the "birth" to her husband and his coworkers, the coworkers became suspicious of the "arrival" of what appeared to be a 10-day-old infant in the household and contacted local law enforcement. The police found the infant, unharmed, at the home of the abductor.

During their investigation, the police also found five weeks' worth of birth announcements from the local daily newspaper in the assailant's home. They learned that she had posed as a child welfare worker and "checked up" on other mothers of infants that had been included in the published birth announcements.

WHAT PARENTS NEED TO KNOW

In a warm and comforting way, health care facility personnel should remind parents of the measures they should take to protect their child. **The following guidelines are good, sound parenting techniques that can also help prevent abduction of infants while in the health care facility where the child was born and once the parents take the child home.**

- At some point before the birth, parents should investigate security procedures at the facility where the birth will take place. They should request a copy of the facility's written guidelines on procedures for "special care" and security procedures in the maternity ward. Parents should know all of the facility's procedures to safeguard the infant.
- Parents should watch their newborn infant very carefully at all times while in the facility. Their infant should always be in their line of sight, even when they go to the bathroom. If they plan to leave the room or go to sleep, they should alert the nurses to take the infant back to the nursery or have a family member watch the infant.
- After admission to the facility, parents should ask about health care facility protocols concerning the routine nursery procedures, feeding and visitation hours, and security measures.
- While at the facility, parents should not give their infant to anyone without properly verified health care facility identification. They should find out what additional special identification is being worn to further identify those health care facility personnel who have authority to handle the infant.
- Parents should become familiar with the health care facility staff who work in the maternity unit. They should know the nurse assigned to them and their infant for all shifts.
- Parents should question unfamiliar persons entering their room or inquiring about their infant, even if they are in health care facility attire or seem to have a reason for being there. If someone seems suspicious, parents should alert the nurses' station immediately.
- Parents should determine where their infant will be taken for tests and how long the tests will take. They should find out who has authorized the tests. If possible, parents should go with the infant to observe the procedure.
- For their records, parents should have at least one color photograph of the infant (full, front-face view) and compile a complete written description of the infant, including hair and eye color, length, weight, date of birth, and specific physical attributes.
- At some point after the birth of the infant but before discharge from the facility, parents should request a set of written guidelines on the procedures for any in-home follow-up care extended by the facility. Parents should not allow anyone into the home who says she is affiliated with the facility but has no health care facility identification. Parents should know what special identification is being worn to further identify those staff members who have authority to enter their home.
- Parents should consider the risk they may be taking when permitting their infant's birth announcement to be published in the newspaper or on line. Birth announcements should never include the family's home address and should be limited to the parents' surname(s).

- The use of outdoor decorations to announce the infant's arrival (e.g., balloons, large floral wreaths, wooden storks, and other lawn ornaments) is not recommended.
- Only persons well known by the mother should be allowed into the home. Mere acquaintances, especially those met during the pregnancy or after the birth, should not be allowed inside. If someone arrives at the home and claims to be affiliated with the health care facility where the infant was born, parents must check identification as described above.

RECOVERY

When the infant is recovered, he or she will be brought by law enforcement to the emergency department of the health care facility from which he or she was abducted. As soon as the infant arrives, medical staff should check the infant for any health-related problems. The infant's previous chart should be reviewed to help establish positive identity through documented skin tags, birthmarks, and so forth. In addition, lab tests should be administered to make a positive identification. Lab tests and footprints, not eyewitnesses, must identify an infant. An infant's facial features can change very quickly, making visual identification difficult. And there is always the possibility that distraught parents will say the infant is theirs, simply to replace their loss.

As soon as the infant is identified, facilities should notify the parents. If media sources have released the fact that an infant has been recovered prior to positive identification, facilities should tell the parents the truth. An infant has been recovered and is being medically assessed. As soon as possible, an identification will be made. It will be natural for the parents to want to go see the infant immediately. Facilities should discourage this. If the infant is not the one that has been abducted, seeing yet another helpless infant will only heighten the parents' anxiety.

Once identification is made (and if there are no medical complications), the infant should be taken by way of bassinet to the mother's room. Accompanying the infant should be a representative of the law enforcement agency in charge of the case, health care facility administration, security, public relations, and, of course, nursing. While there will be an inclination to videotape the reunion, it should be discouraged. It is difficult to maintain a patient's confidentiality and dignity during a videotaping.

After the initial reunion, facility representatives should ask the parents if they would like to hold a press conference. In most cases, media sources will want access to the mother and infant. A controlled press conference is probably the best way to honor this request and protect the mother and infant from overt interruptions during their reunion. Press conferences should be held in rooms large enough to allow everyone to be seated. Press conferences should be videotaped, as should any other public statements made by the parents. In one case, statements made by the mother during the press conference nullified her multimillion-dollar claim for emotional stress for her older child.

Facilities should contact the parents a few days after discharge. They should make sure the infant is healthy and doing well and that the health care facility bill is correct. In one case, the parents had been charged for nursery time during the days of the abduction.

KEY POINTS

- While there is no infant abduction epidemic, there are about 12 to 18 abductions per year nationwide.
- Abductors are most often female and usually meet a certain profile.
- Health care facilities can deter possible infant abductions through various means.
  –use of CCTV, door alarms, and electronic tagging systems
  –staff education (required by the Joint Commission in sensitive areas)
  –parent education
- Each infant should be footprinted and photographed.
- Maternity unit staff members should wear distinctive uniforms, badges, and so on to help the new parent(s) identify them as people authorized to hold or carry the infant.
- The health care facility must have a critical-incident-response plan to prepare for possible abductions.
- The facility should contact local law enforcement, the FBI, and the NCMEC as soon as possible if an abduction occurs.

Appendix 11–A

Self-Assessment for Health Care Facilities

Guideline	Essential/ Recommended	Complies (Yes/No)	Responsible Department
General			
Immediately report persons exhibiting behaviors of potential abductor.	Essential		
Positively identify suspect.	Essential		
Interview suspect.	Essential		
Preserve report and interview records on incident.	Essential		
Alert other birthing facilities in the area when person is identified who demonstrates behaviors of potential abductor.	Essential		
For all attempted abductions,			
• Notify the police	Essential		
• Notify the National Center for Missing and Exploited Children (NCMEC)	Essential		
Proactive measures			
Develop written prevention plan	Essential		
Immediately after birth of infant, attach identically numbered identification bands to infant, mother, and father or significant other.	Essential		
Prior to removal of newborn from birthing room,			
• Footprint infant.	Essential		
• Take color photograph of infant.	Essential		
• Perform and record full physical assessment of infant.	Essential		
Note all these items in infant's medical chart.	Essential		

Guideline	Essential/ Recommended	Complies (Yes/No)	Responsible Department
Require all health care personnel to wear up-to-date, conspicuous color photo identification.	Essential		
In childbirth classes, on preadmission tours, upon admission, during postpartum instruction, and at discharge, distribute guidelines for parents to help prevent facility abductions.	Essential		
Train staff on protecting infants from abduction.	Essential		
While infants are transported within the health care facility, ensure that the following guidelines are met:			
• Only authorized staff members are allowed to transport the child.	Essential		
• An infant is never left in the hallway without direct supervision.	Essential		
• Infants are taken to mothers one at a time.	Essential		
• Babies are always pushed in a bassinet, not carried.	Essential		
Ensure that infants are always in direct line-of-sight supervision.	Essential		
Do not post the mother's or infant's full name where it will be visible to visitors.	Essential		
Establish a policy controlling access to the nursing unit (nursery, maternity, neonatal intensive care, pediatrics).	Recommended		
At the front lobby or entrance to those units, instruct health care facility personnel to ask visitors which mother they are visiting and for how long.	Recommended		
Require a show of the identifying wristband for the person taking the infant home from the health care facility, matching the bands on the wrist and ankle of the infant with the bands worn by the mother and father or significant other.	Essential		
No home address or other unique information should be divulged to the public in birth announcements that			

would put the infant and family at risk after discharge.	Essential
When providing home visitation services, personnel entering patients' homes need to wear a unique form of identification used only by them, strictly controlled by the facility, and known to the parents.	Essential

Physical safeguards

Develop written assessment of risk of infant abduction.	Essential
Install alarms on all stairwell and exit doors on the perimeter of the maternity, nursery, neonatal intensive care, and pediatric units.	Essential
Respond to alarms and instruct responsible staff to silence and reset an activated alarm only after direct observation of the stairwell or exit and the person using it.	Essential
Ensure that all nursery doors have self-closing hardware and remain locked at all times.	Essential
All doors to lounges or locker rooms where staff members change or leave clothing must have self-closing hardware and be under strict access control.	Recommended
Document a needs assessment for an electronic asset surveillance (EAS) detection system, utilizing an EAS infant bracelet that is always activated and tied to video recording of the incident and alarm activation.	Recommended
Install a security camera system.	Essential
Position camera so that it will capture the faces of all persons entering the main entrance of the maternity unit.	Essential

Critical-incident-response plan

General

Develop written critical-incident-response plan for an infant abduction.	Essential
Call NCMEC at 1-800-THE-LOST (1-800-843-5678) for advice and technical assistance	Essential

Guideline	Essential/ Recommended	Complies (Yes/No)	Responsible Department
Nurses in maternity units			
Immediately search the entire unit if an abduction is suspected.	Essential		
Immediately call facility security and/or other designated authority.	Essential		
Protect the crime scene.	Essential		
Move the parents of the abducted child (but not their belongings) to a private room off the maternity floor.	Recommended		
Have the nurse assigned to the mother and infant accompany the parents at all times.	Recommended		
Secure all records/charts of the mother and infant.	Recommended		
Notify lab and place stat hold on infant's cord blood	Recommended		
Consider designating a room for other family members to wait in so that they have easy access to any updates in the case and the parents have some privacy.	Recommended		
Nurse manager or supervisor briefs all staff of the unit.	Recommended		
Nurses should then explain the situation to each mother while the mother and her infant are together.	Recommended		
Assign one staff person to be the single liaison between the parents and facility after the discharge of the mother from the facility.	Recommended		
Hold a group discussion session as soon as possible and require all personnel affected by the abduction to attend.	Essential		
Security personnel			
Call the local police department and make a report if an abduction is suspected.	Essential		
Then call the local Federal Bureau of Investigation (FBI) office or the FBI's Child Abduction and Serial Killer Unit at (540) 720-4700.	Essential		
Immediately and simultaneously activate a search of the entire health care facility, interior and exterior.	Essential		
Assume control of crime scene until law enforcement arrives.	Essential		

Assist nursing staff in establishing and maintaining security in the unit.	Essential
Establish a security perimeter around the facility and assist the nursing staff in establishing and maintaining security within the unit.	Essential
Facility's media plan should mandate that all information about the abduction be cleared by facility and law enforcement authorities before being released to staff members and the media.	Essential
Brief the health care facility spokesperson, who can inform and involve local media by requesting their assistance in accurately reporting the facts of the case and soliciting the support of the public.	Recommended
Call NCMEC at 1-800-THE-LOST (1-800-8434-5678) for technical assistance in handling ongoing crisis management.	Essential
Notify newborn nurseries, pediatric units, emergency departments, and outpatient clinics for postpartum and pediatric care at other local health care facilities about the incident and provide a full description of the infant and the suspected abductor.	Essential

Law enforcement officers

Enter the child's name and description in the FBI's National Crime Information Center's Missing Person File.	Essential
Call NCMEC at 1-800-THE-LOST (1-800-843-5678) to request technical assistance, network with other agencies and organizations, gain assistance in obtaining media coverage of the abduction and coordinate dissemination of the child's photograph.	Essential
Call the FBI's Child Abduction and Serial Killer Unit at (540) 720-4700 for technical and forensic resource coordination, computerized support for case management; investigative, interview, and interrogation strategies, and information on behavioral characteristics of unknown offenders.	Essential

Guideline	Essential/ Recommended	Complies (Yes/No)	Responsible Department
Immediately contact all other birthing facilities in the community and request the retrieval and secure storage of the previous seven days' worth of videotapes or digital disks for review.	Essential		
Consider setting up one dedicated local telephone hotline for sightings and leads or coordinate this function with a local organization.	Recommended		
Consider polygraphing infants' parents, female offender, and her male companion.	Recommended		
Charge abductor.	Essential		
Make every effort to sustain a conviction.	Essential		
Release of information concerning infant abduction should be well planned and agreed upon by the health care facility and law enforcement authorities involved.	Recommended		
Keep family fully informed.	Recommended		
Public relations officers			
Provide facts of case to media and ask for their assistance in releasing that information to the public in hopes of generating leads on the child.	Recommended		
Provide written statement to address callers' concerns over the abduction, especially anxious parents who are planning to have their babies delivered at that facility.	Recommended		
Activate the crisis communication plan.	Recommended		

Chapter 12

Drug Diversion

CHAPTER OBJECTIVES

1. Understand the pervasiveness of the drug diversion problem.
2. Know some of the signs that a person is a drug abuser.
3. Know the various ways to divert drugs.
4. Learn the investigative team concept.
5. Review case studies to learn investigative techniques.

INTRODUCTION

In the quiet stillness of the early morning, a registered nurse (RN) patiently breaks off the security tabs of prefilled syringes of morphine, extracts the precious liquid, refills the syringes with water, and glues the security tabs back in place, leaving these syringes to be used by an unsuspecting nurse. Another nurse has just given a patient a cardiac medication that looked like the pain medication tablet she took herself and charted to the patient. And a certified registered nurse anesthetist (CRNA) has just injected himself with a narcotic and is going into surgery, his patient paying the price of his addiction. Scenes such as these are occurring nationwide every day. Quietly, consistently, drug diversion continues, always compromising the quality of health care.

Substance abuse permeates every aspect of life in the United States. It does not recognize the boundaries of profession or socioeconomic status. Large numbers of nurses, physicians, pharmacists, and other health care workers have succumbed to the temptation and availability of controlled substances. Both the professionals and the institutions involved want the situations handled quietly. Public disclosure of the problem would shake public confidence.

In recent years, national attention has been drawn to the problem of the impaired driver. There are now harsher judicial penalties for driving while intoxicated as well as organizations such as Mothers against Drunk Driving and Students against Drunk Driving.

The material for this chapter was excerpted from Readling & Sells, "Drug Diversion, An Investigative Guide for the Healthcare Professional," 1994, Security Management Institute, 11706 Battery Place, Charlotte, NC.

The problem of impaired health care professionals is at least as serious as, if not more serious than, the problem of impaired drivers. In many situations, nonimpaired drivers can successfully avoid impaired drivers. But can a patient in a health care facility avoid the mistakes or deliberate acts of the impaired nurse, physician, or pharmacist? How would people react if they learned about the pervasiveness of drug diversion among health care professionals?

The problems created by the impaired health care professional range from simple medication or procedural errors to murder through both direct and indirect actions. Nurses take patient medication and leave patients in pain, medications that are potentially dangerous to patients are administered as substitutes for the drugs sought by impaired professionals, and patients die because of impaired physicians' errors.

Several years ago, a CRNA was suspected of diverting controlled substances. An investigation was initiated, and the CRNA was caught leaving the facility with drugs he had diverted from the health care facility. The CRNA was immediately suspended. The administrator feared employment legal action on the part of the CRNA and allowed him to return to work. On the day the CRNA returned, he diverted drugs for his own use and was impaired during a surgical procedure. His impairment cost the patient her life.

The investigation revealed that the lack of proper action on the part of the impaired professional was the proximate cause of the patient's death. The CRNA was charged with second-degree murder, he eventually entered a guilty plea to manslaughter, and the health care facility was exposed to massive civil litigation. What were the costs of not addressing this situation properly? It cost a patient her life, a health care professional his career and his freedom, and a facility an enormous amount of both money and prestige. Could the results have been different? Without a doubt, most of the costs could have been avoided had the health care facility administration recognized the seriousness of the matter and handled the situation differently.

Health care facilities maintain large stocks of controlled substances that are readily available to those who choose to divert them. In the early 1990s, it was estimated that between 6 percent and 20 percent of physicians and nurses were dependent on narcotics, a rate that was 30 to 50 percent higher than that of the general population. That figure may be even higher today due to the influx of a generation of health care professionals that were or remain "recreational" drug abusers. It is safe to say that the percentage of health care professionals involved in substance abuse is at least as high as the percentage of substance abusers in the general population. The problems created by demand and availability are obvious. The health care profession, regulatory boards, and law enforcement cannot afford to be ignorant of the situation.

Security professionals and administrators should be knowledgeable of the problems created by the impaired professional or the loss of controlled substances for self-abuse or other reasons. It is through this knowledge that the administrator will be able to demand vigilance on the part of the staff and will be prepared to deal with the various situations as they arise. It is far easier to deal with an impaired professional on an individual basis than to explain an unnecessary patient death to the press or in a deposition.

Health care professionals themselves are in the best position to police their profession. Physicians, nurses, and pharmacists can and should be trained to recognize abusers and know the methods of diversion. With administration, health care professionals, and investigators working together, diversion of controlled and noncontrolled substances can be identified in the early stages and dealt with accordingly. Appendix 12–A offers text from federal laws that discuss narcotics control in health care facilities.

PROFILE OF AN ADDICTED HEALTH CARE PROFESSIONAL

Because health care professionals have stressful jobs as well as knowledge of and access to controlled substances, they are susceptible to addiction. Many health care professionals begin to abuse drugs through self-medication when they are ill or stressed. Almost always the professionals feel that they are capable of using the drug without becoming dependent. Most of the time, these individuals obtain their medication through various methods of diversion, sometimes with tragic results for both the health care professional and the patient.

Not all health care professionals begin to divert controlled substances for specific reasons, medical or otherwise. These are the professionals that began a pattern of substance abuse in high school or college. They tend to divert controlled substances as either a continuation of an earlier problem or to augment recreational abuse of drugs. Many divert drugs to control the side effects of cocaine abuse. Many divert drugs to counter the effects of alcohol abuse away from the workplace.

Sometimes drugs are not diverted for personal use. For instance, the drugs may be taken for use by a relative or a friend or for resale.

Health care professionals have little trouble noticing the effects of drugs on patients but seem to have difficulty recognizing the signs among themselves. A problem may go undetected because health care professionals are too busy, too trusting, or too isolated from one another. Some of the signs of substance abuse are listed below. These are just some of the more prevalent indicators. No list will ever be complete.

Job Performance

There are several performance-related indicators of substance abuse.

- a decline in overall job performance, including medication errors, charting errors, and a deterioration in handwriting
- increased absenteeism and tardiness
- increased utilization of sick leave
- long periods spent away from the work area, including inordinate amounts of time in a bathroom or lounge
- a tendency to prefer shifts where there is less activity and supervision, including the 3 p.m. to 11 a.m. shift and the 11 p.m. to 7 a.m. shift

Appearance

The appearance of individuals who are abusing drugs may change dramatically.

- They may show less concern for grooming and the state of clothing.
- They may wear inappropriate clothing or change their style of dress. For instance, they might wear long-sleeved lab coats in the middle of summer.
- They may have bruising that they do not explain.

- They may have small puncture wounds on the arms and the back of the hands that they do not explain.
- They may appear sleepy.
- They may have slurred speech.
- They may have discolored pupils.

Behavior

People with substance abuse problems may behave differently.

- They may seem more anxious.
- They may have marked mood swings.
- They may cry or display anger at inappropriate times.
- Their ability to interact with supervisory personnel and peers may change.
- They may have lapses of memory or be forgetful.

Complaints

The substance abuser may often make comments concerning problems in their lives. These problems may or may not be real; the abusers are simply trying to explain their changes in behavior. **Common problems mentioned include**

- marital problems
- financial problems
- health problems
- work-related problems
- problems associated with the recreational use of drugs

Signs Unique to Nurses

While any of the indicators noted above would apply to nursing personnel, other indicators are unique to the nursing profession. **Nurses who are diverting drugs may**

- give more medication than other nurses
- use the maximum amount of medication when other nurses are able to medicate the patients successfully with smaller amounts
- volunteer to give medications quite often
- have an increased amount of waste and breakage
- tend to go to the bathroom or lounge after medicating a patient
- have an increased number of complaints from patients who fail to get relief from medication the nurse administered

Readers take note. The indicators of drug diversion noted in this chapter are simply that—indicators. Many individuals who are not abusing substances have personal or professional problems that would manifest themselves in some of the same ways.

To accuse someone of substance abuse based solely on the indicators would be inappropriate. People should use these indicators only to narrow the list of suspects and focus the investigation.

DRUG INVESTIGATIONS

Health care facilities are large institutions with their own set of protocols and well-defined job responsibilities. The person leading an investigation will soon realize that all professionals on an investigation team have different priorities and expect different outcomes. Seeking consensus can be difficult.

Unlike most security investigations at health care facilities, drug diversion cases may involve many departments. For example, the suspect may work in the nursing department, while the person ultimately responsible for the drugs may head the pharmacy department. The personnel department records the employee's employment status and advises about labor law issues. Security personnel may be involved as the principal investigators or as consultants. And managers are involved because they oversee policies and procedures. It is helpful if administrators have written a policy on drug diversions stating that the health care facility will maintain the integrity of all controlled substances and investigate and pursue prosecution of those diverting drugs.

Before an investigation begins, all members of the affected departments should meet. Each member needs to understand that for the investigation to be successful a close working atmosphere must exist. Each member brings to the investigation special knowledge necessary to resolve the case. The team should achieve an outcome that not only protects the patient but also leads to the identification, prosecution, and, if necessary, treatment of the person diverting from the health care facility.

It is helpful to have a predetermined plan of action. If all members know how they fit in to the investigation, it will proceed more smoothly, without individual bias.

Reviewing and analyzing prior drug diversion cases should help all members to set forth a policy stating the expected role each member will play. All members must appreciate that investigations of this type are charged with difficult emotional, ethical, and legal issues.

METHODS OF DIVERSION

As indicated previously, most of the cases involving the diversion of controlled substances by health care professionals involve self-abuse problems. The diversion may be limited to only a few pills or capsules, may be done regularly or only when there is a physical or psychological need, or may be committed only when the opportunity presents itself. Diversion can occur in every fashion imaginable (Appendixes 12–B through 12–D list some of the successful scams that have been used to divert drugs both internally and externally). As long as people have a need, they will, in most cases, find a way.

Like law enforcement, accounting, and other professions, health care is based on trust among professionals. Most health care professionals do not want to believe that their coworkers are thieves and might have a drug problem.

And because health care professionals are often too busy and overworked, drug diversion goes unnoticed or unaddressed. Most health care facilities have adequate security systems, systems of accounting for controlled substance, and systems of recording patient information. But these systems are rarely cross-checked. They are based on employee trust. Only when someone takes the time to review the records will the diversion be spotted. Thieves are keenly aware of this fact and will use trust and hectic work days as their allies.

This section exposes only the most common methods of diversion. No text can ever be complete. The methods utilized are limited only by the imagination. Though all drug diversion is theft, this section will divide the methods of diversion into different categories: theft, substitution, charting, waste, drug requisition, shorting the patient, and anesthesia.

Theft

In this section, "theft" will be used to describe taking a controlled substance without trying to conceal the act through the manipulation of records or other means. The thief hopes that the item will never be missed or that enough time will elapse to make the identification of the perpetrator nearly impossible.

This method of diversion is generally a crime of opportunity and is accomplished quickly. **The scale of the theft is governed only by the amount of controlled substances available to the thief.**

Pharmacy

Thefts from pharmacy stock usually occur in one of two ways. First, small quantities of drugs may be pilfered from larger drug stocks. Substance-abusing pharmacy personnel can easily accomplish the first type of theft. Small quantities are taken from large stock bottles or drugs packaged in unit-dose systems. This type of theft offers several advantages.

- It is rare that anyone counts the number of dosage units contained in a stock bottle. Even systems that maintain a perpetual inventory count are probably not completely accurate.
- The loss of a few tablets from a large amount of stock will not be immediately noticed (if, in fact, it ever is). If the theft is noticed, the loss will be so small and the number of people having access to the drug so large that nothing will be done about it.
- The loss of a few dosage units from a stock bottle can easily be attributed to a counting error or manufacturer's error, not a theft.

The second method of diversion from a pharmacy involves the taking of large quantities of substances. Generally, thieves take the entire bottle of the drug. The potential for getting caught goes up dramatically when large quantities are taken, but thieves often calculate the risks based on the security of the pharmacy, the inventory control, and the availability of the controlled substance itself.

Typically, Schedule II substances are tightly controlled, both by physical security and limited access. Perpetual inventories are often maintained on these drugs. While these measures decrease the potential for diversion, they do not eliminate it.

Controlled substances in Schedules III through V are often stocked in large quantities and are readily available to those who work in the pharmacy area. Pharmacy personnel will know how and where these drugs are stocked, but so might other people. Maintenance personnel, housekeeping personnel, salespeople, and nursing staff often have this knowledge and can help themselves to the stock.

Suppose that a health care facility has received a shipment of 5,000 diazepam tablets packaged in 100-count bottles. Fifty bottles would be placed on the shelves. With so many bottles in stock, the loss of one or two would not be immediately apparent. The bottles themselves are small and easily concealed. Depending on how long this stock is expected to last, a large amount of this shipment could be diverted over a relatively short period of time.

Prefilled syringes are often targets for theft. Injectable narcotics such as meperidene and morphine are often packaged in this form. Most, if not all, of the prefilled syringes are packaged in plastic flats, with five syringes to a flat. The package will be divided so that each syringe is separated from each other and has a security tab that must be broken in order to remove the syringe in the normal manner.

The factory security system provided can be easily bypassed if a person wishes to do so. The first method is simply to break the security tab and take the entire syringe. This method is rarely seen since the loss of the syringe is quickly apparent.

The remaining methods involve the removal of the contents of the syringes themselves. Content removal is accomplished in basically two ways. The first is to use the applicator that is appropriate for the type of syringe. The prefilled syringe is placed in the applicator, and the controlled substance is injected directly or the drug is placed in a vial or bottle for later use. In either case, the seal surrounding the needle is broken and it is common to see small amounts of fluid around the needle.

The second, and perhaps the most prevalent, method of removing the contents of a syringe involves the use of a second needle and syringe. The needle from the second syringe is used to go through the rubber plunger of the target syringe, and the contents of the target syringe are withdrawn.

Once a person has decided to remove the contents of a syringe, breaching the security of the flat can be accomplished in several ways. First, the back of the plastic flat can be cut and the syringes removed. The security tabs can be carefully removed and reglued after the empty syringe is placed back in the flat.

Second, a sealed package of syringes can be carefully opened. The contents of the syringes are then removed and the box is resealed with glue. The box then can be left to be counted as a sealed box. If the box is not in the pharmacy at the time the theft occurs, it may be returned to the pharmacy to go back into its stock.

This poses additional problems if the diversion is not immediately discovered. The box of syringes can linger in the pharmacy for a period of time and then be reissued to the station that returned the drug or to some other area of the facility.

Also, if the sides of some of the sealed boxes are squeezed, the boxes will bow to the extent that several of the syringes along the outside edges of the box can be removed without breaking the integrity of the seal.

Ampuls pose yet another problem. Most ampuls are shipped in cardboard boxes that are subdivided internally such that each ampul is protected from breakage. The boxes are sealed when shipped. It is not uncommon to find that the seals of these boxes have been broken and that all or a portion of the contents have been removed.

Unit-dose systems are not immune to diversion. In some cases, unit-dose packaging is done in strips. The strips are numbered in descending order and are placed in cardboard boxes for ease of handling and counting. An example of this would be a box containing 25 tablets, each packaged individually. The unit dose numbered 25 is the first visible dose. When it is removed, the unit dose numbered 24 is then visible. A method of diverting these drugs is to open the sealed box and remove some of the units with low numbers.

For example, if the box is opened, unit doses 1 through 15 are removed, and the box is re-sealed, the box appears normal. The box is sent to the floor, and only after the first 10 unit doses are removed are the areas with missing doses visible.

Cocaine, a drug of choice for many people, is expensive. Cocaine powder is often kept in health care facilities, clinics, and dentist offices to use directly or to make solutions to numb areas prior to medical procedures. Since cocaine is a powder, it has to be accounted for by weight. This makes it an easy target for diversion. Taking a few grams from a bottle is a simple task. When considering whether to divert cocaine, thieves have to consider how much cocaine the facility routinely uses and how easily the cocaine can be accessed.

During the interval between receipt of the drug and its recording into inventory, thefts may occur. If proper security procedures are not followed, entire shipments can be stolen. While this type of theft is immediately apparent, the drugs are still gone. Care should be taken to ensure that shipments are immediately moved to secure areas and inventoried.

Nurses' Stations or Floor Carts

Thefts from nurses' stations or floor carts are another area of concern. These thefts occur from both floor stock and the medication ordered for particular patients.

Thefts from nurses' stations are usually committed by health care facility personnel since access is limited and the stations are staffed constantly. Small amounts are usually taken from floor stock since it is not routinely counted and time will pass between the theft and its discovery. Because medications destined for specific patients are forwarded in limited amounts, the potential for discovery is much greater and these drugs are not as likely to be targets for this type of theft.

Another method of diversion seen at nurses' stations is the theft of all or a part of the drugs requisitioned from the pharmacy. In cases where pharmacy personnel are not directly involved in the stocking of the nurses' station or the medication carts, the theft is easily accomplished. The drugs are simply taken. It is also common to find that the sign-out sheet(s) for the drugs are also missing. In some facilities the sign-out sheets are not often reconciled, and if the record noting the receipt of the drug at the station is taken, it is probable that the drug would not be added to the station's inventory. In short, without the sign-out sheet it is conceivable that no one would know that the drugs had ever arrived on the floor.

If the security of the nurses' station and floor carts is not maintained, theft of both controlled and noncontrolled drugs is likely to occur. Health care facilities and nursing homes are constantly filled with visitors, many of whom will take an opportunity to steal drugs if it is presented. Because of time limitations, thieves from outside the facility will often take everything that is available. Many times, the people will not even know what they have taken. They will simply discard what they do not want at a later date.

Theft by outside individuals is easily controlled through good security practices and the locking of floor carts when they are not in use.

Operating Room Suites

Thefts from operating rooms, recovery rooms, and anesthesia areas follow the same patterns as have been noted previously. These areas are particularly vulnerable to theft when they are not in use.

Operating rooms, recovery rooms, and anesthesia areas are utilized for only a limited number of hours on weekdays and only in emergency situations on weekends. These areas are usually supposed to be locked when not in use, but it is not uncommon to find them unlocked. Then a thief can gain immediate access. Once inside, the thief can take what is immediately available through unsecured medication cabinets, medication or anesthesia carts, or other areas. The thief will also have the time to force open the secured areas and take what is there—often the most potent assortment of controlled substances.

Substitution

Theft of controlled substances through substitution is perhaps the most insidious form of diversion. The administration of unknown substances by an unsuspecting nurse can result in unrelieved patient pain, infection, and, at worst, death.

This form of diversion is a calculated, deliberate attempt on the part of the perpetrator to avoid detection. Methods used to divert through substitution can be crude or very sophisticated.

Capsules

Capsules are not sealed. They can be opened by simply pulling the ends apart. The substance inside the capsules can easily be removed and replaced. Any type of powder, including flour, can be put back into the capsules to make them look and feel normal. The capsules are then placed back into the container from which they were removed.

Tablets

Controlled substance tablets are easily substituted when not packaged in sealed unit doses. The tablets are removed from stock bottles, plastic cassettes, or blister packs. Tablets that approximate the original tablets' size and color are put in their place. Anything from aspirin to heart medication has been used to cover diversion.

The person responsible for the diversion is counting on the fact that health care professionals will be too busy to notice the crime. Nurses involved in shift counts may simply glance at the tablets when making counts or taking a tablet from a container to administer.

Injectable Substances

Injectable controlled substances are packaged in one of two ways. The first method is the multidose vial. This is a sealed vial that has a rubber top that allows a needle to be inserted to withdraw the liquid.

The seals of these vials can be violated, and the contents can be removed. The vials are then refilled with a fluid that is the same color as the medication. Anything can be used in the refilling process. Most often, saline or water is used to replace the stolen fluid. Both are common and pose little harm to a patient. The seals are reglued or replaced in some fashion after the switch has been made.

Prefilled syringes are common targets for substitution. Usually these contain some form of narcotic drug. Schedule II drugs are the most likely targets.

Substitution of the fluids contained within the syringes can be accomplished in a number of different ways. The simplest method is to remove the syringe from the flat and put it into an applicator. The contents of the fluid can then be transferred or injected and a substitute solution drawn back in its place without the use of a second syringe. The syringe is then placed back into the flat. Some of the methods used to remove the syringe from the flat and several methods utilized to make the flat appear secure have already been discussed.

To get to the drug inside, a syringe does not have to be removed from the flat. The seals and security tabs do not have to be removed or tampered with. The thief can use a second syringe to make the substitution. The needle of the second syringe is used to puncture the back of the plastic flat containing the syringes. The needle is then inserted into the syringe through the rubber plunger inside the barrel of the syringe. The contents of the syringe are then removed, and the fluid is replaced. The only visible signs of tampering will be the small holes left in the back of the flats. During shift counts, the syringes will be observed to have fluid, and the security tabs will be intact. Only a careful observer will discover the tampering.

It should be noted that at least one manufacturer has placed a metal strip across the back of the plastic flat in an attempt to deter this form of tampering.

Ampuls

Ampuls are considered to be one of the most tamper-proof forms of packaging. It is difficult, but not impossible, to tamper with ampuls.

Ampuls are manufactured to be broken at the neck. If an individual is careful, the ampul can be broken cleanly enough to allow the contents to be removed, a substitute fluid put in its place, and the top glued back on. This form of tampering should be recognizable through visual inspection and should be detected when the ampul is broken open the second time. This is not always the case.

In a rare form of tampering and substitution with ampuls, a needle is used to puncture the ampul. The needle must be heated in order to do this, making the method more time-consuming and cumbersome than most, and thereby increasing the chances of being caught in the act.

Use of Alternative Drugs

Not all forms of substitution require elaborate plans and a great deal of time. Quite often, the patient medication is signed out and properly documented and another drug is substituted for the controlled substance immediately prior to the administration.

For example, a nurse could sign out a Percodan tablet for a patient and document the administration. The nurse could then keep the Percodan tablet for herself and give the patient an oral administration of acetaminophen. The patient would recall getting a tablet, and there would be some analgesic effect.

The same holds true for injectable medications. Noncontrolled injectables such as Nubain and Stadol can be used in the place of Demerol. The patient has no idea what the syringe contained. He or she would only recall receiving a shot. That the shot was not as effective as other shots will probably be seen as another baseless patient complaint.

Charting

Diversion of controlled substances through charting techniques is common in the health care industry. Simply put, a person, most often a nurse, charts the administration of a medication that was not given. The person merely signs out a controlled substance for a patient and does not give it. If the person who signs out the medication for this purpose wants to carry the false documentation through, he or she will also document the administration in the patient's medication administration record and note it in the nursing notes.

Often, the person who is involved in this type of diversion does not maintain continuity among all of the records. Merely signing the drug out on the sign-out sheet is usually sufficient. As long as the drug counts at shift change are correct, this diversion is not readily detected. It is only when someone recognizes that the administrations are not noted on the medication administration record and in the nursing notes that suspicions are raised.

This type of diversion is best done with a patient who requires numerous administrations of a drug and who would not ordinarily be in a position to successfully argue that the administration was not given.

Another method of diversion is falsification of the sign-out sheet. The individual who commits this act either forges the name of someone from the previous shift, noting an administration of the drug during the prior shift, or forges the name of a nurse who is working on the current shift. This method works best when the patient census is high and numerous nurses are involved in administering medications.

Waste

Perhaps the easiest method of diverting controlled substances in a health care facility is the theft of waste. It is common practice for only a portion of an injectable drug to be administered.

The wasting of controlled substances is supposed to be documented and should be witnessed. The person who witnesses the disposal of a medication really does not know what is being disposed of. That witness must take the word of the person disposing of the drug.

For example, a nurse could use a 100 mg Demerol syringe to administer a 50 mg dose. Only half of the syringe's contents are used. The remaining portion of the drug is to be wasted. The nurse who wants to divert the remaining portion of the Demerol either transfers the drug to another container for use at a later time or injects herself with what remains. She then draws water into the used syringe to refill it to the 50 mg level. She has a coworker witness her wasting the leftover "Demerol." She has obtained the Demerol for her own use, the patient has received his medication, and the waste of the "Demerol" has been properly documented.

Many individuals who use this method to obtain drugs create the opportunity for diversion. These individuals will sign out larger amounts of drugs than are required so that waste will be generated. For instance, suppose a patient was scheduled to receive a 25 mg injection of Demerol, and prefilled Demerol syringes were stocked on the floor in 50 mg, 75 mg, and 100 mg strengths. In order to generate a significant amount of waste, nurses could choose a 75 mg or 100 mg syringe. If challenged on their selections, they could state that they had initially misread the order or that they did not see the smaller units.

Another form of diverting controlled substances through waste is the deliberate breakage of ampuls, syringes, tablets, and capsules. In the case of ampuls and syringes, the liquid contents of the items can be removed and replaced with another fluid before an intentional breakage occurs. Witnesses see the broken ampul and the liquid that came from within. The breakage is documented as waste, and the accountability is complete.

This method also works with oral medications that are supposedly dropped or refused by the patient. Care must be taken to ensure that the tablet or capsule being flushed into the sewer system is what it is reported to be.

Drug Requisition

Fraudulent drug requisitions are also a method of drug diversion. This method employs the use of a fictitious requisition to obtain controlled substances. The person who places the requisition must also be in a position to intercept the drugs when they are sent to the floor or unit.

It is most likely that the individual who places the fictitious order will utilize a real patient's name. Thus, if anyone checked, there would be a patient by that name in the area from which the requisition originated. In addition, the patient whose name had been used would be billed for the substance. The pharmacy would have a record of the controlled substance being sent to the floor, and the billing department would bill the patient for the medication. In the complicated world of itemized billing, it is probable that an entry for a drug the patient never received would go unnoticed. The other nurses on the floor or in the unit would not know that the drug had been ordered and would not be looking for the drug.

This method of diversion is not limited to licensed professionals. A unit secretary who works on a regular basis may have the best opportunity to divert drugs in this fashion. This method cannot be used when pharmacy personnel are used to personally stock the carts and floor stock.

Shorting the Patient

This method of diversion combines theft and substitution. It can be easily employed by anyone who routinely administers medication. The method works for both oral and injectable medications.

In the case of injectable medications, one-half or more of the drug is taken by the person diverting the drug. The patient either receives that portion of what is left or receives a combination of the medication and another drug that would tend to potentiate the first.

For instance, if a patient was scheduled to receive an injection of 100 mg of Demerol, a nurse could take half or more of the drug for herself. She could then simply give the patient the remaining amount, or she could add substances like Phenergan or Nubain to the injection. Both of these drugs would tend to potentiate the Demerol and increase its effects. The patient would get both a shot and some relief.

In the case of oral medications, a diversion can occur by signing out more than the patient is given. If the physician's order called for one or two tablets of a given controlled substance, a nurse could sign out two dosage units, keeping one for herself and giving the patient the second.

Shorting the patient can happen in so many different ways. As in the other types of diversions, the actual methods employed are limited only by the imagination.

Anesthesia

Anesthesia is the most vulnerable area for diversion in the health care profession. It is the only area where the system of checks and balances does not ordinarily apply. Couple this with the extensive use of narcotics and the pressures of the profession, and the problem becomes clear.

In other areas of a health care facility, a nurse must have a physician's order to give controlled substances to a patient. This order must be issued before the drugs are sent to the unit. A nurse must document the administration of the drug in several areas, all of which are open to inspection by the nurse's peers and are routinely used in patient assessment. While not perfect, this system has checks and balances. The person who orders the drug does not give it, the person who gives the drug must document the administration, and that documentation is open for inspection.

This is not the case in anesthesia services. Within the health care facilities' formulary, an anesthesiologist or a CRNA may use any and all of the controlled substances available. The individual who administers the anesthesia must decide which anesthesia technique to use depending on the physical state of the patient and the type of surgical procedure to be done. During the surgical procedure, the person administering anesthesia decides when a drug is necessary and what amounts to use. As long as the patient remains stable during the procedure, no one questions the anesthesia technique.

Because of this independence and the numerous methods of administering anesthesia, diversion is relatively easy. Anyone investigating this type of crime must have an understanding of how anesthesia is administered.

Modern anesthesia combines the use of several different drugs to accomplish its goal. Some of these drugs are administered intravenously, others through inhalation. Medication is administered to rapidly put the patient to sleep. Other medication is often administered to induce an element of paralysis to control the muscles during surgery. Other drugs are used to serve as an anesthetic agent, and it is these drugs that raise the most concern.

Some analgesic drugs are in the form of a gas or a vapor. Nitrous oxide is a gas commonly used, and halothane and ethane are induced as vapors. These inhalation agents can be used alone or in conjunction with injectable drugs.

The injectable drugs used in anesthesia for analgesic purposes are some of the most powerful drugs manufactured for use on humans. The list includes meperidene, morphine, fentanyl, Sufenta, and Alfenta.

Diversion from an anesthesia service is easily accomplished by the people who administer the anesthesia. First, these individuals can select a technique that gives them unquestioned access to the drug of choice. Second, the individuals can have all of the medication they might need at their immediate disposal. Third, these individuals are actually charged with the administration of the drug and can give as much or as little as they see fit and still maintain control of the patient. Fourth, the individuals are charged with recording the amount of controlled substances administered to the patient during a procedure. Last, but not least, there is little or no accountability for the amounts of inhalation agents utilized.

Thus, it is easy for individuals administering anesthesia to record that more of a drug was used than was actually used and divert the difference for their own use. The individuals can either simply record fraudulent amounts of the chosen drug or make the fraudulent entries while augmenting the analgesic with the unrecorded use of inhalation agents.

It is also simple for the anesthesiologist or anesthetist to generate significant amounts of waste. Many facilities allow the person administering anesthesia to draw any reasonable amount of medication necessary for a case. Many also have a policy that will not allow medication to be carried over from patient to patient, which requires that any unused portion of the medication drawn for a particular patient be wasted.

It is a simple matter for the individual to draw more than he or she is planning to use. The excess is required to be wasted, creating the perfect opportunity to divert the drugs.

Controlled substances can also be diverted from this area through fraudulent or unnecessary requisitions.

While most facilities require some form of a sign-out sheet to be completed by anesthesia personnel, it is rare that these sheets are ever compared to the anesthesia sheet in the patient's chart. As in most cases, if the count is correct and there is no obvious signs of impairment on the part of the individual, everyone is happy and the diversion can go undetected for a long time.

Diversion cases in anesthesia services are difficult to investigate and even more difficult to prove. These types of cases are best left to investigators who have a background in this area.

CASE STUDIES

The following case studies discuss cases that the authors have investigated. The names of all persons, facilities, and locations have been changed. Any relationship to any person, either living or dead, in these cases is purely coincidental.

Case A

LOCATION: Large teaching health care facility in the Southeast
DEPARTMENT: Coronary care unit (CCU)
DRUG: Nubain, Demerol, morphine
SUSPECT: CCU RN, in her thirties, licensed for 12 years
At the beginning of the Monday 7 a.m. to 3 p.m. shift in a large teaching health care facility, Charge Nurse Anderson counts the narcotics with Nurse Powers of the 11 p.m. to 7 a.m. shift. Both carefully count and document that all narcotics are exact in number and quantity.

At 8:00 a.m. Nurse Smith goes to the narcotic cabinet, unlocks it, and removes an ampul of Nubain 20 mg/ml. As she starts to "pop" the top off the ampul, the top falls off into her hand.

She immediately removes another ampul, and the top "pops" off as it should. She medicates her patient and then confers with Charge Nurse Anderson about the first ampul.

Both carefully examine the remainder of the Nubain ampuls and notice that around the top of the "scored circle" where several of the ampuls would normally be broken, there appears to be a "milky ring." They notify the pharmacy of the problem, and the pharmacy supervisor exchanges the Nubain for fresh stock.

The pharmacy supervisor contacts the director of security, who takes custody of the ampuls. Having the lab perform a comparison of the ampuls to a controlled ampul that has not been tampered with confirms their suspicions. The liquid in the tampered ampuls is saline.

A meeting is held with the nurse managers on the CCU unit, the director of security, and the director of pharmacy. An investigation plan is outlined. The charge nurses on each shift will personally examine all ampuls several times during the shifts and report any unusual findings to both the pharmacy and security directors.

A week passes, and all ampuls appear normal. However, on Saturday night the charge nurse finds an ampul that has been tampered with. She removes it from stock and notes the time of the discovery. She contacts the director of security, who advises her to turn the ampul over to the pharmacy and to check the ampuls every 30 minutes.

The charge nurse later finds an ampul of Demerol 75 mg that appears suspect. She reports her findings and is asked to check the Nubain. She reports that at present the unit is out of stock of Nubain but that a supply delivery is expected at any time. The same events occur during the Sunday night shift. During the rest of the week, all ampuls appear normal. However, the following weekend, the same events occur.

By tracking schedules, the nurse managers are able to determine that only 2 of the 16 RNs assigned to the unit had been working during each incident.

The following weekend, one of these two RNs calls in sick to work. The charge nurse informs the director of security, who asks the charge nurse to check the narcotics each time the one suspect who is working gives medication.

At 1 a.m. the charge nurse notifies the security director that she has discovered a tampered ampul. The security director goes to the unit and has the charge nurse bring the suspect to an office near the unit.

An interview reveals that the suspect has been diverting both Demerol and morphine for over six months. She admits that during that time if a patient was to receive either Demerol or morphine, she would give the patient Nubain instead. (Nubain would offer the patient some relief.) The suspect would then refill the ampul with saline, glue the top on with fingernail polish, and place the tampered ampul back in the box with the remaining Nubain. She would then inject the Demerol into herself.

During the past several weeks, her drug use had become so severe that she would take empty ampuls home, fill them with tap water, and glue the tops back on. She would then have a stock of ampuls ready for use.

At the time of the interview, the suspect admitted to having injected herself with four Demerol 75 mg and two morphine 10 mg during the past four hours.

The suspect was arrested for diversion and given a suspended sentence on the condition that she enter and successfully complete a drug rehab program. While on probation the suspect was arrested for the sale and delivery of cocaine. She was sentenced to six years in the state prison, where she is serving time today.

Case B

LOCATION: Mid-sized health care facility in a suburban area
DEPARTMENT: Medical-surgical nursing unit
DRUG: Darvocet
SUSPECT: Licensed practical nurse (LPN), in her late forties, licensed for seven years

Unit Assistant Perkins went into the medication room to get a fruit drink from the refrigerator for one of her patients. As she entered the room, she saw LPN Davis remove drugs from the bag containing drugs going to the pharmacy for "credit" and place the drugs in her lab coat. Ms. Perkins reported the incident to the head nurse.

The head nurse contacted the security department, and a meeting was held with the security director, assistant director of security, pharmacy director, head nurse, and nursing administrator. A plan was formulated. The assistant director, who was new to the health care facility, would wait in the family waiting area during LPN Davis' shift. The assistant director would be in "plain clothes" and would pose as a family member. From the waiting room, the assistant director would be able to see when LPN Davis entered the medication room.

The drugs that LPN Davis was stealing had been assigned to a patient. These were delivered to the nursing unit daily and were a 24-hour supply. If a patient was discharged early and all the medication was not needed, the drugs were marked "credit," placed in a bag, and returned to the pharmacy. Unfortunately, due to the large volume of patients and medications, the drugs were allowed to accumulate for several days before being sent to the pharmacy.

Early the next morning, the assistant director stationed himself in the waiting room. After the 11 p.m. to 7 a.m. and 7 a.m. to 3 p.m. shift change, the RNs started checking on their patients for the day. The assistant director observed LPN Davis entering the medication room. He was able to go into the hallway. Through the glass window in the medication room door, he saw LPN Davis remove drugs from the "credit bag," place them inside a facial tissue, and put them in her lab coat.

He entered the room, identified himself to LPN Davis, and escorted her to the security director's office. He also notified the head nurse and the pharmacy director. As all parties waited in another office, the security director interviewed Davis. She admitted that she had a drug problem and had been addicted for over four years. She stated that the addiction started after an auto accident. After several surgeries to her left leg, she still was in pain. Her physician had continued to prescribe Darvocet and Tylenol no. 3 for her. Then the physician became concerned that she had no more physical pain and that she simply wanted the painkillers. Instead of suggesting counseling or a rehab center, the physician had simply refused to prescribe the drugs.

It was at that point, two years ago, that Davis began diverting drugs. She admitted that two to four times a week she would steal a supply of painkillers from the credit bag. She rationalized that she was not harming any patients and that the health care facility owed the drugs to her, since she always worked her shift regardless of how much her leg hurt her.

Davis was arrested for drug diversion and placed in a drug rehab program. She was given a suspended sentence. After successfully completing the rehab program, she applied for her license to be reinstated. The state board reinstated her license after a two-year waiting period. She now practices in the same health care facility where she was apprehended.

Case C

LOCATION: Small health care facility in a rural setting
DEPARTMENT: Pediatrics
DRUG: Lortab
SUSPECT: Nursing secretary, in her mid-twenties, employed for two years

In this health care facility, a physician could call in an order to an RN caring for a patient. The nurse would fill out a two-part form and send the top copy to the pharmacy. Upon receipt of the order, the pharmacy would fill the prescription and send the drugs and the top copy of the order back to the nurses' station. The top copy would be matched to the second copy, which had been placed in the patient's chart, and the physician would sign the order the next time he or she came to check on the patient. In addition, the order would be entered into the computer system at the nurses' station. The computer system was connected to the pharmacy so another 24-hour supply could be sent to the patient.

As RN Peterson was checking her patient's chart she discovered a handwritten drug order for Lortab. She became suspicious about the order because the nurse whose signature appeared on the called-in physician's order had been on vacation for over a week and there was not a strength listed for the Lortab. She asked Nursing Secretary Jones about the order. Ms. Jones pulled the order up on the computer and told RN Peterson that the strength was Lortab 7.5 mg.

Nurse Peterson was still suspicious about the order. She contacted the physician, who informed Peterson that he had not called in the order.

RN Peterson informed her head nurse, and together they checked all the charts on the unit. They found four other suspicious orders. In all of these, the orders appeared to have been written by the same person; however, all had different RN signatures. They checked with the RNs and found that none of them had written the orders. They advised the pharmacy director and the security director of their findings.

Several handwritings were checked, and it appeared that the nursing secretary was responsible for the forged orders. The secretary was interviewed and admitted forging orders for eight months. She would write the orders, send the top copy to the pharmacy, and enter the order in the computer. After the drugs were delivered to the nursing unit, she would destroy both copies of the order and delete the order in the computer system. She would then steal the Lortab.

The computer programmers at the health care facility were able to research the drug orders and deletions based upon the secretary's code number. They verified that during the past eight months she had entered and deleted orders for Lortab three or four times a week. Each order was for "1 or 2 every 4 hours for pain." Using that information, the health care facility was able to calculate that the secretary had diverted more than 1,300 units of Lortab. The secretary was arrested for forgery and drug diversion.

Unfortunately for all concerned, the health care facility had failed to conduct a criminal records check of the secretary prior to hiring her. The secretary had two prior convictions for drug possession and one for sale and distribution. She was sentenced to three years in the state prison.

KEY POINTS

- Drug diversion does occur at most facilities daily.
- In many cases, health care professionals who abuse drugs display certain indicators. No one should be accused of drug diversion just because they display these indicators, but the indicators can provide clues in investigations.
- The facility should have a written policy and procedures for dealing with drug diversion.
- All diversion is theft, but a theft may be accomplished through direct theft, substitution, charting, waste, shorting the patient, and other means.
- The Code of Federal Regulation, Part 1300, outlines drug security procedures.

Appendix 12–A

Narcotic Control in Health Care Facilities

STATEMENT OF RESPONSIBILITY

The chief executive of the hospital is responsible for the proper safeguarding and handling of controlled substances in Schedules I through V. Responsibility is delegated to the pharmacy director for purchase, storage, accountability, and proper dispensing within the hospital. The head nurse of each nursing unit is responsible for proper storage and control on the unit.

FEDERAL LAWS AND REGULATIONS

Title 21, Code of Federal Regulations, Part 1301.71 (a), requires all registrants to "provide effective controls and procedures to guard against theft and diversion of Controlled Substances." **Factors to be considered in determining whether a registrant has provided effective controls include the following:**

- .71,b,8 Adequacy of key control system
- .71,b,11 Adequacy of supervision over employees having access to storage areas
- .71,b,14 Adequacy of system for monitoring receipt, manufacture, distribution, and disposition of controlled substances

Title 21, CFR 1301.76 (b) requires notification of the Drug Enforcement Administration (DEA) "of the theft or significant loss of any controlled substances upon discovery of such loss or theft. The registrant shall also complete DEA Form 106 regarding such loss or theft."

Title 21, U.S. Code, Section 842,a,5, reads as follows: "It shall be unlawful for any person to refuse or fail to make, keep, or furnish any record, report, notification, declaration, order or order form, statement, invoice, or information required under this title or Title III."

Title 21, USC, 843,a,4 reads: "It shall be unlawful for any person, knowingly or intentionally, to furnish false or fraudulent material information in, or omit any material information from, any application, report, record, or other document required to be made, kept, or filed under this subchapter or subchapter II of this chapter."

If those responsible for maintaining records are derelict in performing that responsibility, the DEA has authority to prosecute those persons civilly under 21 USC 842,c. Each violation carries a $25,000 penalty, and if the government can show that any violation was committed knowingly there is an additional penalty of up to one year of imprisonment.

The penalty for delivering any Schedule II narcotic drug is imprisonment up to fifteen years and/or a fine of not more than $25,000.

FEDERAL CRIMINAL CODE—TITLE 18 U.S. CODE

18 USC 4 MISPRISION OF A FELONY. Failure to report knowledge of a felony. Punishable by a fine of not more than $500.00 or not more than three years imprisonment, or both.

18 USC 371 CONSPIRACY TO COMMIT AN OFFENSE. If two or more persons conspire to commit any offense against the United States, or to defraud the United States, or any agency thereof, in any manner or more any purpose, and one or more of such persons does any acto to effect the object of the conspiracy, each shall be fined not more than $10,000.00 or imprisoned not more than five years or both.

18 USC 1001 FALSIFY, CONCEAL OR COVER UP. Whoever, in any matter within the jurisdiction of any department or agency of the U.S., knowingly and willfully falsifies, conceals or covers up by any trick, scheme, or device or makes any false, fictitious or fraudulent statement or representation, shall be fined not more than $10,000.00 or imprisoned not more than five years or both.

§ 1301.76 Other security controls for practitioners.

(a) The registrant shall not employ, as an agent or employee who has access to controlled substances, any person who has been convicted of a felony offense relating to controlled substances or who, at any time, had an application for registration with the DEA denied, had a DEA registration revoked or has surrendered a DEA registration for cause. For purposes of this subsection, the term "for cause" means a surrender in lieu of, or as a consequence of, any federal or state administrative, civil or criminal action resulting from an investigation of the individual's handling of controlled substances.

(b) The registrant shall notify the Field Division Office of the Administration in his area of the theft or significant loss of any controlled substances upon discovery of such loss or theft. The registrant shall also complete DEA (or BND) Form 106 regarding such loss or theft.

(c) Whenever the registrant distributes a controlled substance (without being registered as a distributor, as permitted in § 1301.22(b) and/or §§ 1301.11–1307.14), he shall comply with the requirements imposed on nonpractitioners in § 1301.74 (a), (b), and (e).

§ 1301.90 Employee screening procedures.

It is the position of DEA that the obtaining of certain information by non-practitioners is vital to fairly assess the likelihood of an employee committing a drug security breach. The need to know this information is a matter of business necessity, essential to overall controlled substances security. In this regard, it is believed that conviction of crimes and unauthorized use of controlled substances are activities that are proper subjects for inquiry. It is, therefore, assumed that the following questions will become a part of an employer's comprehensive employees screening program:

Question. Within the past five years, have you been convicted of a felony, or within the past two years, of any misdemeanor or are you presently formally charged with committing a criminal offense? (Do not include any traffic violations, juvenile offenses or military convictions, except by general court-martial.) If the answer is yes, furnish details of conviction, offense, location, date and sentence.

Question. In the past three years, have you ever knowingly used any narcotics, amphetamines or barbiturates, other than those prescribed to you by a physician? If the answer is yes, furnish details.

Advice. An authorization, in writing, that allows inquiries to be made of courts and law enforcement agencies for possible pending charges or convictions must be executed by a person who is allowed to work in an area where access to controlled substances clearly exists. A person must be advised that any false information or omission of information will jeopardize his or her position with respect to employment. The application for employment should inform a person that information furnished or recovered as a result of any inquiry will not necessarily preclude employment, but will be considered as part of an overall evaluation of the person's qualifications. The maintaining of fair employment practices, the protection of the person's right of privacy and the assurance that the results of such inquiries will be treated by the employer in confidence will be explained to the employee. [40 FR 17143, Apr. 17, 1975]

§ 1301.91 Employee responsibility to report drug diversion.

Reports of drug diversion by fellow employees is not only a necessary part of an overall employee security program but also serves the public interest at large. It is, therefore, the position of DEA that an employee who has knowledge of drug diversion from his employer by a fellow employee has an obligation to report such information to a responsible security official of the employer. The employer shall treat such information as confidential and shall take all reasonable steps to protect the confidentiality of the information and the identity of the employee furnishing information. A failure to report information of drug diversion will be considered in determining the feasibility of continuing to allow an employee to work in a drug security area. The employer shall inform all employees concerning this policy. [40 FR 17143, Apr. 17, 1975]

§ 1301.92 Illicit activities by employees.

It is the position of the DEA that employees who possess, sell, use or divert controlled substances will subject themselves not only to State or Federal prosecution for any illicit activity, but shall also immediately become the subject of independent action regarding their continued employment. The employer will assess the seriousness of the employee's violation, the position of responsibility held by the employee, past record or employment, etc., in determining whether to suspend, transfer, terminate or take the action against the employee. [40 FR 17143, Apr. 17, 1975]

§ 1301.93 Sources of information for employee checks.

DEA recommends that inquiries concerning employees' criminal records be made as follows:

Local inquiries. Inquiries should be made by name, date and place of birth, and other identifying information, to local courts and law enforcement agencies for records of pending charges and convictions. Local practice may require such inquiries to be made in person, rather than by mail, and a copy of an authorization from the employee may be required by certain law enforcement agencies.

DEA inquiries. Inquiries supplying identifying information should also be furnished to DEA Field Division Offices along with written consent from the concerned individual for a check of DEA files for records of convictions. The regional check will result in a national check being made by the Field Division Office. [40 FR 17143, Apr. 17, 1975, as amended at 47 FR 41735, Sept. 22, 1982]

Appendix 12–B

Physician on Call Scam

This particular scam was reported by a physician who has practiced in both Massachusetts and Georgia. With slight variations, similar scams have been reported from other states. The procedure follows a common format. A physician on call receives a phone call at home from an individual claiming to be a relative of a patient of one of the physician's colleagues (who is not on call). Here are some key points to remember:

- The covering physician is called at home.
- The call comes direct, not through the answering service or hospital.
- The caller is always an intermediary and never the patient.
- There will be a ready excuse (e.g., "no phone at home") if the physician asks to speak directly to the patient.

A plausible story is always presented. The patient (their relative) has had prescriptions for Tussionex in the past and needs one now. There is always a sense of urgency ("very ill," "leaving on a trip"). The caller continues to request Tussionex, even when alternatives are suggested. "Dr. _____ (your colleague) has tried them all, and this is the only one that works."

While other codeine-containing antitussives are occasionally the drug of choice, Tussionex usually is the product requested.

Appendix 12–C

Young Lady in Distress

A New Jersey dentist reported this scam of extreme proportions. A young lady requested an immediate dental appointment due to intense pain. The subsequent examination revealed a complete maxillary denture and only five remaining mandibular teeth, all of which had been previously treated. One incisor was greatly sensitive and obviously the source of much pain. Even though the remaining teeth were little more than roots, the patient explained she was trying to save them for an overdenture. The dentist's suggestion that the painful root be extracted was rejected. The patient explained that when she returned home (to Seattle) her dentist would do what was necessary. She further stated that she had not been able to sleep and that the Empirin-3 she had been taking was ineffective.

A prescription for Percodan was issued. Six days later, the con artist's husband called the dentist to say that his wife's jaw was badly swollen and that she was in extreme pain. The husband further offered that his wife's return to Seattle was delayed due to the death of a close relative. Prescriptions for an antibiotic and more Percodan were given.

The now suspicious dentist began to check with other area dentists and pharmacies. Soon a six-page list of dentists and doctors was compiled—all who had prescribed for the young lady in distress. This clever professional patient had a two-year track record of bilking prescribers throughout southern New Jersey.

Appendix 12–D

New Physician on the Block Scam

A well-dressed, articulate middle-aged man presents himself to a St. Louis chain pharmacy. He explains convincingly that he is a physician who is opening a new practice in the neighborhood. After a brief conversation with the store pharmacist, the new "physician" requests blank prescription forms from the pharmacy in order to write prescriptions for a few of his first patients in the area.

The "physician" calmly writes prescriptions for Tagamet, Lanoxin, Tussend, Dilaudid, and Valium. All required information, including his Drug Enforcement Administration number and the local address of his phantom new practice, is duly provided. The con artist is so convincing and looks and acts so much like a physician that no questions are asked and no identification is requested. The "physician" pays for the prescriptions and is never seen or heard from again.

Unbelievable as it may seem, this new variation of the old chameleon scam did occur. However, a second pharmacist was more alert. When positive identification was required, the new "physician" suddenly had business elsewhere.

Chapter 13

The Controlled Substances Act and Pharmacy Controls

CHAPTER OBJECTIVES

1. Understand what is contained in the Controlled Substances Act.
2. Know the most important security requirements set forth in the Code of Federal Regulations.
3. Understand how Schedule II narcotics are ordered.
4. Know the procedures for receiving and storing narcotics.
5. Be able to explain the controls on dispensing narcotics.

INTRODUCTION

This chapter discusses the scheduling of drugs under federal law. It presents an overview of the definitions and recordkeeping requirements of the Code of Federal Regulations. Most state law is a mirror image of the federal law, but some state laws and regulations may be different. In some instances, states have placed drugs into schedules higher than federal law or have controlled drugs not scheduled by the U.S. government. Facilities must comply with at least the minimum federal requirements, but state law may be more stringent.

Medications utilized in the health care profession fall into one of three categories. First, there are over-the-counter drugs. These drugs may be purchased and used without a prescription. Aspirin, Tylenol, some cold preparations, and numerous other commonly used drugs fall into this category.

Second, there are drugs that can be obtained only by prescription but are not considered controlled substances. These include many antibiotics and birth control tablets.

Third, there are controlled substances. These drugs fall under the provisions of the Controlled Substances Act of 1970 and have been placed under one of the schedules by regulatory action. A controlled substance is a drug, other substance, or immediate precursor that has been included within one of the five schedules of the act. There are three basic factors used to determine how a drug is classified.

1. potential for abuse
2. currently accepted medical use
3. likelihood of dependence, either physical or psychological

199

Specific criteria are used in considering these three factors. Criteria include the following:

- whether some individuals are taking the drug on their own initiative rather than on medical advice, sometimes in amounts hazardous to their health
- whether significant amounts of the drug are being diverted from legitimate channels
- whether there is scientific evidence of a pharmacological effect
- whether there are public health risks associated with abuse of the drug
- whether the drug seems to encourage physiological or psychological dependence
- whether the substance is an immediate precursor of a drug that is already controlled

SCHEDULE I

Drugs in Schedule I meet the following standards:

1. The drug or substance has a high potential for abuse.
2. There is no currently accepted medical use for the drug or substance.
3. The use of the drug or substance is considered unsafe.

The drugs included in Schedule I are generally unavailable to members of the health care profession unless they are engaged in specific research projects.

> Drugs in Schedule I include heroin, LSD, marijuana, mescaline, peyote, and psilocybin.

SCHEDULE II

Drugs in Schedule II meet the following standards:

1. The drug or substance has a high potential for abuse.
2. The drug or substance has a currently accepted medical use in treatment. Some medical uses have severe restrictions placed on them.
3. Abuse may lead to severe psychological or physiological dependence.

The use of Schedule II medications is quite common within the health care profession, particularly in the areas of severe pain relief and anesthesia. Strict recordkeeping requirements are maintained, and the misuse or diversion of these drugs is considered significant.

> Drugs in Schedule II include Amytal, cocaine, codeine, Desoxyn, Dexamyl, Dexedrine, Dilaudid, fentanyl, meperidene, morphine, Nembutal, opium, Percocet, Percodan, Ritalin, Seconal, Tuinal, and Tylox.

SCHEDULE III

Drugs in Schedule III meet the following standards:

1. The drug has some potential for abuse, but the potential is less than for drugs included in Schedules I and II.
2. The drug has a currently accepted medical use.
3. Abuse of the drug may lead to a moderate or low physical dependence or may have a high potential for psychological dependence.

> Drugs in Schedule III include aspirin with codeine, Butisol, Hycodan, Hycomine, Tylenol no. 3 with codeine, Tussionex, and Vicodin.

SCHEDULE IV

Drugs in Schedule IV meet the following standards:

1. The drug has a low potential for abuse relative to that associated with the drugs in Schedule III.
2. The drug has a currently accepted medical use.
3. Abuse of the drug may lead to limited psychological or physical dependence relative to that associated with the drugs in Schedule II.

> Drugs in Schedule IV include Dalmane, Darvocet, Darvon, Diazepam, Equanil, Halcion, Librium, Talwin, Tranxene, Valium, Versed, and Xanax.

SCHEDULE V

Drugs in Schedule V meet the following standards:

1. The drug has a low potential for abuse relative to that associated with the drugs in Schedule IV.
2. The drug has a currently accepted medical use.
3. Abuse of the drug may lead to limited psychological or physical dependence relative to that associated with the drugs in Schedule IV.

Drugs included in Schedule V may be purchased on a signature basis, i.e., the customer shows identification and signs for the drug, from pharmacies. Included in this schedule are cough syrups and other medications with limited amounts of controlled substances.

CODE OF FEDERAL REGULATIONS

The following section will discuss portions of the Code of Federal Regulations (CFR), Title 21, Part 1300 to end, that are important to those charged with maintaining the records concerning controlled substances and to those who have the administrative responsibility to ensure that it is properly done.

Security Requirements

The CFR requires that all registrants shall provide effective controls and procedures to guard against theft and diversion of controlled substances. A registrant is any entity that is registered. A registrant can be an individual, corporation, governmental agency, partnership, association, or other legal entity. Physicians, dentists, veterinarians, and other individuals are considered individual practitioners. Health care facilities are deemed institutional practitioners. Pharmacists are listed in their own category. Health care facilities, physicians, dentists, and pharmacists are all charged with maintaining the security of the controlled substances under their care. The physical security requirements for nonpractitioners are specific, while those placed on practitioners are not.

The CFR states that controlled substances in Schedules II, III, IV, and V shall be stored in a securely locked, substantially constructed cabinet. It does allow pharmacies and institutional practitioners to disperse the drugs throughout the stock of noncontrolled substances if the theft or diversion of the controlled substances is precluded.

Federal regulations for practitioners are not very specific. Industry standards go way beyond what is mandated. Central pharmacies generally have adequate alarm systems, vaults, or limited access rooms where Schedule II substances, as well as other drugs with high abuse potential, are stored.

Access within the pharmacies is limited to those who are actively working within the pharmacies or have a specific reason to be in the area. There are various methods of controlling access to the pharmacy and narcotic vault area. Some options, such as locks, are basic. Card keys and fingerprint and iris readers are more sophisticated choices. The form of access control must be appropriate to the pharmacy operation. If the pharmacy is not open 24 hours a day, 7 days a week, then it needs different access controls than those for a pharmacy that is open all the time. In these cases, the nurse administrator in charge of the facility for the shifts when the pharmacy is closed usually has access and a card key or computer system is probably best. These systems give an account of who entered the pharmacy (by access number) and when that person entered and left.

In addition to access control, the pharmacy needs an external as well as an internal closed-circuit television system. External cameras aimed at the entrance and prescription window should be watched by security. In addition, a camera that lets pharmacy staff know who, if anyone, is at the doorway is beneficial. These cameras, in conjunction with a silent alarm going to security, make the pharmacy safer.

It is also common for the controlled substances sent to nurses' stations and other such areas to be maintained under a double-lock system. This is usually accomplished by use of a double-lock medication cart or in a double-lock system integrated into a medication room.

Notification of Loss or Theft

It is important to note that the federal regulations require that the Drug Enforcement Administration (DEA) be notified of the theft or significant loss of any controlled substances. A DEA form 106 regarding the loss or theft must be submitted.

Records

The CFR specifies that each registrant must maintain the records indicated by the CFR. The required records include inventories, dispensing records, and in most cases, records of the administration of controlled substances.

All of the required records must be readily retrievable. Whether the records are maintained with a manual or an automated system, the registrant must be able to access the required information in a reasonable amount of time, such as 48 hours. If the records cannot be separated, they must be able to be visually distinguished from the other records. For instance, the controlled substance records may be marked, redlined, or identified in some other fashion. Business records showing that someone has been billed for a controlled substance do not meet the accepted standard.

Individual practitioners do not have to maintain records on controlled substances prescribed or administered in the lawful course of professional practice. If, however, the individual practitioner regularly engages in the dispensing or administration of controlled substances and the patient is charged, either separately or as a part of the professional fee, the practitioner is required to keep records of such administration or dispensing.

Individual practitioners and institutional practitioners, including health care facilities, are required to maintain separate inventories and records of Schedule I and Schedule II controlled substances. Inventories and records of the drugs contained in Schedules III, IV, and V can be maintained either separately or so that they can be readily retrieved from ordinary business records.

Pharmacies are required to maintain separate records for all Schedule I and II substances. Pharmacies are also required to maintain prescriptions for Schedule II substances in a separate prescription file. Pharmacy records for the substances within Schedules III, IV, and V can either be maintained separately or be readily retrievable from among other records. Prescriptions for medications within these schedules may be maintained separately or intermingled with other prescriptions. If these prescriptions are placed with other prescriptions, the regulations deem the prescription to be readily retrievable if the letter "C" is written at least one inch high in red ink in the lower right corner of the prescription.

Inventory Requirements

Registrants who are required to maintain records must satisfy certain inventory requirements. Basically, the inventory requirements are that an inventory be taken every two years following the date of the initial inventory. The inventory must contain complete and accurate records of all controlled substances on hand. It must be maintained in a written, typewritten, or printed form.

If a substance is placed into a schedule in the period between inventory dates, the registrant must take an inventory of the substance and then include the substance in the next inventory cycle.

If a registrant is considered to be a dispenser, which is simply a registrant who dispenses controlled substances, an exact count of all substances in Schedules I and II is required. The registrant is allowed to make an estimated count or measure of the substances in Schedules

III, IV, and V if the containers hold 1,000 capsules or tablets or fewer. When registrants have containers that hold over 1,000 dosage units, an exact count is required.

Maintaining Records

Records are required to be maintained on a current basis. There must be a complete and accurate record of each controlled substance received, dispensed, sold, delivered, or otherwise disposed of. The regulations do not require that a perpetual inventory be maintained. The actual dates of receipt or transfer should be used in the records.

Dispenser Records

Records to be maintained by those registered to dispense or conduct research are discussed in the federal regulations. Records for each controlled substance must include

1. the name of the substance
2. each finished form of the substance and the amount contained in each commercial container
3. the number of each container received, including the date received and the name, address, and registration number of the entity from whom the shipment was received
4. the number of units dispensed, including the date of dispensing, the name and address of the person to whom it was dispensed, and written or typewritten name or initials of the person who dispensed the controlled substance

Records must also be maintained on the number of units disposed of in any other manner.

Order Forms

A DEA form 222—an order form—is required for each distribution of a substance in Schedule I or II. Health care facilities and pharmacies must obtain their Schedule II drugs by using this form.

The form is in triplicate. One part of the form remains with the purchaser, one remains with the supplier, and one is sent to the DEA. Only one item can be entered on each line of the form, and each different finished form or size of container must be entered on a different line. For instance, morphine injections of two different strengths must be entered on different lines.

The regulations require that the name and address of the supplier be on the form. Only one supplier can be listed on a individual form. The form must be signed and dated by the person authorized to order the drugs.

The forms provide a space on which to note the date of receipt of the Schedule II substances ordered and to provide a check against the amount ordered and the amount received. The orders should be checked and the date of receipt noted on the form. The purchaser must retain a copy of the form for two years, keeping it apart from all other records.

Prescriptions

Prescriptions for controlled substances may be issued by an individual practitioner who is authorized to prescribe controlled substances. A medication order in a health care facility is not considered to be a prescription. For a prescription to be valid, the prescription must be issued for a legitimate medical purpose by a practitioner acting in the usual course of his or her professional practice.

It is interesting to note that the CFR requires that the pharmacist who fills the prescription be satisfied that the prescription is valid. If a pharmacist has doubts about the legitimacy of a prescription, he or she is not required to fill it. In fact, if a pharmacist fills a prescription that he or she knows is not valid, the pharmacist is subjected to the same penalties as the person who issued the prescription. A pharmacist is not required to blindly fill a prescription. The pharmacist has the right to refuse to fill any prescription that seems suspect.

There are certain requirements for prescriptions for controlled substances. They all must be signed on the date of issuance. Each must bear the name and address of the patient. The name, address, and registration number of the practitioner must appear on the prescription.

Only written prescriptions are permitted for Schedule II drugs. On oral prescription for a Schedule II drug can by issued in an emergency. The quantity of the substance that can be prescribed this way is limited, and the prescribing practitioner must forward a written prescription to the pharmacy within 72 hours.

A prescription for a Schedule II drug cannot be refilled. In the event that a Schedule II prescription can only be partially filled, the remaining amount on the prescription must be dispensed within 72 hours. Partial filling of a Schedule II prescription is approved for patients in long-term care facilities provided that certain requirements are met.

Prescriptions for substances in Schedules III, IV, and V can be either written or oral, in which case the prescription must be reduced to written form by the pharmacist. Prescriptions in this schedule can be refilled. They are valid for six months and can be refilled up to five times if so authorized by the issuing practitioner. Refill information can be maintained either manually or through automated data processing systems.

If a manual system is employed, refill information must be placed on the back of the original prescription. This information will include the date of the refill, the initials or signature of the pharmacist who refilled the prescription, and any information about partial refills.

A physician may increase the number of refills originally authorized. This information must also be noted on the back of the original prescription. These increases may not exceed the five-refill or six-month limit of the original prescription. After six months' worth or the maximum number of dosage units allowed by the original prescription are dispensed, a new prescription must be issued.

An automated data processing system employed to maintain refill information must meet certain requirements. The system must be able to provide on-line retrieval by video display or hard-copy printout of the original prescription order information. There must be an auxiliary procedure in place in case the computer system malfunctions.

The system must also be able to provide on-line retrieval of the refill history for Schedule III and V prescription orders during the past six months. The refill information entered into the system must be documented by the pharmacists. Any such computerized system must also be capable of producing a printout of any refill information that the pharmacy is required to maintain. The federal regulations specify what information must be included in these printouts.

Prescriptions issued for medications in Schedules III, IV, and V may be transferred between pharmacies. Once a prescription has been filled, it may be transferred once to obtain refills. Information is transferred between the pharmacies, and the original prescription is voided in the pharmacy that filled the prescription.

Prescriptions may be issued for drugs in Schedule V, but in most cases these medications can be purchased directly from a pharmacist without a prescription. Restrictions determine how much and how often these medications can be sold to an individual.

Administration Records

Since most facilities charge for the controlled substances administered, records must be maintained to account for these drugs. Record systems vary from facility to facility, but some information is kept by all facilities: the name and strength of the drug given, the date, the time of administration, the patient's name and room number, the name of the physician who authorized the administration, and the name or initials of the person who administered the drug.

Most often, these administration records are not intermingled with business records or patient charts. However the records are maintained, they must be able to provide a record showing how a drug got to the recipient of the drug.

All the recordkeeping systems required by state and federal law have one central purpose: to track controlled substances from the point where they are manufactured to the point where they are dispensed to the ultimate user. As the drugs move, different people are held responsible for the control of the drugs. Manufacturers, wholesalers, pharmacies, and health care professionals are all held accountable at different times. The best defense against theft and diversion is a consistently applied recordkeeping system that is monitored for accuracy. A good recordkeeping system can help identify or even prevent drug diversion.

PHARMACY CONTROLS

Each day, thousands of doses of drugs are administered in a health care facility. The responsibility for tracking and controlling all medications ultimately lies with the person holding the DEA license. In most cases, the license will be in the name of the health care facility, and an administrative officer will be issued a power of attorney for the health care facility, making him or her the official registrant. The administrative officer and head pharmacist will be responsible for all recordkeeping required by the DEA. All DEA records—including all records of purchasing, selling, destroying, and administering narcotics—must be retained for at least three years.

Purchasing Schedule II Drugs

Schedule II narcotics are ordered on DEA form 222. The DEA order forms are ordered from the DEA by using form 222a. A maximum of three books (containing seven order forms each) may be ordered at any one time.

When ordering Schedule II drugs directly from a manufacturer or wholesaler, form 222 must be completed. The front of the form must contain the company name, address, and date. The number, size, and name of packages needed must be indicated. Changes cannot be made by voiding the line and rewriting the entry. If a mistake is made on the form, the entire form must be voided. If a form is voided, it must be retained with the completed forms.

After all ordered items are entered on the form, the number of items ordered must be entered at the bottom of the form in the "Number of lines completed" section. All forms must be signed by the official registrant. The last copy of the 222 form is retained. The first two copies are sent to the manufacturer. (The copies must be intact, with the carbon between them.)

Receiving and Storing Schedule II Drugs

When Schedule II drugs are received, they should be taken to a licensed pharmacist for processing. The packing slip or invoice should be matched to the form 222. The amount received and the date should be matched to the purchaser's copy of form 222, and the drugs should be counted. If for some reason a drug is not received as ordered, an explanation should be noted on the packing slip and the form 222. After the count is verified, the drugs can be entered into the health care facility's inventory and placed in the separate Schedule II narcotics vault.

All Schedule II drugs must be stored under lock and key, in a separate area away from the other schedule drugs. Adequate controls prohibiting access to the Schedule II drugs by anyone other than a licensed pharmacist must be in place. If a pharmacist is in the Schedule II room and must leave, even for a few minutes, the area must be locked. Records of all Schedule II drugs should be treated with the same degree of security as the drugs themselves.

Dispensing Schedule II Drugs

Accurate dispensing records of Schedule II drugs must be maintained. As stated above, all DEA records must be retained for three years. This holds true for records of dispensing.

If the drugs are dispensed to a nursing unit, the pharmacist should note the date and unit receiving the drugs on a perpetual inventory form. The pharmacist should note the theoretical count, i.e., ledger count, and then perform an actual physical count to be sure the two match. The pharmacist should not assume that the theoretical count is correct. Each time a Schedule II substance is dispensed, a physical count should be taken. If the theoretical count and the physical count do not match, the pharmacist should investigate to resolve the discrepancy.

If the drugs are dispensed by sale to another licensed entity (e.g., health care facility, physician's office, or drugstore), the same controls should be in place. The pharmacist should record the transaction on form 222. The two copies received from the requesting entity are separated, and the carbon and copies are reversed. The purchasing institution is listed as an alternate supplier. The official registrant must sign the form. The supplier's copy is then retained, and the DEA copy 2 is mailed to the regional DEA office. The Schedule II drugs are then taken out of stock and a new count number is noted for both the theoretical count and physical count of the supplying entity.

At least once a month, an audit should be conducted on Schedule II drugs on hand. The auditing pharmacist should enter the correct count in both the theoretical and actual "on hand" columns and date and sign the form.

Destruction of Schedule II Drugs

Occasionally there will be a need to destroy expired Schedule II drugs. Drugs received back into stock from the nursing unit as well as expired drugs still in the pharmacy are handled the same way. The drugs are listed in an Expired Schedule II inventory. The drugs are then listed on a DEA form 41 in triplicate, and a cover letter explaining the request for destruction is sent to the regional DEA office. Destruction may take place in one of three ways. First, upon receipt of instructions and permission from the DEA, the drugs may be destroyed. The destruction must be witnessed by a pharmacist and one other person who is not assigned to the pharmacy department. Second, DEA representatives may ask for the drugs to be sent to them for destruction. Third, DEA representatives may require that a DEA representative come to the site and witness the destruction. After destruction has taken place, a copy of the DEA form 41 is signed and returned to the regional office.

Drugs in Other Schedules

While controls on those substances in Schedules III, IV, and V are less stringent than controls on Schedule II drugs, accountability is still required. There are no specific requirements as to how a recordkeeping system is established as long as two criteria are met.

1. The pharmacy can account for the drugs. In the event that the pharmacy is audited, the pharmacy can provide a pill-by-pill accounting of the controlled substance from the time the substance entered the facility until it was consumed by the patient.
2. The records can be produced in a reasonable period of time. In other words, the records are readily retrievable.

Unexplained Loss or Diversion

In the event of an unexplained loss or actual diversion, the pharmacy should notify the appropriate law enforcement agency and the DEA. Notification of diversion is reported to the regional DEA office on form 106.

Audit Committee

A functioning audit committee can be a valuable tool in preventing drug losses. This interdisciplinary committee should comprise representatives from pharmacy, nursing, security, and quality assurance. These representatives monitor any reports of packaging errors, review a sampling of the medication administration records and nursing notes, and inspect forms for possible forgery and unusual medication trends. Any unusual findings should lead to further investigation.

Robberies and Burglaries

Due to the inherent danger of working in a narcotic delivery system, pharmacy employees should receive training in dealing with robberies and burglaries. The use of closed-circuit television, access control, and silent alarms will help prevent these acts. Doors to the pharmacy should always be kept locked, and a pass-through should be used at the prescription window. The staff should be trained to not resist in the event of a robbery and to be as observant as possible. In the event of a robbery or burglary, staff should contact security immediately and be careful not to disturb the area. Only security personnel (and emergency medical personal to treat anyone injured) should be allowed into the area.

Pharmacy staff should also be familiar with scams that con artists have used to get controlled substances. Appendix 13–A lists some of these scams.

The manner in which narcotics are delivered to the nursing units must receive special attention. In many facilities, non-narcotics are sent to the nursing units via a pneumatic tube. Narcotics are delivered to the units by a pharmacy technician. The narcotics are placed in a plain paper bag (the narcotics for each unit are packaged separately) and put in a push cart. The technician takes the bags to the units. The technician should never leave the cart unattended and should make sure someone at the unit opens the bags in the technician's presence and signs for the drugs.

In some facilities, the nurse manager for the unit must come to the pharmacy and sign for the narcotics. While this system is probably more secure, it takes valuable nursing time away from the patients.

Automated Computerized Dispensing Systems

Automated computerized dispensing systems allow a practitioner to enter a personal identification number and patient room number and select the drug needed. The computer will then open only the drawer containing the drug requested. The computer will ask the practitioner to confirm the inventory on hand both before and after the practitioner removes the patient's drugs. When computerized dispensing systems are in place, individual computer codes should be carefully protected. In addition, the dispensing units should be serviced regularly to ensure that they operate properly.

KEY POINTS

- The Controlled Substances Act of 1970 classifies drugs based on potential for abuse, current accepted medical use, and likelihood of dependency.
- The Code of Federal Regulations, Title 21, Part 1300 to end, spells out the necessary security requirements for a facility working with controlled substances.
- The pharmacy must have stringent controls on all drugs, especially Schedule II drugs. There must be controls on ordering, receiving, dispensing, and destroying Schedule II drugs.
- All thefts and significant losses must be reported to the DEA.
- Because of the nature of pharmacy inventory, pharmacy staff must be trained in dealing with robberies and burglaries.

Appendix 13–A

Various Scams

THE TRAVELING PHYSICIAN SCAM

An insidious scam, used repeatedly, throughout several Midwest states, involves a clever and audacious professional patient who had learned to mimic a foreign accent and mastered medical nomenclature related to his scam. By using the phony accent, the con artist could claim to have misunderstood should any problem develop.

The format varied little from town to town. The con artist would arrive in town in a metropolitan community and rent a motel room there. Using local phone books, he would plot a list of suburban pharmacies that would become his targets. Using the fake accent, he would make calls to the drug stores and the scam would begin.

He made attempts to order a variety of prescription drugs for a phantom patient. The pitch was usually the same: "Hello, this is Doctor [strange name]. I need your help. A short while ago, I just happened to be at a local service station [or garage, automobile agency, etc]. A young mechanic had been badly burned in a gasoline explosion. Of course, I did what I could before the ambulance arrived. When I returned to my office the young man's wife called nearly hysterical. Her husband has refused to be admitted to the hospital because of a lack of insurance. He is now at home and in pretty bad shape. I agreed to see the young man as soon as I can. In the meanwhile, the wife will be coming to your store. Please have the following ready for her." At this point, an order is given for a variety of medications and materials appropriate for severe burns. Then, almost as an afterthought, "Oh yes, he is probably in terrible pain. He will need some _____."

Dutifully the "doctor" then provides his office address (usually a large medical complex) and a DEA number. Within minutes after completing his final call, the con artist begins to deliver his girlfriend (the "patient's wife") to each store that has agreed to cooperate. Once all the prescriptions are collected, all non-narcotic materials are discarded. The analgesics are immediately sold to local street dealers. By the day's end, the con artist and his friend are safely out of that town and on their way to the next.

EMPLOYEE SCAMS

Several cases of major controlled substance diversion have been reported to the Bureau of Narcotics and Dangerous Drugs recently. In each of these cases, an employee of a physician, dentist, or pharmacy had been involved in the diversion. The employee ordered controlled substances through regular drug distributors using the practitioner's DEA registration number and diverted the drugs when they were delivered. The employer was charged and paid for the drugs.

Although employers must trust employees, failing to develop adequate controls and accounting systems can result in drug losses. Any registrant who delegates ordering, receiving, and storage of controlled substances should periodically review drug orders, receipt records, and inventory to ensure that all controlled drugs are accounted for. The review should include verification that the specific drugs and quantities ordered are those that are actually used in the professional practice.

In another case, a trusted office manager of a physician placed drug orders requested by the physician and paid the bills. When she resigned and moved to another state, the physician saw his monthly bill with a wholesale drug company in the East drop considerably. When the physical requested receipts for the previous four years, he discovered his office manager had been diverting controlled drugs for her personal used or for illicit sales for the past four years. Over 16,000 dosage units of controlled substances had been diverted. In addition to such drugs as Xanax, diethylpropion, diazepam, halcion, and Vicodin/ES, large quantities of Stadol injectable were diverted. The reported value of the loss exceeded $17,000.

One case involved a dentist's wife who was also his office manager. In addition to products actually used in the practice, she ordered "diet pills" for her personal use. The dentist was unaware of the diversion until the wife was admitted to treatment for substance abuse.

In another case, a pharmacy technician who had learned the procedure for placing orders to a wholesaler diverted 64,000 dosage units of Tylenol no. 4. The technician checked in orders and would meet the delivery person, process the orders, and take the drugs he had ordered for his personal use to his vehicle. The receipt records were destroyed at the time the drugs were diverted. The monthly statement was not reconciled with daily receipt records, so the thefts were not detected for a long time.

Chapter 14

Nursing Units

CHAPTER OBJECTIVES

1. Understand security controls, administrative records, and inventory controls for Schedule II narcotics.
2. Understand how the physical placement of the nurses' station affects security.
3. Know how to handle a patient's personal property on the nursing unit.
4. Know about security-related problems that occur in the nursing unit.

INTRODUCTION

In this chapter, "nursing unit" will mean all locations where a patient receives care, including inpatient, outpatient, and clinic settings. Areas with their own specific security risks (e.g., emergency departments and psychiatric units) are discussed in separate chapters.

This chapter will focus on how to control the narcotics the patients need to relieve their pain, how the physical design of the nurses' station can impact security, and what security can do to assist patients with specific security issues.

NARCOTIC CONTROLS

As stated in Chapter 13, recordkeeping is the key to controlling Schedule II drugs. This recordkeeping requirement extends from the pharmacy to the nursing unit, all the way through to the moment when the drug is administered. This section will discuss the various security and recordkeeping functions needed to control Schedule II drugs.

Ordering Schedule II Drugs

While some health care facilities still use a control sheet for each Schedule II drug, most use a 24-hour perpetual inventory control sheet. This control sheet lists all the normal Schedule II drugs available on the unit in floor stock. The quantity of each Schedule II drug in floor stock is determined by previous use and estimated future need. This quantity is then considered the "par level" for the drug. By use of a 24-hour perpetual inventory sheet, the pharmacy will be able to stock the nursing unit back to par level at predetermined times. The pharmacy can subtract the usage from the par level and distribute to the nursing units the proper amount to bring the unit back to par level.

Administration of Schedule II Drugs

All Schedule II drugs must be kept on a double-key control system on the nursing units. Generally, two keys are necessary to open the Schedule II storage cabinet. While it is best that only one registered nurse carry the keys to the narcotics per shift, this usually proves to be impractical on a busy nursing unit. In most cases, one of the narcotic keys is locked in a medication cabinet and the other carried by the head or charge nurse. Any nurse needing to enter the narcotics cabinet will need to get the key for the medication cabinet from the head or charge nurse and then secure the second key from the cabinet.

When a patient needs a Schedule II drug, the nurse removes the drug from the cabinet, signs the drug out by patient name on the perpetual inventory sheet, and initials the sheet. At that point, the nurse should subtract the amount removed from the perpetual inventory count. Once the drug is administered, the nurse should note the drug, quantity given, and time in the patient's chart, usually in the nurse's progress report.

Discarded Schedule II

If a patient is given only a partial dose of the Schedule II drug, the remainder of the dose must be wasted. The administering nurse must have another licensed person witness the destruction of the medication, usually by expelling it into the drain of a sink. Both nurses must sign the perpetual inventory sheet noting the amount administered to the patient and the amount wasted. **Under no circumstances should a nurse cosign a waste report without physically witnessing the wasting procedure.**

If any Schedule II drugs are on the nursing unit at or past their expiration date, the drugs should be returned to the pharmacy. All nurse managers should periodically check their floor stock to ensure that expired drugs are pulled from stock at once. For medical and liability reasons, a patient should never be given an out-of-date drug. The drugs should be listed as "returned to pharmacy" on the 24-hour perpetual inventory, signed by two nurses, and taken to the pharmacy, where a new supply will be issued to replenish the stock to par level.

Inventory Procedures

At the change of each shift, one nurse from the incoming shift and one nurse from the outgoing shift should count and verify the Schedule II drug inventory. Both nurses should count the drugs to avoid the possibility of false counting. Both nurses should then sign the 24-hour perpetual inventory form. If a discrepancy occurs in the count, every attempt should be made to explain the shortage (e.g., a drug was given and not signed out correctly). If the shortage cannot be explained, the nurse manager should inform the pharmacy and the security department.

At the end of all three shifts, the nurse manager should verify that each shift count was completed and signed by two nurses. The nurse manager should then sign the inventory form and forward it to the pharmacy to be used for stock replenishment and retention.

DESIGN OF NURSING UNITS

There are probably as many designs for nurses' stations as there are health care facilities. However, the four most popular are the pod design, the intersection design, the straight hall design, and the horseshoe design. All of these designs have benefits and drawbacks.

Pod

In a pod design, the patients' rooms are in areas similar to small cul de sacs off a common hallway. This design offers excellent privacy and noise control for the patient. But none of the patient rooms are visible from the nurses' station—a drawback for security.

The nurses' station is usually centrally located in the middle of a large common hallway. Ceiling-mounted security mirrors can help nurses monitor the hallways. Security cameras can be added, but they are rather expensive. From a security standpoint, the pod design is probably the least desirable.

Intersection Design

In this design, the nurses' station sits at the corner of two intersecting hallways. This design usually gives the nurses a view of several patient rooms as well as the hallways. Patients with a specific security need may be placed in the rooms visible from the station. Security cameras would increase security for units with intersection designs, but they would not be as expensive as those needed for the pod design.

Straight Hall

In a straight hall design, the nurses' station is placed against the wall in the middle of a hall. Straight hall designs offer some of the same security features as intersection designs, but there are fewer patient rooms near the nurses' station. This design is usually found in older facilities with very long corridors, which can mean that nurses must do a lot of walking to get from one room to another. The primary security device used with straight hall designs may be timed delayed crash bars on stairwell doors. These sound an alarm for up to 15 seconds before releasing the door. Facilities should check with local fire officials prior to installing such devices.

Horseshoe Design

Horseshoe designs are usually found in intensive care areas. The nurses' station is located at the open end of a horseshoe formed by a series of rooms. This design is excellent for small nursing units. All the patient rooms are close by and all are in the nurses' line of sight. Horseshoe designs afford very good security for patients having special security needs—second only to the security provided by locked-down units.

Personal Space for Staff

Regardless of the nursing unit design, staff need a comfortable lounge area where they can shower, dress, and eat. The area must contain a locker in which each staff member can store personal belongings. Staff should be instructed that even though the facility is furnishing them with a locker for their use, the facility maintains the right to open and inspect the locker (or desk, file cabinet, or any other container) at any time, regardless of whether the staff member is present. This policy should be put in writing and distributed to all staff. Countless times, staff members have been caught hiding facility narcotics, alcohol, or weapons in their lockers.

PATIENT PROPERTY

One problem that seems to plague all facilities is the loss or theft of patient belongings. But most claims can be prevented. As soon as a patient comes onto a unit, the nurse conducting the assessment should list all of the patient's belongings. Valuables (e.g., watches, rings, neck chains) should be given to a family member to take home for safekeeping.

If the facility must accept responsibility for the patient's valuables, the items should be inventoried by two staff members, secured in an envelope for patient valuables, and placed in a secured area, usually the safe in the business office. Chapter 17 discusses this subject in more detail.

Some patients will want to wear their wedding bands or engagement rings. Nurses should wrap surgical tape around the rings to keep them from slipping off and keep other staff members from seeing how valuable they are. Patients or their family members should sign a release of liability for any valuables they refuse to send home. A copy of the release should be placed in the patients' charts.

Some facilities take the extra step of having a representative of security visit the patient. During the visit, the security representative discusses not only the patients' valuables but also security and parking at the facility. In most facilities, reductions in staff make this commendable approach impossible.

PATIENT ELOPEMENT

If a patient is mentally competent and decides to refuse or discontinue treatment, most facilities attempt to have the patient sign an "against medical advice" form. The form simply states that the attending physician is advising the patient that it is in his or her best medical interest to stay and receive treatment and that the physician has notified the patient of the possible result of refusing the treatment.

Some patients—sometimes because of mental illness or medication—will leave their room without permission.

Many times the nursing staff will call security and ask them to stop the patient. How should security representatives react? What can they do to stop a patient from leaving? Having a predetermined code system can help. Consider these examples of how a code system might operate at one facility. Medical staff can use these codes as shorthand when speaking with security about a patient.

- **Level 1.** A nonphysician suggested that the patient be detained. Security should use only verbal skills to keep the patient from leaving.
- **Level 2.** Security should use verbal tactics and "soft hands" to persuade the patient to stay. The patient has seen a physician, and his or her ability to make decisions is impaired. A physician must make this determination.

- **Level 3.** Either a patient has been seen by a physician who has deemed the patient to be a threat, or the patient has been served with involuntary commitment papers and is under a court's jurisdiction. Security may use more drastic measures, including physical restraint, to prevent a level 3 patient from leaving.

> **Security representatives and other facility staff should remember that unless patients are deemed incompetent by a court or deemed a threat to themselves by a licensed physician, they have the right to discontinue medical care and leave a facility.** More than one facility has been sued for false imprisonment and assault for keeping a patient at the facility when the patient wanted to leave.

WANDERING PATIENTS

The responsibility for patient care lies with the medical staff first and foremost. They are responsible for monitoring the patients and knowing their whereabouts. If a patient is missing, then it is appropriate to summon security to assist in locating the patient.

After having been notified that a patient is missing, security dispatch should notify all officers to be alert for the patient. A description of the patient and the last place he or she was seen should be given over the radio, but the patient's name should not be given over the radio unless the officers have earpieces for their radios. No one else should hear the name. If the nursing staff determines that using the patient's name will assist in persuading the patient to return to the unit but the officers do not have earpieces, then only the patient's first name should be transmitted.

Security should search all common areas of the facility's interior, such as the lobby, waiting rooms, food service areas, and restrooms. At the same time, officers should check the boundaries of the property, then continue the search by moving inward toward the buildings. Likewise, all connecting buildings (e.g., a medical office building connected with a skywalk) should be searched.

Once the patient is found, security should notify the nursing unit. Unless the patient is in danger (e.g., starting to cross a street), security should wait for the patient's nurse to arrive on the scene. Too often, the sight of a uniform will scare or anger a confused patient. The patient's nurse should be the one to approach the patient because the patient will probably know the nurse.

If the patient is not found, security should notify nursing when all areas have been searched. Nursing should then contact administration, family members, and various agencies as per facility policy.

PATIENT SITTING

When a patient has become verbally abusive and threatened to leave or to assault staff, emergency departments will ask security representatives to patient sit. Sometimes security will be asked to stand by while the patient is being treated, a process that may last several hours. Most security departments simply cannot afford to take one officer out of service for several hours. If this situation arises often, facilities should consider hiring an officer to be stationed at the emergency department.

PATIENT RESTRAINTS

Security may be asked to assist in restraining an unruly patient by holding the patient while medication is administered, staying in the room, or placing leather restraints on the patient. Regardless of the type of restraint, patient restraint is a medical procedure. The medical staff must request the restraint, be in control of the restraint, and document the restraint in the patient's medical chart. Too often, medical staff give up their control to security. This should never happen.

After the patient is safely restrained, both nursing and security should debrief each other. What did they do well? What did not go so well? In addition, both nursing and security representatives should fill out an incident report stating the reason for the restraint, the names and titles of all who assisted in restraining the patient, and the injuries that anyone, including the patient, suffered during the course of the restraint.

Both medical staff and security should develop "game plans" for different scenarios involving unruly patients. These training sessions should help both the medical staff and security to know how to act when situations arise. They should determine who will talk to the patient, who will hold the left arm, and so on, before the patient is approached.

Facility staff should remember that patient restraint is a medical procedure that is necessary to treat the patient. Restraints are never punitive. Anyone who uses excessive force in restraining a patient should be disciplined severely.

VISITOR RESTRICTION

At times, patients request that particular people be banned from patient rooms. Usually these requests stem from disputes between spouses or between boyfriends and girlfriends or from custody situations concerning a minor and estranged parents. It is extremely difficult to guarantee a patient that someone can be kept out of the health care facility. Health care facilities are large complexes with multiple entrances and exits.

Security can take several courses of action. First, if the patient already has a restraining order issued by the court, a copy of the order should be given to security. Security should verify that the order is still in effect by calling the court of jurisdiction.

Second, the patient should sign a visitor restriction form (Exhibit 14–1). This form serves several functions. The patient must read and sign the statement saying that he or she is requesting that a particular person or certain persons not be allowed to visit and that the security department take reasonable means to ensure that the person not be able to see or talk to the patient. The patient agrees to appear in court and testify that the security department is acting on his or her wishes. The form also states that the patient may rescind the request at any time before the restricted person comes onto the property and that the request to rescind the order must be in writing.

Once the visitor restriction form is completed, a copy of the form—along with a description of the restricted visitor—should be posted in the security office. The existence of the restriction should be noted to all officers coming in to duty on subsequent shifts. Security pa-

Exhibit 14–1 Request for Visitor Restriction

I, _____ request that _____ not be allowed to visit me
          (patient's name)

while I am a patient at _____. I understand that this request can be reversed
                        (facility name)

by me upon giving notification to the security department and realize I am responsible to docu-

ment this change in writing prior to the visitor's arrival at the facility. I accept all legal responsi-

bility for this request and agree to testify as deemed necessary by _____ re-
                                                                    (facility name)

garding my support of their actions to prevent the visit.

_____   _____
Patient signature   Witness signature

_____   _____
Date   Date

(ADDRESSOGRAPH PLATE OR LABEL)

---

trols of the patient's unit should also be increased. The reception area should also note the restriction in the inpatient computer system. The nurses' station should be made aware of the restriction. With all groups working together, the patient's wishes should be fulfilled.

As an extra security precaution, the patient's name can be omitted from the patient registry and the patient's room phone number listing. The patient can also be listed under an assumed name. If needed, plain clothes security personnel can be stationed across the hall from the patient. Having plain clothes officers usually works better for this type of situation since the stationing of uniformed officers tends to indicate the location of the patient.

PATIENTS WHO ARE PRISONERS

Patients who are under arrest or who are in prison and come to the facility for treatment pose an unusual set of challenges for the security department. While the patients are under the jurisdiction of law enforcement or the courts, they still should be treated with the same dignity as all patients.

Security should be trained to understand that if the patient is under arrest or in the custody of the state, security representatives (unless they are also sworn law enforcement officers) cannot take custody of the patient and keep the patient from leaving. The law enforcement agency must supply someone to stay with the patient.

Under guidelines of the Joint Commission on Accreditation of Healthcare Organizations, the law enforcement officer staying with the patient must be informed of the facility's emergency codes, the location of the nearest fire exit, and what to do in an emergency.[1] The fact that these instructions were given to the law enforcement officer should be noted in the patient's chart.

Exhibit 14–2 offers a sample of the directions a facility might provide a law enforcement officer posted to guard a prisoner at the facility. Exhibit 14–3 is a sample facility policy on prisoner patients.

Exhibit 14–2 Sample of Directions to Law Enforcement Officials Posted at Health Care Facility

- The hospital requires that all inpatient prisoners be guarded **at all times** by the custodial agency responsible for the prisoner. Exceptions, such as prisoners released on their own recognizance or on a medical furlough, will be reviewed, in advance, by hospital security and the custodial agency.
- The admitting department will notify hospital security and the hospital administrator of every admission of an inpatient prisoner to the hospital and will provide a daily roster of all inpatient prisoners.
- Hospital administration and the hospital public relations department will coordinate their efforts to ensure that any press releases regarding prisoners are appropriate and in accordance with the prisoner's rights and hospital policy.
- The hospital security department will be responsible for coordinating check-in and checkout (including change or shift and relief) procedures for all police and corrections officers assigned to prisoners admitted as inpatients to the facility and will coordinate any security issues with the involved agency.
- When assigned by external law enforcement and corrections agencies, officers are to remain within the prisoner's room on the inpatient units. In intensive care units (especially if the patient is in critical condition) the officer may sit outside the door of the prisoner's room. Officers are to leave the prisoner's rooms only when relieved or on request of the physician or other appropriate health care provider.
  - If the officer on duty is asked to leave the room of the prisoner, the officer will assume the position to maintain visual contact with the prisoner but be of sufficient distance away to protect the prisoner's right to confidentiality.
  - If bed curtains must be drawn or the door must be closed, the officer will assume a position that will prevent the prisoner's escape.
  - The officer will reenter the room of the prisoner as requested by the physician or other appropriate health care provider or on departure of the physician or health care provider.
  - If the inpatient prisoner goes into the operating room (OR), the officer must remain in the room until the patient is anesthetized. Then the officer must leave the OR and wait outside the room.

- When the prisoner is transferred to the recovery room, the officer will accompany and remain with the prisoner.

Exceptions to the provisions requiring the officer to be present in the prisoner's room can be made due to the physical conditions in the room or infection control considerations. Exceptions will be approved by the senior management team of the hospital, including hospital security, administration, nursing, and the attending physician. Information on the reason for the exception should be shared with security and nursing personnel, and the duration for such exception should be noted. The decision should be reevaluated on a daily basis.

- External officers are to comply with all hospital policies.
- All officers, when coming on duty, must read the universal blood and body fluid precautions and correctional officers policies.
- All hospital personnel will be made aware that surgical and other medical instruments (as well as kitchen utensils) can be used as weapons by inpatient prisoners. Every possible precaution will be exercised to make such instruments inaccessible to the prisoner.
- The hospital security department will assist external police or correctional officers as appropriate when requested. The hospital security department does not assume responsibility for the custody of the prisoner. In the event of an extreme emergency that incapacitates the assigned external officer, the hospital security supervisor will be responsible for assigning personnel to protect patients, staff, and visitors pending arrival of appropriate relief coverage.
  Hospital security does not provide relief coverage for external officers for purposes such as meals or personal breaks.
  In the event that a patient prisoner expires while at the hospital, hospital security will assist the external officers to gain access to the morgue or transfer the body to the coroner.
- To provide protection for physicians, nurses, hospital personnel, visitors, and other patients and to prevent the escape of the inpatient prisoner, the external officer shall use external restraints (which may include handcuffs or leg irons) unless they directly interfere with required medical care. The use of restraints must be approved by the patient's physician and must be used in compliance with hospital policy on the safe use of restraints.
- Inpatient prisoners who must leave their bed and room for any purpose, such as visits to ancillary treatment areas, must be accompanied by the assigned external officer.
- Law enforcement and corrections officials will not interrogate or conduct official proceedings involving an inpatient prisoner unless the attending physician is informed and grants consent. This provision ensures that the inpatient prisoner is medically able to participate in such activity.
- No visitors shall be allowed in the room of the inpatient prisoner except those authorized by the custodial agency. The custodial agency, rather than hospital personnel, is responsible for screening all visitors. Admission of any representative from the press requires explicit consent of hospital administration.

Exhibit 14–2 Sample Facility Policy on Prisoner or Inmate Patients

This policy offers guidance on the security and care of patients who are prisoners or inmates. This policy is primarily directed toward inmate or prisoner patients who are admitted to the hospital. If inmates or prisoners are going no further than the emergency department for outpatient treatment, security personnel on duty need only be notified of their presence. No further action is necessary.

POLICY

1. Definitions
   –Inmate: an individual who has been sentenced by a court of law and is serving a sentence with the state department of corrections
   –Prisoner: an individual who normally has not been sentenced and is not in custody of the state department of corrections but is in the custody of a local, state, or federal law enforcement agency
   –Corrections officer: a security officer employed by the state department of corrections
   –Law enforcement officer: a police officer employed by a local, state, or federal law enforcement agency
2. The degree of security will vary with the type of inmate or prisoner. A minimum of one corrections or law enforcement officer will accompany any inmate or prisoner at all times, even during outpatient treatment in the emergency department.
3. Inmates will be preadmitted whenever possible. Admissions, emergency department, will notify security whenever an inmate or prisoner is on the premises being treated or admitted.
4. "Safed" rooms (rooms stripped of any objects that could harm the patient or staff) will be used except when an inmate or prisoner
   –requires intensive care
   –has an infectious disease
   –is in labor
   –requires long-term transitional care
5. The corrections facility of a law enforcement agency will be responsible for
   –preadmission
   –legal arrangements for the custody of a newborn

PROCEDURE

1. Corrections officers or law enforcement officers must accompany the inmate or prisoner to the designated treatment area along with the hospital security officer. If the inmate or prisoner goes beyond the emergency department for any reason, such as testing, he or she is to be transported in a wheelchair with a sheet covering handcuffs, leg cuffs, and so on, so as not to arouse attention from other staff, patients, or visitors.
2. The correction facility or law enforcement agency must provide a photo and physical description of the inmate or prisoner (if available) to hospital security, while the individual is on hospital property, as soon after arrival as possible, only if the inmate or prisoner will be treated beyond the emergency department.
3. All external inquiries regarding the inmate or prisoner must be directed to the accompanying corrections officer or law enforcement officer.

4. The corrections officer or law enforcement officer must wear photo identification at all times (if available). If the individual is an inmate in the state department of corrections, he or she will wear photo identification at all times, as well.

5. When the accompanying corrections officer or law enforcement officer wears a firearm, he or she will be required to be in uniform or wear some type of identification on an outer garment.

6. Staff must remove the sharps box and telephone from a room housing an inmate or prisoner. In consultation with the corrections officer or law enforcement officer, staff must also remove anything else in the room or treatment area that could be used as a weapon.

7. Staff must order meals for the inmate or prisoner and the corrections officer or law enforcement officer.

8. Staff must remove their name tags when caring for the inmate or prisoner.

9. Staff must notify the switchboard operator and volunteer office of inmate or prisoner presence. Information about inmate or prisoner presence is not given out to anyone.

10. Staff must identify themselves to the corrections officer or law enforcement officer and introduce other staff assigned to the inmate or prisoner.

11. Staff may request that the corrections officer or law enforcement officer be present during care of the inmate or prisoner.

12. The corrections officer or law enforcement officer must remain inside the room with the inmate or prisoner under most circumstances.
    –No other patients will be placed in the room with the inmate or prisoner.
    –When it is not practical or possible for the corrections officer or law enforcement officer to be in the room with the inmate or prisoner, the officer remains outside the door.

13. If the inmate or prisoner requires surgery,
    –The corrections office or law enforcement officer will accompany the inmate or prisoner to the preoperative holding area.
    –The corrections officer or law enforcement officer may use a "bunny suit," i.e., a full-body disposable suit.
    –The corrections officer or law enforcement officer may leave the operating room after the inmate or prisoner is under general anesthesia. If the inmate or prisoner is given a local or regional anesthesia, the corrections officer or law enforcement officer will remain with the inmate or prisoner during surgery and be dressed in the appropriate garb.
    –The corrections officer or law enforcement officer will remain with the inmate or prisoner as soon as he or she is moved from surgery to the recovery room

14. The corrections officer or law enforcement officer will accompany the inmate or prisoner to all procedures.

15. A copy of the inmate's or prisoner's medical records, progress notes, discharge instructions, and discharge summary will be sent to the correctional facility or law enforcement agency upon request.

KEY POINTS

- Nursing unit staff must strictly control narcotics in the unit.
- The design of the nursing unit can affect security in the unit.
- If staff personal items are stored adequately, theft in the unit may be reduced.
- Security representatives can assist nursing staff with locating patients who have strayed, restraining patients, restricting visitors, and handling patients who are prisoners.

REFERENCE

1. Joint Commission on Accreditation of Healthcare Organizations, *Comprehensive Accreditation Manual for Hospitals* (Oakbrook Terrace, IL: 1996).

Chapter 15

Laundry Security

CHAPTER OBJECTIVES

1. Understand why laundry and linens areas need to be monitored carefully.
2. Learn the kinds of theft involving laundry and linens.
3. Know the various ways to have a secure laundry system.

INTRODUCTION

To write about security in health care facilities and not discuss controlling laundry and linens would be inexcusable. While health care facilities use a large volume of laundry items, few facilities have developed a security program to curtail the theft of laundry and linens. To control theft, facilities must control the use and movement of linens. Facilities must carefully examine each step in the movement of laundry and linens, from vendor order to pickup of soiled linens.

VENDOR ORDER

In most facilities, a manufacturer's representative (i.e., salesperson) will visit the laundry manager regularly. **The purpose of these visits should be threefold.**

1. Representatives should check current laundry and linens for durability and to make sure the manufacturer's cleaning instructions are being followed.
2. Representatives should help the laundry manager to place an order for replacement items.
3. Representatives should tell the laundry manager about new products, special deals, and so forth.

The relationship between the representative and the laundry manager sometimes becomes clouded. A laundry manager, having to juggle multiple tasks and manage a large department, may relinquish inventory control to the representative. The mandate from the laundry manager to the representative is simple: to keep a sufficient supply of laundry on hand and not exceed the laundry purchase budget. That may sound like a good plan. The laundry manager has one less task to deal with, and the representative has frequent access to a major account. However, one facility found out this seemingly good plan can turn into a bad situation.

A laundry manager for a health care system became very friendly with a representative. They frequently had lunch together and socialized with each other away from work. The representative told the manager that he needed to make his yearly sales quota and asked the manager to place a large order. The representative told the manager that if a large order were placed, the facility would qualify for a big discount. Because the facility would need some of the items anyway, the laundry manager proceeded to place an order that was almost three times the norm.

When the items arrived, it soon became apparent to the laundry manager that he did not have enough room to store the items. The representative was contacted. The representative told the manager that the items could be shipped to the company's regional warehouse and delivered as needed. The items were then shipped to the warehouse.

No new orders were placed for several months. During that time, the representative came by the laundry frequently and checked on inventory. During each visit, the representative and manager socialized and went to lunch. The representative continually assured the manager that he (the representative) was keeping track of the inventory.

Approximately six months after the large order was placed, the manager placed another order for the same items. He sent the order to the representative. The representative contacted the manager, explaining that the representative had discovered an excellent deal on the needed items. He stated that a smaller health care facility had made a large purchase and in the time between the order and the delivery of the items the health care facility had been bought by a competitor. The manager at the smaller facility was told that the new corporate owner bought laundry items from a group purchaser and wanted to cancel the outstanding order.

The representative told his friend that he could get a great deal on these items. His plan would be for the representative to purchase the items from the smaller facility himself and then resell them to the laundry manager for his facility. The plan sounded good to the laundry manager, so he placed the order, paid the representative, and stocked the items.

What the laundry manager did not know was that he had just repurchased most of the large order that had been stored in the manufacturer's regional warehouse. During the time between the initial storage of the items and the resale, the representative had been keeping phony inventory control records. In fact, the laundry manager had forgotten completely about the items being stored. This fraud would have cost the facility over $50,000 if a laundry employee had not been terminated for cause. During an exit interview, the employee talked about the overly friendly relationship between the representative and the manager and how the representative acted as if he were the employee's supervisor. A subsequent investigation uncovered the above facts.

As this case illustrates, the laundry, like any other department, must have a system of checks and balances, especially in the placing of orders and authorizing of invoices.

SHIPPING AND RECEIVING

The most common problem security consultants see in shipping and receiving areas is lack of separation of duties. Facilities that use an off-site laundry are especially vulnerable to losses because the driver of the laundry delivery truck usually pulls his or her own orders, loads the truck, and is solely responsible for the delivery process.

One facility learned a costly lesson by having this type of system. Operating on an anonymous tip, the security department began following various laundry trucks as they left the central laundry. This particular off-site laundry served three health care facilities in the same city and 20 physician offices and clinics. During the investigation, the security department discovered that one-third of the laundry that had been loaded on the trucks was being dropped off at a small storage unit. The drivers were then selling the laundry and linens to ambulance services and nursing homes in the area. Upon interviewing the drivers, it was learned that this type of theft had been going on for at least three years. The estimated loss to the facilities was over $100,000.

> When using off-site laundry services, make sure that there are controls on who pulls and loads the delivery trucks. Make sure the drivers have the opportunity to count their load and sign for the load. Make sure that signatures are obtained at the points receiving the laundry and some point spot checks are conducted.

The same types of thefts can occur when soiled laundry is returned from the facility to the laundry. There should be a central loading area at the facilities where the soiled laundry can be weighed as it is loaded on the truck. In the same manner, the weight should be checked when the soiled laundry is accepted at the laundry facility.

LAUNDRY FACILITY

Regardless of whether the laundry is done inside or outside the facility, basic security precautions must be taken. If the laundry area is not staffed 24 hours a day, seven days a week, make sure there is a working security and fire alarm system. These systems should be checked at least monthly.

Another security item normally overlooked in the laundry is control of keys to the laundry area, the linens storage areas on the patient care units, and the delivery trucks. One facility discovered that the laundry drivers were coming back to the laundry on weekends and "borrowing" the laundry trucks to use in their part-time moving business. The trucks' mileage should be recorded every day, and these entries should be checked for discrepancies. For example, if the delivery route is 20 miles per day but a mileage check reveals the truck was driven 35 miles a day, the question of "why" should be raised.

When new laundry and linens are received, the items should be moved to a secure stamping area. All facility laundry and linens should be stamped with the facility name and logo at this location. Stamping deters theft and can be a form of public relations.

It is especially important to stamp scrubs. If they are stamped, area facilities can meet monthly to return the scrubs that roving physicians have left at the wrong facility. This process can save thousands of dollars annually.

PATIENT CARE AREAS

Most facilities lose thousands of dollars' worth of laundry in patient care areas each year. Part of the problem is inventory control on the units. How much linen is needed? Some facilities deliver set amounts—the par level—of linens to patient care areas on a regular basis, regardless of use and patient census. High inventory increases the likelihood of theft. Par level deliveries can also increase staffing costs because deliveries are made on a daily basis. The better method is the as-needed system. Someone on the patient care unit is responsible for placing an order to the laundry for needed items. Naturally, there are defined procedures for this type of system.

First, the linens must be stored in a central area on the unit. The storage area should be large enough to keep the laundry and linens in an orderly, easy-to-count fashion.

Second, the storage area must be secured and, if possible, located away from elevators and stairways. Facilities should keep the storage areas secured (including closing doors to the areas). Scrubs, lab jackets, and smocks must be controlled to prevent their use by someone abducting an infant or impersonating a health care professional.

In some facilities, visitors can be seen going into the storage areas and removing items and taking them to patient rooms. What happens to these items? It really is anyone's guess.

Third, access to the laundry must be denied to ambulance services. When one of these services transports a patient to the facility, the service and the facility swap the service's soiled linens for the facility's clean linens. The swap is supposed to be on a one-to-one basis. Most facilities do not monitor these swaps. In a vast majority of facilities, these services will take out multiple sets of linens. In one facility, security officers noted that on each trip, one particular ambulance service was taking out anywhere from six to eight sets of linens for each item it brought in. A full investigation was initiated, and a security camera was placed in the linens room. Over the following month it was discovered that the service was stealing between $2,500 and $4,000 per week in linens. The service was storing the stolen linens at the service's warehouse. The linens were being used for its operation. Subsequent subpoenas proved that the ambulance service had not purchased any linens in over five years of operation.

Some facilities have purchased automatic dispensing machines to control scrubs and linens. These dispensing machines are similar to computerized drug dispensing machines. Staff members use their facility identification cards to open the machine. They then note the number of items and, if applicable, the number of the patient they will be caring for while wearing the scrubs. While these systems can track the issuance of such items, they do not control theft or the more serious problem of infection control if staff members wash their scrubs at home.

Fourth, the laundry must have a procedure in place to respond quickly if unforeseen events lead to a rapid change in patient census. For example, if a disaster occurs, the facility will need more linens than it normally has on hand. The laundry managers must keep a sufficient emergency stock of laundry and linens on hand in case of an emergency. The laundry manager should always be included on the emergency call list.

KEY POINTS

- Laundry and linens are targets for theft.
- To control theft, security procedures must be in place for each step in the laundry process, including ordering, receiving, storage in the general facility area, delivery to medical units, storage on the medical units, and pickup of soiled linens.

Chapter 16

Food Service

1. Understand the most common ways food and supply theft occurs in the food services department.
2. Know policies to prevent food and supply theft.
3. Understand basic cash control procedures for the food services department.

INTRODUCTION

Most food services departments are large, well-organized entities. A variety of staff—from dietitians to dishwashers—are needed to handle the enormous workload. Food services departments must process millions of dollars of food supplies yearly. Given the size and scope of a food service operation, if controls are not in place, theft can run rampant. Many departments lose thousands of dollars in food each year. They also lose supplies: cooking utensils, plates, cups, etc. at an alarming rate.

Food and supplies are stolen from the food services area and in other departments. Most patient care areas have a small nutrition station with soft drinks, juice, crackers, and other supplies for patient use. Likewise, many departments order food items from food services for department use. To have coffee, sugar and creamer packets, and soft drinks in a department is quite normal. Employee theft of these items can quickly add up.

To prevent these types of thefts, each department must have a strict procedure for ordering, receiving, and distributing food items. To ensure that departments are frugal, they should develop a strict budget for food items and be held accountable for the budget. If a department desires a catered function, a separate catering request should be completed and authorized by an administrator if the cost is over a predetermined amount.

The first step in controlling theft in the food services department is conducting an operational security audit. Following are some key areas to be reviewed during this audit.

ACCESS CONTROL

How accessible is the storeroom and refrigerator area? Are these areas locked when a supervisor is not in attendance? Leaving these areas open invites theft and can lead to health department violations.

Are exterior doors in these areas and exterior doors to the department pinned? Are all the locks in good working order? Is there a key control system? How often are locks rekeyed? Is the department locked when no one is present?

Controlling access to the department is vital—the first step in controlling theft. All department keys should be marked "Do not duplicate," and there should be a secure sign-in and sign-out system for departmental keys. Locks should be changed or an area should be rekeyed after a key-carrying employee leaves the organization.

Facilities should prohibit employees from parking their vehicles at or near exit doors and trash dumpsters. Food service employees should park in designated spaces with all other facility employees. Too often, employees carry food items out in boxes or bags to their vehicles or place these items in the dumpster, then pick them up later.

POLICIES/PROCEDURES

Is there a policy addressing food theft? Having a set policy may deter theft.

Is there a policy prohibiting giving leftover food to employees? If this is allowed, chronic overcooking will become commonplace. Many facilities that decided to stop giving employees leftovers saw their food costs drop dramatically soon afterward. In some cases, investigations have shown that entire families had been living on food brought from the facility, including bulk condiments.

Is there a bag check policy or locker inspection policy (see Appendix 16–A)? Is there a rule that only clear plastic bags may be used for trash removal? Security and administration should conduct spot checks of containers coming into and going out of the facility. Removal of food items without authorization should be treated as any other theft.

OPERATIONS

Does food services management authorize all invoices for payment? Do managers spot check items marked "received" on a regular basis? Are orders for food items placed by materials management rather than food service personnel? Do separate personnel order, receive, and store food items? Is there a policy prohibiting visitors in the food service cooking and storage areas? Is the weight of food items checked (a 35-pound box of lettuce could turn out to be 5 pounds lettuce and 30 pounds water and ice)? Are vendors giving the department proper credit for food items they pick up?

CASH CONTROL

Two areas constantly plague food service departments: theft of money and underringing purchases. Proper accountability is necessary to control theft of cash. Only one cashier should work out of each cash drawer. In this manner, the cashier can count and sign for the beginning cash in the drawer, have exclusive access to the money, and be responsible for accounting for all sales through the register. The cashier and a supervisor should count the ending cash together and fill out a cashier's daily report (see Exhibit 16–1).

During the day, excess cash can be removed from the register by the cashier and supervisor. When doing so, both should sign an "excess cash" note that is placed in the register (see Exhibit 16–2). After the cashier closes for the day and the money is counted, the cashier's deposit should be placed in an envelope, sealed, and signed. The envelope should identify the cashier, register number, and time. This envelope should be placed in a safe until the bank deposit is made. At some facilities, food service deposits are taken to the business office and put with other hospital deposits. It is best that the food services deposit be made separately, not mixed with other business deposits.

From time to time during a cashier's shift, the food service director and supervisor should check the register. To do so, they bring the cashier a new till and remove the old till. They remove the detail tape from the register and balance the register. Does the register balance within an acceptable amount (usually within a dollar)?

In most cases when a register is over, the cashier has been making a bank. To do so, the cashier calculates what a particular meal costs in advance. Say the total is $4.25. When someone comes through the line with that meal, the cashier tells the customer $4.25 but does not ring up the sale. The cashier simply puts the money in the register. During the shift, the cashier may place a coin in a designated location, say under the $5 bills, to help keep track of the overage. At the end of the shift, the cashier simply counts the number of coins and re-

---

Exhibit 16–1 Cashier's Daily Report

TODAY'S DATE _____	CASHIER NAME _____	REGISTER # _____

BEGINNING CASH $ 100.00

TOTAL SALES   1100.85 (ending register reading minus beginning register reading)

SUBTOTAL   1200.85

LESS VOIDED SALES   12.15 (must be cosigned by a supervisor at the time of the void)

LESS COURTESY SALES   60.00 (list by department and attach)

LESS NEXT-DAY CASH   100.00 (verified by a supervisor)

CASH FOR DEPOSIT $ 1028.70 (amount placed in deposit envelope)

SIGNED _____   _____

      CASHIER   SUPERVISOR

Exhibit 16–2 Excess cash pickup

REGISTER # _____   CASHIER _____

DATE _____   TIME _____

AMOUNT PICKED UP $ _____

BY _____   TITLE _____

SIGNED _____   _____
　　　　　CASHIER　　　　　　　　　　　　　　SUPERVISOR

moves the same number of units of $4.25 from the register. This type of theft is common when cashiers are allowed to work out of an open till (i.e., do not have to shut the register between sales).

Likewise, checks can cause losses. Cashiers should be allowed to accept only checks that are authorized by the supervisor. If cashiers are permitted to authorize checks themselves, they could use the food service register to "kite" their own loans, placing personal checks in the register and removing cash. When accounting for the day's deposit, the cashier deposits the cash and removes the check. The next day, the cashier places another personal check with the current date in the register; therefore, their personal check is never presented for payment to the bank.

Courtesy meal tickets can also result in losses. Most registers have a key that denotes that a sale is being paid for by a courtesy ticket. The used courtesy ticket should be register validated, signed by the person receiving the meal, and placed in the register. These courtesy tickets should be tightly controlled and signed out by food service by number and quantity to the various departments authorized to use courtesy tickets. If courtesy tickets are not tightly controlled, food service departments can find themselves giving away an unexpected number of free meals.

Another constant problem is underringing of friends' food. For instance, a friend of a cashier might come through the cashier's line with an $8 meal and be charged just $2. Several methods can reduce these losses.

- The cashier area must be constantly supervised.
- Closed-circuit television can show the food items presented to the cashier and the sale price display area.
- Totals for sale-specific register keys can be compared against the food prepared plus any waste. Say that a food preparation area made 100 portions of a daily special, the cashier rang up 85 portions of the daily special, and waste (leftovers) accounted for 6 portions. What happened to the remaining 9 portions? Were they rung up as another item by mistake? Were they rung up at all? This method can be an effective audit if only one register is used. If multiple registers are used, it becomes more difficult but can still be effective.

KEY POINTS

- Food theft can cost a facility thousands of dollars every year.
- Access to storage areas, trash disposal, shipping, and receiving must be controlled so that food theft is more difficult.
- The facility should have a policy that prohibits giving food away to employees.
- There must be security controls for the cash register area.

Appendix 16–A

Bag and Locker Check Policy

POLICY

At XYZ Regional Medical Center, all containers are subject to inspection by management personnel and security or special police officers. These checks ensure that the appropriate item removal authorization form is present when any health services property is removed from hospital premises.

Unfortunately, a few employees are stealing from our facilities. Security experts estimate that $2,600 is stolen per bed, per year, from hospitals nationwide. Eighty percent of the thefts were done by employees. Our facilities alone could lose $2 million per year.

PROCEDURE

All containers—including duffel bags, tote bags, briefcases, purses (larger than a small billfold), grocery bags, lunch pails, and trash bags—may be checked. If hospital property is found in any of these containers without the appropriate authorization form, the employee will be asked to accompany the management representative or security officer back to the employee's supervisor to get the form filled out. Employees who refuse to cooperate in this process will face serious disciplinary action. A security officer will never put his or her hands into one of these containers. The officer will ask the employee to open the container. If appropriate, the employee will be asked to remove the item from the container.

In the same manner, please be mindful that all corporate furnishings and equipment (i.e., desks, lockers, file cabinets, and so forth) are subject to the same administrative inspections. If such an item is to be inspected, the employee will be contacted by his or her supervisor and asked to open it.

If the employee refuses or is not available, the item will be opened by plant engineering, special police, and the employee's supervisor. If an employee-owned lock is broken, the corporation will replace the lock. The contents of the locker, desk, or other item will be inventoried and turned over to the employee's supervisor for safekeeping until the items can be given to the employee.

We ask you to remind your employees about this policy and to ask their cooperation if they are stopped for a bag check by security or management representatives. For several months, we have been informing new employees of this procedure. There may be employees in your department who may not know about it.

237

Chapter 17

Business Office, Medical Records, and Human Resources Security

CHAPTER OBJECTIVES

1. Learn that having secure business offices, medical records departments, and human resources departments is as important as having secure direct patient care areas.
2. Know the most common security issues in the business office area, medical records area, and human resources department.

INTRODUCTION

The business office, medical records department, and human resources departments do not have direct patient care areas. However, they can have a major impact not only on the care a patient receives but also on the patient's and public's view of the facility. Breach of patient and employee confidentiality, theft, impaired staff, and other problems can tarnish the facility's image. Security personnel often forget that security breaches in these areas can have a major effect on the health care facility.

BUSINESS OFFICE

The business office normally comprises many different operations: registration of patients; admission of patients; financial planning for, and collection of, patient account payments; and patient valuables security. In most facilities, the business office may have satellite locations. At the emergency department and in outpatient services some business offices functions—patient registration and payment or insurance information collection—are performed. Since the business office handles not only large volumes of cash but also patient valuables, basic robbery prevention techniques must be instituted.

Physical Security

The cashier area must be secured to prevent both external and internal thefts. Access must be limited to those who work in the area. The best method to control the access is the use of

239

card access and card egress. With this card system, the cashier cannot "buzz" someone into the area. If the area is difficult to access, robbery is deterred.

The counter between the cashier and the customer, as well as the cashier window, should be constructed of bullet-resistant material. To further aid in preventing someone from simply reaching over the counter and taking money from the cashier's money drawer, the cashier counter should be at least 42 inches high and 24 inches wide. The cashier's money drawer should be located below counter height to prevent someone from seeing the drawer from the customer side of the counter.

Like the cashier area, the safe room must be protected. The safe should be located in a room that does not have a wall adjacent to a hallway, to another department, or to the outside. The room should not have a drop ceiling, and the door should be solid cord and fire rated.

Electronics

The use of electronics can dramatically increase the security of the business office. As noted above, electronic access control helps secure the cashier and business office area. It is good to have a record of who came into and went out of the cashier areas and safe room. Other electronic devices offer additional security.

- **Closed-circuit television (CCTV).** Cameras should be mounted so that they film the entrances and exits of the business office, cashier stations, and safe room. Additional cameras can be used to help secure the financial counselors' offices. Due to the nature of financial counselors' jobs, they can be at risk for assault.
- **Burglar and panic alarms.** The business office should be secured when not open, and it should have its own burglar alarm. Likewise, each cashier station, the safe room, and the financial counselors' areas should have silent panic alarms. Care should be taken when mounting these alarm buttons to keep them from accidentally being activated. All alarms should be monitored by security and checked weekly.

Cash Security

The location of the business office affects the security of its cash. More facilities are locating the business office away from the main facility in an office building. In many cases, the facility leases the space in the office building. To facilitate adequate security of this department, the lease agreement should establish the type of security that the lessor will provide and when the security department of the health care facility should be called. Many times, departments located away from the main campus are considered to be "on their own" when it comes to security matters. The security department should at least conduct a security audit of the off-site office and present the findings to both health care facility and building management.

Adequate screening of employees is essential to keeping cash secure. All employees, especially those handling cash and other valuables, should be screened closely. The screening process is discussed under "Human Resources."

Once good, honest employees have been hired, the facility must be sure that there are adequate controls in place to keep these employees honest. One facility found out that an employee with an impeccable record had been stealing from the facility for almost a year. The employee finally confessed to stealing thousands of dollars and stated that the cash system was so uncontrolled that she was surprised that everyone in the department was not stealing. Is lack of control an excuse for theft? Of course not, but sometimes the temptation is just too much.

Each cashier should receive, count, and sign for a cash till at each shift. The cash drawer should remain locked unless the cashier is handling a transaction. If the cashier leaves the area, the drawer must be locked and the cashier should take the key. If the cashier is relieved for a meal or break, the relieving cashier should have his or her own money till.

Keys to the cash drawers must be secured. All locks should be changed periodically or when an employee is terminated.

If the cashier receives a large amount of money during a shift, some of the money should be pulled from the drawer, counted by both the cashier and supervisor, and placed in an envelope (see Exhibit 16–2 for a related form). The envelope should be sealed and placed in the safe, with the amount written on the envelope. This practice can help reduce the chance of a large cash loss from either external or internal sources.

At the end of the shift, the cashier should gather all related documents and the cash drawer and balance the drawer with the verification of a supervisor. Upon completion of the balancing, the cashier and supervisor should prepare a deposit for the day (see Exhibit 16–1 for a related form). All discrepancies should be investigated.

There should be adequate locker space away from the cash area for the storage of personal items. Purses, briefcases, and coats should not be permitted in the cashiers' area. Too often, these items are used to transport stolen cash.

The cash drawers should be audited periodically to ensure that all money is being received and accounted for properly. In one case, a health care facility learned that a cashier was crediting her boyfriend's account for payments made by other patients. In another facility, a cashier was cashing her own check in the cash drawer. Every day, she removed the previous day's check and put a new check in the drawer. She was getting a continuous free loan at the health care facility's expense because her check never went to the bank for payment. Needless to say, a cashier should never be allowed to cash his or her personal check.

PATIENT VALUABLES

In most facilities, the business office is responsible for the safeguarding of patient valuables. The business office usually comes in possession of the valuables in one of two ways. If the patient is admitted through normal procedures, the admitting clerk will first ask if the patient can send the valuables home with a family member. If this is not possible, the admitting clerk will, along with the patient, inventory the valuables, place them in a patient valuable envelope, and fill out the front of the envelope—primarily patient identification information. The valuables and the inventory sheet are then placed in the envelope, and the envelope is sealed. The patient is given the claim check portion from the envelope. During discharge, the patient presents the claim check and identification, and the valuables are returned. If the patient expires or is too ill to pick up the valuables, the valuables should be released to the person listed as the patient's closest relative on the admitting form.

The other way the business office may come to be in possession of patient valuables is when a patient is admitted through the emergency department. If a patient is alert and accompanied by a family member, then the family member is usually asked to take the valuables. If this is not possible, then the procedure described above is followed. If the patient is alone or unconscious, two staff members should inventory the valuables and fill out the valuables envelope. The staff listing the valuables should not jump to conclusions. For instance, a ring that is yellow may not be made of gold. Staff should record it as a "yellow metal ring." The patient claim check is then included in the patient chart. If the medical staff feel that the patient will be discharged shortly, they can hold the valuables in a secure area. When the patient is discharged from the emergency department, the valuables can be retrieved from the discharging nurse.

If the patient is admitted, the valuables are normally sent to the business office. There, the valuables envelope is logged in and placed in the safe. Normal retrieval procedures are followed. At the change of each shift the patient valuables envelope should be inventoried by patient name. This inventory can help ensure that all patient valuables are present.

MEDICAL RECORDS

While most medical facilities advertise that they offer higher-quality care than their competitors, most health care facilities in a given area offer comparable care. What the facility is really selling is trust. Patient comments like "this is my hospital, and they always take care of me" are common. But just as the manner in which patient care is rendered is vital, the confidentiality of the patient's medical records is paramount. Too often, information from the medical records of highly visible people has appeared in the tabloids. Even if the breach of confidentiality is not that severe, countless patients have had their medical history and current condition laid open for public review.

While breaches of confidentiality can occur in many areas of the facility (the most common is colleagues talking about a patient in an elevator with the public present), the most sensitive area is medical records. The medical records area must be secure, with controlled access. Those who work in the medical records area should sign a confidentiality agreement when hired and on each anniversary of their hire.

Access to the records should be on a need-to-know basis. Naturally, the attending physician and primary nurse should have unlimited access. But what about others who want access for a limited time? For example, the security director may need to review the medication administration record if he or she is investigating a possible drug diversion case. In these situations, staff should be allowed access to only the needed section.

The medical records department is best secured by having an attendant on duty to screen those requesting access. This person can also assist those seeking a medical record and let the requesting person know when the record will be available. In larger facilities, a wait of one to two days to locate a record and have it transferred to the viewing areas is not uncommon.

As stated above, access to the medical records department and especially the storage area must be controlled. The best access methods are electronic. Using card access, palm print access, or other electronic forms of identification, it is easy to discontinue access when employees stop working at the facility.

Care should be given to securing the medical records storage area itself. The area should have a fire suppression system and, if it is not attended 24 hours a day, an intrusion alarm. These alarms can be monitored by security, or if no security department is available, the switchboard. Entrances to the department and storage areas should be monitored by CCTV.

Some facilities store out-of-date medical records off site. This type of storage area should be as secure as an on-site area. It should be visited daily if possible to ensure that the area is secure and there have been no attempts at forced entry.

Staff should also consider record security while the patient is being treated. Whether the patient is an inpatient or outpatient, care should be given to control public access to the record. Too often, a patient's medical record is left lying on the counter of a nurses' station with no one present, or the record is left in the patient's room. These actions can lead to possible legal action if the patient's confidentiality is breached.

HUMAN RESOURCES

Just as a patient has the right to have a confidential medical record, employees have the right to have a confidential personnel record. Access to the working area of the human resources department should be controlled. This working area should be separate from the public areas.

Too often, a person applying for a position has overheard an employee discussing a private matter. Any discussions with an employee about employment issues should be held in a private area. Cubicles are not private areas.

Who should have access to an employee's personnel record? Naturally, the employee, administration, human resources, and the employee's supervisor must have access. But what about others? Should a manager of a separate department have access? Should the security department have access? The answer depends on the reason for the access request. If an employee has requested a transfer to a new area, the manager of that department may need to review the employees' work history. Security may need to review the items in an employee's record during an investigation. To minimize conflicts, those seeking to review an employee's record should request permission in writing, stating the reason for the review, to the vice president or others designated by the vice president.

The areas for storing employee personnel files should have the same level of security as medical records areas. There should be access control, a fire suppression system, and an intrusion alarm in use after hours.

The human resources department must make every effort to ensure that good, honest employees are hired. As noted above, hiring departments must call the applicant's references, do an extensive criminal record check, and screen applicants for drugs. Unfortunately, most facilities do a rather poor job of checking an applicant's past criminal record. They usually check with the local police. If no record is found, the applicant is cleared. This is a better approach: the facility should check the county or counties and state or states in which the applicant has lived or worked for at least the past five years. Some states permit a medical facility to use the state's criminal record repository for checking criminal records. While this method may be easy, quick, and inexpensive, it is not thorough enough. The various counties in a state are required to report all guilty verdicts of felony charges to the state repository. However, reporting misdemeanor convictions is usually voluntary. If would be easy for someone to have a clean record with the state repository but a lengthy criminal record at the county level.

> One nursing home learned a costly lesson about checking criminal records. It hired a nursing assistant without checking the person's background. It was not until the nursing assistant severely beat an elderly patient that her past was investigated. They learned that the nursing assistant had recently been released from prison for child abuse and had a history of violent crimes.

Most new hires undergo a health and drug screening. Facilities most often use the standard drug screen used by the Department of Transportation (DOT). While this screen is acceptable for most nonmedical personnel, it is not adequate for those having access to controlled substances. The standard DOT screen will not record any use of synthetic narcotics—those most likely to be abused by health care professionals. Morphine and Demerol are the most abused drugs, but neither of these will be picked up on a standard DOT test. All health care professionals should receive a separate test for determining whether these synthetic narcotics are present.

To assist employees who are undergoing problems, the human resource department should either establish an employee assistance program (EAP) or contract for this service with an outside agency. The EAP can be a valuable resource for good employees with outside problems that are affecting their job performance. Some EAP departments have formed partnerships with other departments to further assist the employee. For instance, the facility's security department may assist in keeping an estranged spouse away from the facility. Or the EAP can try to arrange a short-term loan through pastoral care for employees with financial difficulties. Having facility departments work together to help an employee is an idea that is long overdue.

The security department should know all human resources policies, especially those regarding violence in the workplace, preemployment drug testing, random drug testing, fitness for duty, administrative inspections (checks of bags, desks, lockers, etc.), employee theft of facility property, employee theft of patient property, employee theft of narcotics, unauthorized possession of a master key, unauthorized copying of any facility key, and use of drugs or alcohol during or just before work.

KEY POINTS

- The primary security issues for business offices are access control, the use of electronic security systems, cash security, and security of patient valuables.
- The primary security issues for medical records areas are confidentiality of patient records, access control, key control, and record storage.
- The primary security issues for the human resources department are access control, confidentiality of employee records, and record storage.

Chapter 18

Emergency Department Security

Rick J. Flinn

CHAPTER OBJECTIVES

1. Understand the extent of emergency department violence.
2. Know the reasons for emergency department violence.
3. Describe the security responses necessary in the emergency department.
4. Know what a training program for security and nursing staff personnel for the emergency department would entail.

INTRODUCTION

Today, many people seek medical treatment because of injuries from intentional and random acts of violence. The emergency department (ED) is typically the first place that victims of violent acts go. Despite the challenge of managing the physical and emotional aftermath of violence, all too often, ED staff also find themselves in harm's way when aggressors follow patients to the health care facility. This problem demands a proactive, collaborative approach by all EDs, whether they are located in a rural, suburban, or urban environment. Unfortunately, no individual or community is immune from this national epidemic.

The early teachings of Dr. Martin Luther King, Jr., made violence a major issue for the nation's leaders. He stated that "the choice today is no longer between violence and nonviolence. It is either nonviolence or nonexistence."

In this chapter, violence will be defined as the use of physical force—to injure, abuse, or kill—against others or oneself. People who commit such acts of violence may come from a variety of socioeconomic backgrounds. Many people have the potential for violence, making this societal dilemma widespread, multifaceted, and extremely complex. Violence manifests itself in many ways, including assault, suicide, murder, terrorism, rape, child abuse, spouse battering, gang-related crime, and aggressive driving that leads to injury.

THE PREVALENCE AND COSTS OF VIOLENCE NATIONWIDE

The Bureau of Justice reports that every U.S. citizen has a 75 percent chance of becoming a victim of an actual or attempted assault. This translates into over 1.5 million assaults in the United States each year. These acts of violence have different outcomes depending on the intent, degree of physical force, and specific response of the victim. Unfortunately, death is too often a result. Despite some favorable regional trends across the country, there are still over 20,000 murders annually. Clearly, homicides and suicides continue to be a leading cause of premature death.[1-3]

Many Americans live with the physical and emotional consequences of senseless violence. Whether people are victims of an aggravated assault during a robbery, a forcible rape, or an extended period of spouse battering, their physical and psychological scars may never mend. These scars affect the individual, family members, coworkers, friends, and the community at large.

This multifaceted dilemma knows no geographical boundaries and is not limited to one socioeconomic group. Both victims and perpetrators can be found anywhere. One of the more staggering trends is the prevalence of youth violence in rural and urban regions. By the middle of the 1990s, the number of juvenile arrests for crimes of violence had increased by nearly 50 percent.[4] Clearly, the expanding presence of organized gangs in cities, towns, and neighborhoods has precipitated this surge in violence, especially among youth. Other factors contribute to the incidence of violent acts and crime: poverty, unemployment, drug and alcohol abuse, racism, firearm access, parental absence, dysfunctional relationships, and the absence of traditional, positive values. Unsurprisingly, no one solution will clear up this tragic, complex problem.

The impact of violence on our communities' health is huge. Traumatic injury is the fourth most common cause of death in the United States. In recent studies, individuals were reported to be more likely to present to local EDs as a result of injuries associated with violent acts than because of trauma related to motor vehicle crashes. Actually, even some automobile crashes are a result of intentional acts of aggression. On a national level, aggressive driving violations (e.g., tailgating, weaving) have risen an average of 7 percent yearly since 1990. During a six-year study by the AAA Foundation for Traffic Safety, at least 218 people were killed and another 12,610 injured when drivers acted on their anger.[5]

More common than road rage is the use of firearms during acts of aggression. Seven states have identified firearm violence as the leading cause of traumatic death. Many forecasters predict that firearm injury will be the primary cause of injury-related death in this country by 2003. Health care facility EDs have been left to repair the damage. Despite the high mortality rate associated with firearm injuries, nearly 60 percent, there are many survivors, and they must endure prolonged hospitalizations, extended rehabilitation, multiple complications, and reduced autonomy. During the recovery, many individuals incur enormous medical expenses and often lose wages. A conservative estimate is that firearm injury costs our society over $20 billion each year.[6]

Clearly, the costs of violence extend beyond the physical and emotional wounds. Violence results in crowded EDs, a changed atmosphere in inpatient units, increased risk for health care personnel, and significant societal costs. Annually, violence costs the nation $400 billion. Specifically, the cost per crime-related injury is almost $41,000.[7]

WHO MAY BECOME VIOLENT IN AN ED?

Trauma bays across the country are filled with victims suffering from intentional trauma, both penetrating and blunt. Factors that can lead a person to commit a violent act include

- fear of the unknown
- a threat to self-esteem or sense of physical well-being
- a threat to goals and expectations
- a threat to personal space
- a reaction to an intense situation or a series of situations gradually escalating in intensity

There are also factors that increase the likelihood that a person will be aggressive on a given day.

- use of alcohol or drugs
- current or past mental disorder
- anger associated with the mental condition
- stress related to an injury or illness
- behavioral changes associated with the disease or injury (e.g., closed head injury, acute psychiatric condition, seizure disorder)
- annoyances at institution (e.g., prolonged wait times, uncomfortable waiting area, open access for general public)
- personal issues (e.g., losing work time, having to get child care)
- presence of criminal gangs
- history of domestic violence

Persons who commit violent acts within EDs can be categorized into several groups. First, there are spouses or significant others whose acts of domestic violence have sent their partners to the ED. The incidence of domestic violence has reached disturbing levels. Even given the fact that domestic violence is often unreported, there are approximately 2 million to 4 million American women battered each year. Actually, studies have shown that 20 to 30 percent of women who seek emergency care have been in or are still in an abusive relationship. This patient group is highly vulnerable to repeated acts of abuse, especially if there is a perceived risk of discovery during the care. It is not uncommon for the battering spouse to accompany the patient and even continue the abuse through intimidation, verbal ridicule, or physical attack. The violence could be directed at the patient or at the health care worker attending to the patient.

Second, there are homeless or mentally disturbed individuals who do not necessarily have any medical reason for being in the ED and use the waiting room and treatment areas as a platform for acting out. Often these individuals are simply looking for shelter or attention. Confronted regarding their presence or asked to leave the facility, they may respond aggressively.

Third, there are patients or family members under the influence of alcohol or mood-altering drugs. Their judgment may be so impaired that they challenge authority, confront other visitors, or defy institutional policies. Patients under the influence of alcohol and other drugs create a real challenge. The health care team must manage these patients' clinical problems while being acutely aware of the potential for verbal and physical outbursts.

Fourth, there are persons frustrated with long waits for care. Patients with less urgent conditions often have to wait longer in an emergency department than patients with urgent conditions. Lack of communication between provider and patient or relative contributes to the anxiety and stress related to episodic illness and injury as well as delays.

Fifth, there are psychiatric patients who are a threat to themselves or openly threatening to others. Health care workers may respond to violent psychiatric patients by using various approaches, including chemical or physical restraint and seclusion. Loss of control may precipitate attacks against the nurse, physician, or security officer. Just the process of administering medications or interviewing may compel the person with a mental condition to attack.

Sixth, there are gang members, both patients and visitors. Depending on the area, opposing gang members may be treated in the same department, creating a high risk for violence. Not only the victims but also other gang members may be present in the ED. Rival gang members frequently follow the injured person to the health care facility and resume the feud on the facility's property.

THE PREVALENCE AND COSTS OF VIOLENCE IN AN ED

Workplace violence is on the rise and affects EDs, which are the workplaces of many Americans. Workers' family crises may spill into the ED. For instance, health care workers may be harassed, threatened, stalked, or injured while on the job because of an irate significant other. And angered employees may display aggression as a result of a work-related incident. Too many employees and managers have fallen victim to a coworker who is out of control.

> The Bureau of Justice reports that 8 percent of all rapes and 16 percent of all aggravated assaults occur in the workplace. Homicide continues to rank second among causes of work-related deaths. Unfortunately, 49 percent of assaults occurring in the workplace are against health care workers. An ED nurse is six times more likely than another person in the workplace to suffer from a violent act.[8]

In 1994, the Emergency Nurses Association conducted a comprehensive survey of EDs to determine the prevalence of violence and learn about facility responses, both reactive and proactive. Each health care facility reported a rise in violent acts within their EDs. Sixty-seven percent of respondents said that staff members had suffered an emotional or physical injury following an act of violence within the work area. Verbal abuse and physical assaults, with or without a weapon, were occurring routinely, even daily. Actually, 11 percent of the surveyed EDs required a security response to manage a violent patient or visitor in more than 25 incidents per month. These findings validated the perceptions of many practitioners and leaders within the field. Fortunately, the survey ignited a concentrated attempt to improve the safety of clinical staff, patients, and family members. President Clinton discussed the problem at a State of the Union address during the mid-1990s, highlighting the need for a collaborative approach. "We must all work together to stop the violence that explodes in our emergency rooms," the president said.[9]

ADMINISTRATORS AND SECURITY EXPERTS RESPOND

The increasing threat of violence in EDs has intensified the challenge for health care facility administrators, security professionals, and ED managers to ensure a secure and safe environment. No one strategy or plan is right for every health care facility. EDs throughout the country have instituted a broad range of security measures. As early as the beginning of 1993, a study by the American College of Emergency Physicians found that several health care facilities were beginning to think proactively about ED security. The survey results showed that 52 percent of respondents were using panic alarms, and 31 percent of EDs maintained 24-hour security coverage. Any security plan or initiative should be researched well; cost-effectiveness is critical in today's health care environment.[10]

THERE ARE SOME KEY SECURITY MEASURES THAT EVERY ED SHOULD CONSIDER

- dedicated security officer coverage
- access control
- enhanced visibility of ED entrances
- use of metal detectors
- duress alarms
- guest services programs
- closed-circuit television (CCTV)
- seclusion rooms
- nonviolent crisis intervention training
- visitor control
- restriction of weapons by security and law enforcement during restraint
- separation of patients based on acuity
- debriefing of staff after critical incidents

All of these measures will lead to a safer work environment. Security personnel and administrators must decide on the best approaches for their EDs.

Security Assessment

The initial step in planning a security program is assessment. The determination of an individual health care facility's level of risk or vulnerability is critical and serves as the foundation for deciding the type of enhancements needed. An in-depth review of design, operations, trends in violent activity, policies, staffing, crime rates, and demographics truly assists in identifying problem areas and determining the degree of threat to personnel, patients, and visitors.

A large midwestern ED used the following factors to gauge their overall risk and create a case for a proactive security plan:

- location (e.g., urban, rural)
- ED personnel's perception of risk
- volume and acuity of psychiatric patients
- prevalence of drug and alcohol use among ED patients

- average length of stay in the ED
- statistics regarding regional and national ED violence
- weapon use, gang activity, and other crime within market area
- trauma center designation (e.g., level one, level two)
- frequency of security incidents and response
- proportion of patients arriving with penetrating trauma as compared with percentage of patients arriving with blunt trauma
- proportion of patients arriving with intentional trauma as compared with percentage of patients arriving with nonintentional trauma
- number of victims of violence in the ED
- frequency of staff assaults
- overall design and layout of the ED and adjoining properties (e.g., parking lot, corridors)

Obviously, the risk assessment may require some time and effort, but it will support and help focus security's efforts to prevent violence in the ED. Once the initial security plan is in place, risk assessments should continue to be conducted periodically to determine the need for policy, system, or design changes. Lastly, representatives from security, facilities, public and guest relations, administration, and the ED must collaborate when planning, implementing, or evaluating any program or security modification.

In theory, the strategies to achieve the most secure and safe ED fall into three distinct categories: design, personnel, and policies. Based on the risk assessment, a variety of security measures within these categories are available and should be considered for inclusion in a comprehensive security approach.

Design

The design of an ED plays a major role in ensuring effective traffic flow of personnel, patients, and visitors. Typically, design features will help staff deter as well as respond to violence. Clearly, a collaborative, well-planned design will be the first step in preventing an untoward incident. Security professionals must be a part of any renovation project, as well as new construction, in order to address visibility issues, access control, blind spots, technical requirements, and any other issues.

Waiting Areas

Violence often occurs in ED waiting areas. It is not uncommon for a conflict between visitors or a domestic dispute to erupt in the waiting room. Stress levels may be high. Staff must monitor the waiting areas constantly, institute rounds, and talk with family members and significant others in an effort to relieve the anxiety associated with sudden illness or prolonged waiting times.

> The waiting area should be comfortable and allow privacy. Adequate seating, public telephones, vending machines, functional televisions and VCRs, noise control, informational materials, and clean restrooms can keep visitors at ease and minimize their tendency to migrate from the area.

Many EDs are separating the pediatric population in an effort to manage noise. Others install aquariums to distract people. In addition, a separate quiet or grieving room can be a great addition when handling awkward situations or managing the distraught family following the news of an untimely injury, illness, or even death.

Entrances

Depending on the risk assessment findings, many EDs have or are considering improved protection at key portals of access. Clearly, access control through electronic keypads or card readers is almost a must when protecting the clinical area from unauthorized entry. Most of today's EDs have separated the ambulatory and ambulance entrances, making control of access more complicated. Each access area must be incorporated into the plan, and special consideration must be given to how appropriate entry is managed. Intercoms, CCTV, or escorts may need to be used in order to meet both the safety and customer services imperatives. Safety glass enclosures for triage areas and security stations will help departments at risk for weapon use at the primary entrances. These measures give the staff peace of mind but are costly and will make the facility seem less friendly to customers. Controlled access is a primary strategy for most EDs and should be incorporated into the health care facility's plan for traffic control and after-hours entry to other patient care areas.

Panic Alarms

Duress or panic alarms should be strategically placed at reception areas, triage stations, registration cubicles, treatment areas, and seclusion rooms to enable the staff to summon security. Often this notification is silent and is routed directly to a central or decentralized alarm panel that is monitored 24 hours a day. This immediate, prioritized summons for assistance is easy and quickly alerts the security personnel that a potentially dangerous situation exists in a particular place. Focused attention should be given to areas where an exchange of currency occurs (e.g., financial counselors' offices). Duress or panic alarms can be extremely useful in isolated treatment areas, such as fast track or express care.

Metal Detectors

Metal detectors are gradually becoming more popular as EDs refine their approaches to maximizing security within their individual units. Obviously, the presence of a weapon or firearm during a volatile incident can lead to tragedy within seconds. During 1996, Barnes-Jewish Hospital in St. Louis, Missouri, detected 9,107 potential weapons in routine screening using both fixed and hand-held metal detectors. Despite the fact that only four handguns were recovered, over 6,300 sharp objects were held or confiscated. Each item was deemed capable of injuring personnel or others. Interestingly, over 230 individuals refused the screening, perhaps because they were carrying a weapon. The goal of most programs incorporating metal detection screening is to ultimately persuade individuals to avoid carrying weapons through the front door. Signage provides a critical warning and must be clearly visible to the public (see Figure 18–1 for a sample sign). If metal detection screening is employed, the approach must be consistent and show no bias. At Barnes-Jewish Hospital, all patients and visitors are screened initially or following acute intervention. The traffic flow must be streamlined so that persons cannot bypass or divert the process, unless the patient is unstable. It is

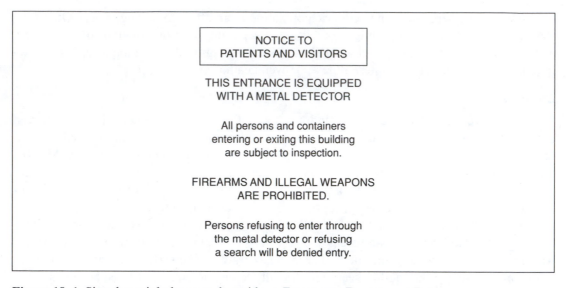

NOTICE TO
PATIENTS AND VISITORS

THIS ENTRANCE IS EQUIPPED
WITH A METAL DETECTOR

All persons and containers
entering or exiting this building
are subject to inspection.

FIREARMS AND ILLEGAL WEAPONS
ARE PROHIBITED.

Persons refusing to enter through
the metal detector or refusing
a search will be denied entry.

Figure 18–1 Sign that might be posted outside an Emergency Department Entrance.

highly recommended that unstable and ambulance-transported patients be scanned using a portable wand once they are settled in the treatment area. Finding a nine-millimeter handgun while resuscitating a trauma patient can be quite alarming to the entire team.[11]

The drawback to any fully operating metal detection system is the staffing requirements. The passage of patients and visitors through the metal detector must be supervised, and the officer needs to be prepared to manage the discovery of lethal weapons. In addition, policies must be clear regarding the handling and return or confiscation of legal and illegal items. Despite the fear of negative public response, most EDs have had minimal complaints. Service-oriented communication and explanations play a huge role in soliciting the public's and medical staff's endorsement. In addition, local law enforcement should be consulted and incorporated into the response plan upon discovery of a illegal weapon. Exhibits 18–1 through 18–3 contain a sample policy and procedure sheet on metal detectors and searches, a metal detector statistical sheet, and a metal detector property receipt.

Seclusion Areas

Seclusion areas may need to be included in the physical layout of the ED, depending on the number of psychiatric patients that come through the ED. At a minimum, certain treatment rooms should be flexible enough in design to allow removal of sharps and other hazards in order to accommodate an irrational, confused, or dangerous patient.

New construction often allows the opportunity to create a dedicated seclusion room to manage agitated prisoners, patients with behavioral disorders, and violent patients under the influence of alcohol or other drugs. These rooms should be equipped with a high, solid ceiling, shatterproof lighting, a recessed nurse call system, a video camera, padded walls, lightweight furniture (when appropriate), a two-way door, and an outside locking mechanism.

Audiovisual Systems

Audiovisual systems are key components to an effective design for today's EDs. As departments renovate or expand, more and more square footage require surveillance. On a rotational basis, each segment of the ED should be monitored by security personnel on site or at a remote command center. In the absence of an actual security presence, CCTV can be an extremely valuable surveillance tool. Obviously, no one person or team can be in all places at all times. Cameras should be widespread and placed in a manner to ensure maximum visibility. Areas deemed critical include entrances, triage, the security and reception area, registration, the waiting room clinical work station, blind corridors, the seclusion room, and the immediate exterior, such as parking areas, ambulance decks, helipads, and so forth. The CCTV system should be microprocessor-based to provide maximum flexibility in sequencing, rotation, and call-up capabilities. To ensure maximum benefit, consideration should be given to recording capabilities, color, zoom lenses, and wide-angle views.

Lighting

A simple design feature for EDs is exterior lighting. Good lighting consistently serves as an effective deterrent to criminal activity. ED personnel and others find a well-lighted area comforting when they approach or leave the facility. Typically, this is a low-cost option that will reap optimal benefits for the organization.

Personnel

The placement of trained security personnel is a critical consideration during the development of any comprehensive security plan. Regardless of the approach, staffing is by far the greatest expense and requires the most justification. Whether the department utilizes off-duty police officers, contracted security, or in-house personnel, salaries must be an integral component of the proposed budget. In addition, backup coverage through bike patrols or other security responders is essential.

Security officers assigned to the ED should be well known to the staff and viewed as permanent members of the emergency care team. All efforts should be made to avoid frequent rotation of security personnel, to ensure consistency and better working relationships. Selected personnel must have strong backgrounds in safety and security in order to maximize their success and overall contribution in this fairly volatile and stressful arena. Security officers must be knowledgeable about the business of emergency care and fully understand their role in personnel safety, property protection, and guest services.

In order to enhance the officer selection process, many security directors are beginning to utilize a multidisciplinary interview team that includes security personnel, physicians, ED managers, and other pertinent clinical staff. This approach can help to truly determine a match between candidate and department. In addition, the entire team is vested in making selected security officers succeed in their new role.

Exhibit 18–1 Metal Detector/Searches—Policy and Procedure

	Issued By:	Policy #:
	Prepared By:	Revision #:
	Approved By:	Effective Date:
Subject:		Page of

POLICY STATEMENT

To ensure that no person(s) is found to be in possession of a weapon, dangerous device, or contraband, all persons entering the hospital shall be subject to search as a condition of entry to property. Persons refusing search will be denied entry to property.

INTENT AND SCOPE

The intent of this policy is to provide a safe environment for health care delivery. This procedure applies to all visitors, patients, and employees entering the property. Exception or deviation from this policy may be made in the best interest of the facility and its patients, provided the intent is observed.

GENERAL INFORMATION

The metal detector will be in operation 24 hours a day, 365 days per year.

PROCEDURE

1. The metal detector will be placed at the entrance of the emergency department or other areas designated by the director of security and approved by the associate administrator.
2. A security officer will be present during the period of operation.
    *   All persons entering the emergency services areas will be required to pass through the detector unless medically unqualified to do so.
3. Signs will be placed at entrances to the hospital announcing that a metal detector is in operation and that person(s) entering the hospital will be required to pass through the metal detector as a condition of entry. Entering any hospital entrance will constitute consent to a reasonable limited search. Signs will indicate that persons refusing to comply with instructions to enter the hospital through a detector-monitored entrance may be denied entry.
4. Erected signs will set forth the following information:
    *   The hospital reserves the right to inspect the contents of all packages or articles entering or being removed from the hospital.
    *   Firearms and illegal weapons are prohibited.
    *   Metal detector(s) are in operation and person(s) refusing search may be denied entry to the hospital.
5. Weapons, dangerous devices, contraband, and suspected stolen hospital property will be retained for disposition with law enforcement authorities.
    *   Security lockers will be maintained for the purpose of storing legally possessed items (i.e., knives, legally prescribed drugs, hand luggage or purses that have not been subject to search, and legally possessed firearms).
    *   Person(s) refusing search of hand luggage or purse may check such hand luggage or purse with the officer in charge of the metal detector, or his or her designee. On completion of hospital business, the checked hand luggage or purse will be returned to the person originally checking the hand luggage or purse. Such transactions will be recorded using a claim check system.

Courtesy of Tarrant County Hospital District, John Peter Smith Hospital, Fort Worth, Texas.

Exhibit 18–2 Metal Detector Statistical Sheet

Place completed form in officers' daily report box.

Date: _____

Duty Hours		Total Visitors	Number of Patients/ Visitors Screened	Number of Weapon(s)		Number of Illegal Weapons	Officer Name/ID
				Retrieved	Returned		
T H I R D S H I F T	0000–0200						
	0200–0400						
	0400–0600						
	0600–0800						
F I R S T S H I F T	0800–1000						
	1000–1200						
	1200–1400						
	1400–1600						
S E C O N D S H I F T	1600–1800						
	1800–2000						
	2000–2200						
	2200–2400						

Courtesy of Tarrant County Hospital District, John Peter Smith Hospital, Fort Worth, Texas.

Security officers in the ED have many different responsibilities.

- patrolling the clinical area
- monitoring the external perimeter (including ED parking areas)
- controlling facility and department access
- protecting assets
- escorting personnel to psychiatric units and remote sites (e.g., parking lots)
- managing metal detection screening
- securing confiscated or surrendered weapons
- assisting with violent patients and visitors
- monitoring CCTV surveillance
- collecting patient valuables

Exhibit 18–3 Metal Detector Property Receipt

Date _____   Time _____

Name _____

Address
    Street _____ Apt. # _____

    City_____ State_____ Zip _____

PROPERTY RECEIVED:

_____

_____Will Not Be Held Responsible for Property or Items Retained in Excess of 15 Days.

                          Owner's Signature _____ Date _____

                          Claimant's Signature _____ Date _____

    Receiving Officer's Signature and Identification # _____ Date _____

    Returning Officer's Signature and Identification # _____ Date _____

Courtesy of Tarrant County Hospital District, John Peter Smith Hospital, Fort Worth, Texas.

- helping to restrain patients
- investigating criminal acts internally
- providing lost visitors with directions
- documenting security incidents and violent acts
- managing hostage situations and bomb threats
- interfacing with local law enforcement, fire protection districts, and regional emergency medical services
- assisting with helicopter safety and landings
- participating in health care facility safety programs
- securing the facility during disasters

In addition to handling these key responsibilities, security personnel need to be very flexible and adopt a "whatever it takes" attitude. In many situations, the health care security professional is the first contact for patients and visitors who seek service from the institution.

The number and type (armed, unarmed, power of arrest, uniformed) of security officers varies and should be based on the level of risk for the specific ED. In addition, the security officer's scope of responsibility is a major determinant of the staffing plan. For example, an ED that utilizes metal detection, maintains decentralized monitors for unit-specific CCTV, and responds to the clinical area for patient restraint has a significant need for coverage by several providers. Larger facilities and institutions with significant risk for violence routinely require at least 24-hour coverage.

Security Uniform versus Street Clothes

The security officer's image is an important consideration in every institution. Most EDs have adopted the uniformed approach in the hopes that a visible security figure will deter violence.

Armed Security versus Unarmed Security

The decision to employ armed security officers, with arrest power, continues to be controversial. Depending on the results of the department's risk assessment and the security officer's post duties, the decision may be less complicated. Those who oppose using armed personnel argue that weapons may be misused and personnel injured if an irrational person confiscates the weapon. If the decision is to arm all or part of the security force, proper training, licensure, and policy generation regarding weapon handling in clinical interactions is critical. In addition, the power of arrest may be very beneficial in some institutions. Despite the constitutional restrictions, arrest power may be important for certain on-site personnel to have and may provide further deterrence. Often, shift supervisors serve in this role and are trained according to regulatory directives.

Training

Training is an integral component of every security officer's job. The International Association of Healthcare Safety and Security recommends a basic program of 40 hours of training, including discussions of security and health care facility organization and procedures, public relations, communication strategies, surveillance, access control, asset protection, security equipment and systems, safety policies, legal issues, self-defense, treatment of disturbed or agitated individuals, and use of weapons. All ED personnel and security officers must learn nonviolent crisis intervention (including proper restraint techniques).

Due to the growing violence in EDs, many states are regulating minimum training requirements. For example, the 1993 California Assembly Bill 508 states that

> All health care facility employees regularly assigned to the ED shall receive on a continuing basis . . . security education and training related to: personal and general safety, the assault cycle, predictors of violence and aggression, characteristics of aggressive and violent patients or visitors, verbal and physical techniques to defuse or avoid violent behavior, strategies to avoid physical harm, restraining techniques, appropriate use of medication as a chemical restraint, and access to support programs, i.e., Critical Incident Stress Debriefing, Employee Assistance Program, following assaults.

A well-trained team can prevent violent assaults by recognizing when a patient or visitor is likely to become violent, controlling factors leading to anxiety and frustration, and defusing a situation through effective communication skills. Recognition of the individual who is at risk for a violent outburst is critical. Persons who begin to be impatient display some consistent behaviors. Trained staff will be on the lookout for individuals who speak in an angry way, seek attention, have a threatening attitude, and use degrading language. In addition, staff should watch persons who are pacing, seem tense, or are under the influence of alcohol or other drugs. Once a potentially violent person is identified, the security officer and clinical staff have a "window of opportunity" to defuse the situation. Nonviolent crisis intervention training endorses the following simple approach to defusing a potentially violent situation: listen, empathize, clarify, solve problems, and close. In addition, other straightforward verbal or behavioral strategies can assist when confronting the angry customer: maintain eye contact, respect the individual's "personal space," move slowly, plan an escape, personalize the contact, allow reasonable choices, apologize when appropriate, clarify limitations, remain calm, and be prepared to react. Training is an invaluable part of any comprehensive security program.

Policies

The solidification of any security plan includes adopting policies and practices that will compliment the design and personnel resources. These policies provide structure and direction while ensuring a consistent approach to maintaining a safe work environment.

Visitor Control

Visitor control policies are debated as clinicians and security personnel attempt to balance the patient and family needs with the safety requirements necessary to secure the department. Every ED should adopt and endorse a consistent visitor policy. The policy should include the number of visitors allowed, age restrictions, exceptions, and responsibilities for enforcement. Clearly, the security officer must understand the exceptions to avoid conflict, misunderstandings, and customer dissatisfaction.

Ideally, each individual in the clinical area should wear an identification badge. Simple color-coded or dated visitor passes can be an effective addition to any program.

Communication between Security and Nursing

A system identifying several levels of security response can be very helpful when situations begin to escalate. Each level is associated with certain types of situations and desired security responses. Exhibit 18–4 shows a sample policy on levels of security. This policy approach helps clarify both responsibilities and expected outcomes of any security response.

Victims of violence pose a unique challenge for most departments in the health care facility. Persons suffering from sexual assault, penetrating trauma, or gang-related violence create an identifiable risk for the institution. Once these persons are identified, it is prudent to restrict information regarding their whereabouts to the public and media. A clear policy highlighting communication, visitor restrictions, telephone privileges, and compliance can prevent further violence within the health care facility. It is imperative that the family is identified and is supportive of the rationale and process. Law enforcement officers have valuable information to assist security personnel in determining the need for this restrictive policy.

Documentation

Another key policy issue that deserves attention is the process for documenting, reporting, and tracking violent acts within the clinical area. The number of verbal and physical assaults against health care workers is grossly underestimated due to inconsistent reporting. In fact, many clinical staff, especially emergency care providers, do not even think to report incidents. Many nurses and physicians believe that the abuse, both verbal and physical, is a component of the job! A concise, factual approach for identifying incidents of violence should be developed in each facility. Local, regional, and national data are essential to measuring the

Exhibit 18–4 Sample Policy on Levels of Security

Level One

Designated when:

- There is little or no threat present in the emergency department.

Security measures:

- Security officer is posted at the emergency department entrance to provide surveillance.

Level Two

Designated when:

- A patient is admitted to the emergency department who is a victim of violence.
- Agitated or hostile family members accompany a patient to the emergency department.
- Persons arrive who have indicators that arouse suspicion such as drugs and/or drug paraphernalia, or multiple alias names.
- An object is sighted that has the potential to be used as a weapon (a baseball bat, brass knuckles, etc.).

Security measures:

- The person noting the threat informs the security officer and the head/charge nurse.
- The security officer informs the security supervisor of the potential threat.
- If the person is a victim of violence, the patient is placed on protective status. The social worker explains the protective status designation to the patient's family and obtains the name of three designated visitors and one clergy. All other family members are asked to leave.
- The security officer, security supervisor, and the head/charge nurse assess the situation and determine if additional measures are warranted.
- The head/charge nurse informs the nursing and medical staff in the emergency department of the threat, if appropriate.
- The security officer closely monitors all persons entering the area. All persons other than designated visitors are referred to the security officer, who informs those persons that there is no information on the patient and asks that they leave.

Level Three

Designated when:

- A victim of violence is admitted to the emergency department who is attracting a great deal of media and/or community attention.
- Multiple family members arrive who are having difficulty controlling their behavior.
- Overt or covert threats have been directed at the staff, security, and/or visitors.
- Two victims of violence who were injured in the same incident are admitted to the emergency department.
- St. Louis police officers advise the staff that the patient or visitors have a history of disruptive or violent behavior.

Security measures:

- The emergency department security officer and the head/charge nurse are alerted by the person noting the threat.
- The administrator on duty (AOD) is notified and arrives at the emergency department.
- The security supervisor and the security dispatcher are notified, and additional security officers are requested. The supervisor will respond to assess the circumstances.

continues

Exhibit 18–4 continued

- Additional security personnel report to the emergency department and are assigned duties by the security supervisor.
- The social worker and/or the AOD approach the persons who are presenting the threat and attempt to arrive at resolution. When appropriate, the persons who present the threat are asked to leave the area. If they refuse to leave, they are detained for the St. Louis police.

Level Four

Designated when:

- The security supervisor, the AOD, and the head/charge nurse have determined that a level three situation is escalating out of control, and the persons presenting the threat refuse to leave.
- A gun or knife is sighted.
- An act of violence occurs in the emergency area.

Security measures:

- The head/charge nurse and all emergency department staff are informed of the level four security designation.
- Bystanders are removed to an area of safety. The persons presenting the threat are taken to the quiet room, and all staff members proceed to the treatment area. All access doors to the treatment area are locked.
- If not present, the AOD is notified and arrives at the emergency department.
- If not present, the security supervisor is notified, and additional security personnel are requested. Additional security officers are posted under the direction of the security supervisor.
- The persons presenting the threat are removed by security officers upon the authorization of the security supervisor.
- The security supervisor or his designee notifies the St. Louis police department.
- An emergency medical service ambulance may be diverted only by order of the AOD/attending physician/charge nurse.

---

magnitude of the problem and soliciting the necessary resources for reducing the risks associated with emergency care.

Clearly, experience has enlightened security and clinical personnel on the violence associated with EDs. However, regardless of the facts, many departments struggle to convince health care facility administration to support a dedicated security program in the ED. It is imperative that facility leaders collaborate to "sell," develop, implement, and maintain a proactive security program that tries to anticipate and prevent violence, not just respond to it. A facility must protect its greatest assets—its staff members and customers.

CONCLUSION

Violence will continue to be a major concern for EDs in the next century. An individualized, strategic, collaborative, and proactive security plan is important. No one security measure will create a totally risk-free department, yet a combination of well-planned strategies will reduce acts of aggression and make staff, patients, and visitors feel safer. Without hesitation, the time to act has arrived.

KEY POINTS

- Securing the ED involves a team approach.
- Violence takes many forms, from spousal abuse to gang-related shootings.
- Health care facilities, and in particular EDs, should be "safe havens," but often they are not.
- A security assessment should be made of an ED at least annually.
- Good ED design can reduce the potential for violence.
- Electronic security equipment can assist in deterring and preventing violence.
- ED staff and security officers should learn techniques for defusing violence.
- Nursing and security must communicate clearly about security matters.

REFERENCES

1. C.W. Schwab, "Violence: America's Uncivil War," *Journal of Trauma 25,* no. 5 (1993): 657–663.
2. J. Fox, *Homicide Trends in the United States* (U.S. Department of Justice—Bureau of Justice Statistics, 1998), 2–15.
3. New York Times News Service, *Crime Rates Dropping Nationwide* (February 1998): 2–15. www.crl.com.
4. T. Morganthau, "The Lull Before the Storm," *Newsweek* (December 4, 1995): 40–42.
5. J. Vest, L. James, W. Cohn, and M. Thorp, "Aggressive Driving and Road Rage: Dealing with Emotionally Impaired Drivers," *www.drivers.com* (July 17, 1997): 1–20.
6. W. Max and D. Rice, "Shooting in the Dark: Estimating the Cost of Firearm Injuries," *Health Affairs 12,* no. 4 (1993): 171–185.
7. T. Miller, M. Cohen, and S. Rossman, "Victim Costs of Violent Crime and Resulting Injuries," *Health Affairs 12,* no. 4 (1993): 186–197.
8. G. Warchol, "Bureau of Justice—National Crime Victimization Survey," *Bureau of Justice Special Report* (1998): 1–8.
9. Emergency Nurses Association, *Violence in the Workplace* (1995): 1–23.
10. F. Jackson and R. Flinn, "The Emergency Room View on Violence," *Security Management* (1994): 25–30.
11. 1996 Barnes-Jewish Hospital Annual Report.

Chapter 19

Psychiatric Unit Security

CHAPTER OBJECTIVES

1. Know the various types of psychiatric units.
2. Understand how security may be used in psychiatric units.
3. Recognize the key security issues for psychiatric units.

INTRODUCTION

Hospitals use many different names and organizational structures for psychiatric units. Each structure has strict licensing requirements.

- **Behavioral sciences unit.** One that treats all levels of patients, those admitted on both a voluntary basis and an involuntary basis. The only general exception are those deemed criminally insane.
- **Therapeutic community.** Normally treats only patients admitted on a voluntary basis. Usually, these units will not accept patients that have a potential for violence.
- **Adult (or juvenile) full (or partial) services.** These programs are normally either full (all day) or partial (part of a day). In these programs, the patient normally does not stay overnight at the facility but receives treatment during normal business hours.

Regardless of the type of program offered, the psychiatric unit—like the emergency department (see Chapter 18)—is an area where security can truly work hand in hand with caregivers to assist the patient. The psychiatric unit should have a direct communication link to security in an emergency. Security personnel should be trained by the unit staff on how to respond and assist in an emergency. There are many ways that security may assist in patient care in a psychiatric unit.

- They often assist in patient restraint, keeping patients from hurting themselves or others.
- If the patient is committed involuntarily, security normally escorts the patient and the law enforcement officer with custody of the patient to the psychiatric unit.
- Security may be called upon to help train staff in methods of verbal de-escalation or search techniques.

- Security may be asked to assist in securing the psychiatric unit and to provide security during recreation and patient walks around the property.

This chapter will discuss key security issues in psychiatric units. While reading the chapter, readers may think of additional ways that security can be utilized in psychiatric units.

EMPLOYEE SCREENING

The facility must make sure that employees hired to work in psychiatric units do not have any history of violence or sexual offenses. Initial background checks should be performed at the hiring stage (see Chapter 17). In addition, employees working in this sensitive area should have their criminal background rechecked at least every three years, or if circumstances warrant.

EMPLOYEE TRAINING

After the proper employees have been selected, the facility must provide training for the employees. The facility should not rely on the fact that an employee has worked at another facility and should have received adequate training there. The facility will be held accountable for staff training and education, regardless of the employee's previous training, if an incident occurs. A psychiatric unit's employee training program should cover certain important topics: patient confidentiality, abuse and neglect, recognition and de-escalation of aggression, elopement risks, and suicide risks.

Patient Confidentiality

Unfortunately, those who seek treatment for mental or emotional problems are still viewed negatively by some people. It is absolutely essential that staff understand and adhere to the facility's confidentiality policy. All employees working in the psychiatric units should re-sign the hospital's confidentiality statement during their review each year.

Many psychiatric units assign code numbers to patients. If someone calls or comes to the unit to see or inquire about a patient, only those who have been given the code number by the patient will gain access or information. If the patient has a protracted stay, the code number should be changed at least every 30 days.

Abuse and Neglect

The psychiatric unit, like the rest of the facility, must have a policy against any form of patient abuse or neglect. Abuse and neglect can be defined in many ways (see Chapter 26).

At the least, abuse consists of kicking, slapping, pushing too hard, making any sexual contact, and using profanity or making insults. Likewise, the inappropriate use of physical restraints and withholding of food, drink, or proper clothing cannot be tolerated.

All staff must understand that working on a psychiatric unit can be extremely stressful. The staff must feel comfortable talking with their supervisor if they feel the stress is more than they can tolerate. Some staff may need to accept a temporary transfer away from the unit, especially if a particular patient has singled out the staff person for verbal or physical abuse.

Recognition and De-escalation of Aggression

All unit employees must be trained in recognition and de-escalation of aggression. There are several nationally recognized organizations that offer such training and can provide "train the trainer" sessions, thereby making it possible for the facility to have a "certified" trainer at the facility.

Elopement Risks

All employees must understand that the possibility of patient elopement is always present. Closed-circuit television (CCTV) can help deter patient elopement. Many facilities use CCTV, with motion detectors installed within the cameras, to survey hallways after "lights out." If a patient opens his or her door or leaves his or her room, the motion detector will alarm staff. The motion detector keeps staff from having to watch the cameras at all times. Most facilities with motion detectors also utilize a VCR to record alarm activity.

Another area where elopement is always possible is during exercise or recreation. Most facilities allow patients to "earn" the right to exercise by walking in a group around the campus. They are, of course, escorted by staff members during the walks. The staff must always be in direct contact with the unit and security in case either or both are needed. Many facilities use either cell phones or radios to maintain this contact.

Suicide Risks

All staff must understand that the risk of patient suicide is always present. They should be trained to know what chemical substances a patient could ingest in a suicide attempt. Such items as paint and paint thinner, cleaning supplies, and air fresheners should be eliminated from patient care areas. Windows on the unit should be kept closed and locked (check local fire ordinances). Patients who have earned the privilege of participating in group walks should be monitored closely to ensure they do not leap into the path of a vehicle.

UNIT ENVIRONMENTAL DESIGN

Security into and out of the unit must be maintained. A barrier of protection should exist between the patient care unit and the hospital's common areas. A barrier could be several sets of locked doors, a reception area, or a waiting room. Anyone should have to go through several steps to enter or leave the unit.

The nurses' station should be designed to help keep staff and patients safe. It should be self-contained and accessible through a locked entrance. Even in this secure area, staff must be vigilant in keeping sharp objects (e.g., pens, pencils, scissors) out of sight. The location of the nurses' station must afford staff a clear view of all hallways, either by direct line of sight or with the use of CCTV. Staff should be aware that water fountains, pay phones, paintings, and almost all recreational items can be used as weapons.

The unit itself should be reviewed to make sure that all electrical outlets are secured with tamper-proof screws and that all shower rods and air vents are the "break away" type. In addition, all doorways should open into the common area, preventing patients from barricading themselves in a room. All furnishings on the unit should be flame-retardant and either constructed of lightweight material or bolted to the floor. This will prevent the furniture from being set on fire and/or being used as a weapon.

The design and settings of interview and treatment rooms should be reviewed. Furniture should be arranged so that the staff member sits between the patient and the doorway. This gives the staff member quicker egress if the patient becomes violent. The doors to all interview and treatment rooms should open into the common area and not into the room. The rooms should be equipped with emergency alarms, and the staff should carry pocket alarms going to the nurses' station that can be used in an emergency. Some interview rooms are separated from an adjoining office by a two-way mirror. In the other room, staff can observe interviews being conducted and can quickly assist if there is a violent episode.

PREPARATION FOR FIRES

All units should be equipped with a fire suppression system. This system should be linked to the facility's main system but activate only sprinkler areas in the psychiatric unit. Staff should have preassigned duties during an actual fire or fire drill. They should decide in advance who will be stationed at the doors, who will notify the patients, where the patients will go, and what accounting procedure will be used to ensure that all patients are present. The fire alarms on the unit should be secured to prevent patients, especially those in juvenile units, from setting off the alarms.

Staff should carry keys to the unit entrance, windows, patient rooms, and interview and treatment rooms. They must be drilled on the time it takes them to "unlock" the unit, and a definite evacuation plan must be established.

SEARCHES

The unit must have a formal search policy that addresses search upon admission, upon return from off-unit activity, and at any time there is a reasonable suspicion that a weapon or contraband is present. During the admission process, the patient must be told that in addition to weapons and drugs, the following personal items are prohibited: ties, belts, knives, letter openers, scissors, any smoking material, and any other items that the staff believe could be used as a threat to the patient or others.

Searches should be conducted by at least two staff members. All items confiscated from the patient must be listed on a patient valuables inventory form and either stored for safekeeping or sent home with a family member.

During a search, staff must check the patient and all containers, i.e., suitcases, purses, etc. Staff should also open the tops of all containers such as hair spray and shaving cream dispensers to ensure that drugs are not hidden in these containers.

WEAPONS

The unit must have a policy prohibiting weapons from being brought onto the unit. Most locked units have a "gun box" located outside the door. Law enforcement officers can place their weapons inside the box, lock the box, and retain the key while doing their business on the unit.

Staff must understand that many items can become weapons. Ashtrays, clipboards, keys, books, and furniture can all be used as weapons. Plastic spoons, forks, and knives must be used on the unit. Drinking containers and serving utensils should also be made of plastic.

RESTRAINTS

The facility must have a policy on who can initiate a patient restraint. Many units ask the physician of record to write a standing restraint order. If a patient must be restrained, all concerned must remember that a patient restraint is a medical procedure, not a punitive action. If security staff are called to assist in the restraint, they must be instructed and supervised by a medical staff member who also is taking an active part in the restraint.

Patients can be restrained using sheets, leather restraints, or restraint clothing. They can also be placed in a seclusion room. This room should be completely empty, with padded walls and floor. The ceiling should be secure and not of a "drop-type" construction. If a patient is placed in a seclusion room, he or she should remain under observation.

After a patient restraint event, those involved with the restraint should spend a few minutes critiquing the event. Was there anything that could have been done to avoid having to restrain the patient? Did anyone become angry during the restraint? Was the correct restraint method used? Remember, restraints are a medical procedure and should ultimately help the patient.

VISITATION

The unit must establish a visitation policy that is appropriate for the types of patients on the unit. The patients and their family members must understand that all visitors to the unit are subject to search. Too often, weapons or drugs are brought to patients by visitors.

KEY POINTS

- There are several different types of psychiatric units.
- Employees of these units must be thoroughly screened.
- Staff should be trained to recognize and avoid abuse or neglect of patients and to recognize the steps of aggression.
- The unit's physical design should be considered to assist in reducing the potential for assaults and other threats of violence.
- Security can assist on these units by helping with patient restraints, detecting weapons, and escorting law enforcement to the units.
- These units must maintain high levels of confidentiality and control visitation.

Chapter 20

Home Care

CHAPTER OBJECTIVES

1. Understand what steps may be taken to reduce home health employee theft.
2. Know the steps to take prior to a visit to increase staff security.
3. Know the steps staff can take during travel to the home to be more secure.
4. Understand what security procedures should be followed during a home health visit.

INTRODUCTION

There is no doubt that home health care is a major component of an integrated health care system. As lengths of stay in health care facilities decline, managed care organizations place more emphasis on outpatient and home care.

Under the traditional patient care delivery system, the patient comes into a controlled environment, but in home health, the caregiver goes into an unknown and sometimes uncontrolled environment. Certain security issues arise in home health care, including staff stealing from patients, staff getting into automobile accidents, staff getting robbed, and staff confronting violence in the patient's home. How can the health care security professional address these issues effectively? The first step is to recognize that these problems occur. Specific mention is even made of home health care in the Occupational Safety and Health Administration's guideline 3148. Likewise, there have been countless articles in home health journals concerning security. However, in most cases security professionals will spearhead education in this area. This chapter will help security professionals to address these issues. The chapter will be divided into two sections, internal security issues and external security issues.

INTERNAL SECURITY ISSUES

Employment-Related Issues

The employment screening process is critical to security in home health care. Most home health agencies utilize a variety of staff in delivering care, depending upon the need and medical condition of the patient. Nonlicensed personnel assist patients in minor nonmedical needs, such as bathing or dressing. Certified nursing assistants care for minor medical needs.

271

Licensed practical nurses or registered nurses handle more advanced medical care. When hiring licensed personnel, home health care agencies must verify that the applicants have a current and valid license. However, even licensed personnel may not be honest.

In one case, a registered nurse working for a home health agency was stealing personal checks from patients and writing these checks to friends. Upon investigation, after this person had forged thousands of dollars in checks, the agency discovered that the nurse had nursing licenses in multiple states and was licensed in no less than five different names. The nurse left town prior to being arrested and escaped prosecution. The agency not only suffered adverse publicity but was sued by the victims, who claimed negligent hiring, supervision, and retention.

Regardless of the status of the employee, a thorough criminal background check must be completed. Most states require that a home health agency conduct a criminal background check on home health workers. Most agencies conduct these checks through state criminal history repositories. There are problems in conducting these checks.

- In many states, it takes a long time to receive the criminal check back from the repository.
- In most states, counties are required to communicate to the repository only felony convictions and not misdemeanor convictions. Therefore, a state criminal check may not reveal that a person was convicted of misdemeanor assault or petty theft. The agencies should also conduct a criminal record check of all the counties in which the person has lived and worked for the past five years. While this may seem like a time-consuming and costly process, it could help the agency escape problems in the future.

Home health care agencies sometimes subcontract with temporary agencies for employees. In most states, contracting with a temporary agency does not relieve the home health agency from the responsibility for conducting a thorough criminal background investigation. Likewise, in most states, home health agencies are required to conduct the preemployment background check themselves, not through contract with an investigation agency. Agencies should consult with their attorney concerning their requirements under the law.

Employee Misconduct

Most home health workers receive little if any day-to-day supervision. While most employees do an excellent job, incidents (e.g., stealing supplies, padding mileage, recording visits that never took place) do occur. It is critical that these incidents be investigated with the help of law enforcement if necessary. In addition, the agency must administer fair, consistent discipline.

> In one facility, a nurse aide was selling her patient's visit schedule to an organized group that would show up at a patient's home unannounced. They would claim that the physician had requested the visit and would then collect money from the patient. In several cases they also stole property from the patients. In another case, a home health nurse was stealing drugs and other supplies from the agency. Because the agency did not control its supplies well, she was able to commit these thefts for a period of several years before being discovered.

Patient Visit Issues

Planning for a safe patient visit begins with teaching staff to identify and avoid potential problems. Prescreening visits and visit scheduling will help reduce potential problems.

Prescreening

All patients should be thoroughly screened prior to a visit. Any history of drug abuse, domestic violence, or other problems should be noted. The area where the patient lives should also be evaluated. Does it have a lot of crime, especially violent crime? Health care workers may want to ask a member of the local police department to accompany them to homes in high-crime areas or with potentially violent patients. Home care workers with agencies that are part of an integrated health care system can ask for assistance from members of the health care facility's security department instead.

It is important that the health care worker have specific and clear instructions to the patient's home. If possible, the employee and a supervisor may want to visit the home at the same time of day as the visit will occur. They can see the area and talk with the patient and learn of anything that might endanger the health care worker.

Scheduling

Even though the visits are scheduled, to help ensure safety and efficiency, it is best to call the home just prior to the visit. If the home is in an area known for high crime or drugs, health care workers should schedule the visit for as early in the day as possible. In addition, on the way to the home, they should contact the local police and let them know they are going to the area and will call them from the home.

Other Safety Tips

Staff members should be provided with a cellular telephone. The agency should have sound policies governing the use of the phone. For example, a policy that states that the phone should be used only when the car is parked in a secure area, except in an emergency, is valid. There have been numerous times an agency has been sued after a staff member trying to drive and talk on the cell phone at the same time had an accident. The policy should spell out how many minutes of air time per month staff are allowed to use for personal calls.

Staff should keep all equipment in a nursing bag in the trunk of the vehicle when the equipment is not in use. They should carry only the supplies needed for that day's visits.

Staff should be discouraged from wearing jewelry or carrying purses. They should carry only a small amount of cash and a driver's license.

EXTERNAL SECURITY ISSUES

Staff Security on the Road

Most home health care workers are dedicated professionals who care deeply about their patients and strive to deliver quality medical care. But they must remain safe. Staff should learn to trust their instincts. Whenever they feel that they are not safe, they should leave the area and call their supervisor. Team meetings to discuss safety and security should be held regularly. Managers should encourage staff to talk openly and freely about their concerns.

Most home health staff spend at least 50 percent of their time traveling between the office and patients' homes. They need to receive documented training on security away from the office. One excellent video for this type of training is distributed by Communicorp in Lombard, Illinois, and called Away From the Office: Personal Safety for Homecare Professionals.

Staff should be given the following instructions:

- Keep the vehicle doors locked at all times.
- Keep the windows up. If they must be lowered for ventilation, make sure only the driver's window is lowered one-half inch or less.
- Keep the vehicle in good working order. Have it checked regularly by a trusted mechanic. Also, keep an eye on the gas gauge, filling up when there is at least one-quarter of a tank left. Attempt to fill up at your regular service station where you know and trust the surroundings.
- When going to your vehicle, have your keys in your hand prior to going outside. Walk straight to the vehicle, staying aware of your surroundings. Upon reaching the vehicle, look under the vehicle and in the interior of the car before entering. Enter and quickly lock the door behind you.
- Watch the traffic as you are en route. If you feel you are being followed, drive to the nearest safe haven (e.g., police department, fire station, public area) and call the police.
- When arriving at the patient's home, park in a well-lit area if at or near dark. Observe the area closely before exiting the vehicle. Are there groups of people who make you feel uncomfortable? Are you being watched? If anything makes you feel uneasy, leave, call the patient, and ask that a family member meet you at your car. If you still feel unsafe, call the office and reschedule the visit.
- Make sure everything you need for the visit is already in your carry bag. Do not be caught off guard, bent over looking in your trunk with your back exposed and unprotected. Again, preplanning the visits is vital for safety.
- Exit your vehicle quickly, locking the door and carrying the keys in your hand. Walk confidently to the patient's front door, constantly looking around.
- When reaching the patient's door, listen for signs of trouble. If you hear an argument, leave at once. If everything sounds normal, ring the bell, listening to make sure it is

working. As you wait for the door to be answered, recheck the area. If no one answers the door in a reasonable period of time, do not search for the patient. Do not knock on other doors. Instead, go back to the vehicle and call the patient using the cellular phone. If you get no answer, leave the area at once. Call the office, and ask the police to investigate. Never enter a patient's home without someone greeting you. There have been numerous instances where a home health worker walked into a burglary, domestic assault, or other dangerous situation.

- Drive defensively. If you are involved in an accident, stay in the car until the police arrive, unless it is unsafe.[1]

Carjacking

Carjacking is on the rise. Women traveling alone are especially vulnerable. Since home health care staff spend so much time on the road, they should learn special security tips related to carjacking.

- Always keep your doors locked and windows rolled up.
- Always be observant of the road and people around the vehicle. Try to travel in the middle lane, and always leave at least a car space between you and the car in front when stopping at a red light. This space will give you some maneuvering room in case of an attack. Be especially observant for individuals loitering at street corners. One of the commonly used tactics is to throw a brick through the passenger window. As the driver shields him- or herself from the flying glass, the suspect reaches in the vehicle and grabs items from the front seat. Any item that must be carried in the vehicle should be placed under the dash, on the floor of the passenger front seat. This will keep the item from being visible to outsiders.
- If your vehicle is bumped from behind, stay in the vehicle. Most carjackers work in teams. One will bump your car with a vehicle. When you exit to observe the damage, another member will jump into your car and drive away.
- Never stop to assist at an accident scene unless the police are there. Likewise, never pick up a hitchhiker.
- Preset the speed dial on the cellular phone to the police (911 in most areas).

On the Street

In many areas, staff members travel by public transportation to the patient's home. Instruct staff to stay alert while on the street.

- When using public transportation, try to sit across from the door, close enough to escape if necessary, but far enough away so that thieves cannot reach in and grab your belongings. When waiting for the bus or train, keep the nursing bag on your shoulder with the flap toward your body. Beware of pickpockets!
- Know ahead of time where you need to get off the bus or train.
- When walking on the street, keep your head up while maintaining eye contact with people. Do not stare, but let people know you see them.

- Walk in the middle of the street when possible. Avoid blind corners, alleys, hedges, vacant lots, and so on.
- Walk around crowds. If necessary, cross the street to avoid walking through a group.
- Avoid lengthy conversations with people on the street. Do not get caught up in answering people's questions. Keep your mind on your surroundings. Never give out personal or business information.
- When entering elevators, stand at least five feet away from the doors when they open. Make sure the elevator is safe (level and working) before entering. If someone in the elevator makes you feel uncomfortable, exit quickly and wait for the next elevator. Refrain from using the stairways. They are soundproof and offer little chance of escape.
- Along the route, note the location of pay phones and safe havens.
- If at any time you feel you are being followed, quickly walk to the nearest business and call the office and the police.

In the Home

Due to the nature of home health, staff members are in homes and privy to family problems and activities. Staff members should avoid lengthy discussions about family problems and never take sides on an issue. Sometimes, however, staff members can find themselves in the wrong place at the wrong time.

Domestic Disputes

Home care employees should not attempt to intercede in a family argument or conflict. These situations can become violent in seconds. At the first sign of trouble, staff members should leave the home and inform the family that a return visit will be scheduled. Staff members should never try to referee a situation.

Firearms

Many of the homes that staff members visit will have firearms in them. It is not uncommon for patients to keep firearms beside their beds. During previsit conversations, the agency should instruct the patient that all firearms must be secured prior to a visit. If a firearm is present when the staff member arrives, the staff member should tell the family that for the visit to continue the weapon must be secured. If the weapon is not secured, the staff member should leave.

Use of Drugs or Alcohol

Both drug and alcohol use present problems for home health staff. If staff members see illegal drugs in a home, staff members should leave at once and call the office. The patient must be informed that no other visits will be made unless the person using illegal drugs leaves during the visit. A supervisor should accompany the staff member during the next visit and explain to the patient and family that if illegal drugs are present during future visits, visits will be discontinued and the police notified. Likewise, if there is excessive use of alcohol by a family member during the visit, staff should leave and schedule another visit, during which they should be accompanied by a supervisor.

Large Groups in the Home

Many home health workers tell stories of visiting homes where large groups of people are sleeping on the floor and couches and trying to recover from the previous night's party. Many recount stories of groups having sex and using drugs while they are present. Sometimes, multiple generations of family members may live at the same residence. With too many people and too much confusion, rendering care may be impossible. If this is the case, the agency must inform the family that some of the members must leave the home while the visit is taking place.

Talk It Out

Staff members should be encouraged to leave homes if difficult situations arise. Sometimes it is better for them to offer an excuse rather than just walking out. Some excuses will serve well.

- The staff member left a piece of equipment in the car or at the office.
- The employee received notice of an emergency on the beeper and must go to another patient.
- The employee feels sick and must leave.

CONCLUSION

The mission of home health is to deliver quality medical care. No one wants a staff member to neglect this responsibility. However, a staff member's safety should never be compromised. If a particular situation is too dangerous, the agency should contact the physician and social services to see if other arrangements for care can be made.

The security professional will find more challenges in the area of home health as medical care becomes more decentralized and home health care grows. Security professionals would do well to ride along with home health staff members and learn firsthand about the variety of situations they encounter.

KEY POINTS

- There are both internal and external aspects of home health care security.
- Agencies interviewing applicants for home health care positions should do thorough criminal history background checks.
- Home health care patients should be prescreened to see if they may be violent.
- Staff should be able to adjust the time of day or night that visits are made to assist in their protection.
- Staff must be taught security techniques to use while on the road, on the street, and in the home.

REFERENCE

1. J. Moran, *Away From the Office: Personal Safety for Homecare Professionals* (Lombard, IL: Communicorp, 1995). Videotape.

Chapter 21

Bomb Threats

CHAPTER OBJECTIVES

1. Know how to minimize the likelihood that a bomb will be placed at a facility.
2. Understand why planning is the key to a successful bomb threat assessment.
3. Know how to train switchboard operators on what to do if a bomb-related call is received.
4. Understand how to evaluate the call.
5. Know proper facility search procedures.
6. Be able to evacuate an area effectively.
7. Be able to properly conduct a debriefing session.

INTRODUCTION

LOCATION: Large urban medical center in metropolitan area
DATE/TIME: January 10, 1998, 2:00 p.m.
CALL RECEIVED AT SWITCHBOARD: "There is a bomb in the building. It's going to explode in 20 minutes."

LOCATION: Mid-sized medical center on the East Coast
DATE /TIME: June 15, 1998, 1:30 p.m.
CALL RECEIVED AT SWITCHBOARD: "You let my father die. Now a bomb will blow all of you to hell."

LOCATION: Small rural hospital
DATE/TIME: November 25, 1998, 9:00 p.m.
CALL RECEIVED AT SWITCHBOARD: "There is a bomb in one of the mechanical rooms. It will go off in 2 hours. Get the patients out; they don't deserve to die. I only want to destroy the hospital." A few minutes later, a call is received at the local police department emergency number: "Get the patients out of the hospital; there is a bomb in the building."

How should facilities respond to each of these calls? Which is most likely to be real?

Unfortunately, hundreds of bomb threats are called in to medical facilities each year. Fortunately, very few are real. How the facility reacts to the calls has a direct bearing on not only the safety of patients, visitors, and staff but the likelihood of other calls being received. Is it possible to reduce or eliminate bomb threat calls?

- Facilities can never totally eliminate these calls, but there is much facilities can do to reduce the frequency of the calls.
- There are no absolutes in evaluating bomb threat calls, but preplanning and understanding the characteristics of serious bombers and hoaxers can help determine the proper course of action.

The facility can reduce the chance of a call being made by reducing the chance that a real bomb could be placed in the facility. If a hoaxer knows that the facility has taken steps to prevent the possibility of a real bomb being placed, he or she will be less likely to place a call, knowing that the call will not produce dramatic results.

How can a facility prevent a bomb from being placed in the facility? Staff education and planning for a call are the keys. For instance, all staff should always be vigilant, keeping closets locked, being observant for any foreign object that is not accounted for, and calling security (not touching the object) if a foreign object is present. In patient care areas, staff should recognize which patients' family dynamics could lead to violence. Administration should make sure that trash is removed from public areas in a timely manner and that restrooms are checked frequently.

The perimeter of the facility should be secure. Trash dumpsters should be locked, closed, and set back from the facility. All deliveries should be supervised, and all points of access should be controlled. Security should maintain a high profile and frequently patrol common areas of the facility.

If a call is received, knowing how to react can reduce the chance that future calls will come in. In addition, proper planning can help a facility continue its routine business with as little interruption as possible after a call comes in.

THE PLAN

Without a comprehensive plan, the facility has only two choices: (1) ignore the call or (2) panic. A comprehensive plan should help facility leaders make rational decisions. The facility must have planned, orderly responses to these calls.

There should be a comprehensive bomb threat plan that has been distributed to all managers (see Exhibit 21–1 for a brief sample bomb threat procedure from a health care facility). Since it is expected that the plan will be used infrequently and there is employee turnover, the plan should be reviewed at least every six months in a managers' forum. The plan should be developed in conjunction with local law enforcement. If the facility is located in an area that could be determined to be a site of political or social unrest, state and federal law enforcement should be contacted for their input.

A complete plan should name the responsibilities of key personnel. In addition, the plan should delegate authority to one person. This person should be the staff member most knowledgeable about the plan and bomb threats. Normally the coordinator of the event is either the

Exhibit 21–1 Sample Bomb Threat Procedure

In the event that a bomb threat is received by the hospital, it is important that standard procedure be established for personnel to follow. The following five-phase program is intended to minimize the dangers of a bomb threat.

   I. **Receipt of Warning.** It is anticipated that threats will be received by the hospital switchboard. For this reason, a form has been prepared for the operator to use in the event of a bomb threat. However, all department heads and clinical directors should be aware of some basic procedures when a call of this type is received.
   - Prolong the conversation as much as possible.
   - Be alert to distinguishing background noises such as music, voices, aircraft, and so on.
   - Note any distinguishing voice characteristics.
   - Ask where the bomb will explode and at what time.
   - Note if the caller indicates knowledge of the hospital by his or her description of the bomb's location.
   - Make a written note of everything the caller says.

   As soon as the call is received, the following people should be notified:
   - The security department, which will notify the police and fire departments by dialing 911
   - The administrator on call or the administrative coordinator if at night, or during the evening

   Experience has shown that publicity generates threats, and for this reason publicity should be limited.

   II. **Search Procedure.** The police will assume control of the situation as soon as they arrive. They should be taken to the security office to direct the search.
   - The police and fire departments will need the assistance of qualified employees. The administrative officer will utilize security officers and maintenance employees to assist in the search.
   - The building will be divided into sections, with specific personnel assigned to search each section. Public areas such as lobbies, stairwells, restrooms, and so on should be covered first. The last places searched should be areas that are locked and unavailable to the public.
   - If you find what appears to be a bomb, **Do not touch it.** Clear the area quietly and obtain professional assistance. Isolate the object as much as possible by closing doors.
   - Do not tell patients or visitors about the bomb threats. If they are aware of the threat, assure them that all is well.

   III. **Evacuation.** The senior administrative officer, chief of the medical staff (or an alternate), and the senior police department official on the scene should decide together whether to evacuate all or part of the hospital.

   IV. **Communications.** The security office will serve as the communications center. All reports from search teams should be called in to this area. An administrator (or nursing supervisor during off-hours) will be available to answer calls and control general activities from this location. The administrator on duty may move the control center if more space is needed for secretarial support.

continues

Exhibit 21–1 continued

V. **General Information.**
- When a nursing floor is notified of a bomb threat, staff should immediately close doors to patient rooms. Staff should stand by for specific instructions.
- Any threat received by the hospital will be assumed to be legitimate. Evacuation will be used as a last resort due to the threat it poses to the welfare of patients.
- It is the responsibility of all employees to react to this type of situation in a calm and professional manner. The welfare of patients depends upon prompt action by employees.

administrator or the security director. The plan should also appoint alternates for off-hours and weekends. While all managers should have copies of the plan for response to a bomb threat call, the coordinator and alternates must have recent copies readily available. These plans must be in an easy-to-read checklist format.

In addition to establishing the responsibilities of key personnel, the plan should establish the location of a command center as well as name an alternate location. Most facilities establish the command center in one of three locations: the security command center, the administration board room, or an office adjacent to or near the emergency department. The command center must be easily accessed by outside authorities and be large enough to accommodate emergency personnel and coordinate the search activities. Phones, facility floor plans, and emergency power must be provided in the command center.

THE CALL

Most bomb threat calls are received through the facility switchboard. However, it is not uncommon for a call to be received in one department. If a call is received in a department, it may provide a clue as to the validity of the call. Have there been any patients or family that verbalized any threats, or has an employee recently been terminated? The main difficulty with calls being received in one department is one of training. It is almost impossible to train all employees, especially with facility turnover, on how to properly receive and process a bomb threat call. Inservices can help, but the key is training the managers.

If the call is received at the switchboard, the operators must be trained in how to process the call. They should have a preprinted checklist visible at their station (see Exhibit 21–2). For example, the operators should speak in a clear, calm voice and try to keep the caller on the line as long as possible. While doing so, the operator should be able to alert other operators about the nature of the call. If one-party taping is permitted in the state, the call should be audiotaped. The call should also be traced if possible. The operator should try to write down the caller's exact words and listen for an accent and other speech characteristics and background noises. The operator should try to solicit as much information from the caller as possible. What type of bomb is it? What does it look like? Where is the bomb? (The operator should try to get as exact a location as possible.) When will the bomb explode? Why did the caller plant the bomb? All of these bits of information help determine if the call is a hoax or real.

Exhibit 21–2 Bomb Threat Call Checklist (To Be Completed by the Person Receiving the Call)

Time/date received _____   Time/date reported _____

How reported   _____

Exact words of caller   _____

Questions to ask:

1. When is the bomb going to explode? _____

2. Where is the bomb right now?   _____

3. What kind of bomb is it?   _____

4. What does it look like?   _____

5. Why did you place the bomb?   _____

6. From where are you calling?   _____

Description of caller's voice:

Male _____ Female _____ Young _____ Middle aged _____ Old _____

Accent _____ Tone of voice _____ Background noise _____

Is voice familiar?   _____ If so, who did it sound like?   _____

Other voice characteristics _____ Time caller hung up _____ Remarks _____

Name, address, phone of call recipient: _____

For the most part, **real bombers do not call.** But if they do call, operators will know it. Real bombers will usually be calm, since the peak of emotion for the bomber is placing the bomb, while the hoaxer's emotion peaks during the placing of the call. The real bomber will usually give details about the location of the bomb. Likewise, the bomber will be proud of the bomb and may elaborate about the type and size of the bomb. Remember, the bomber is a criminal who has chosen a particular type of weapon to commit a crime. The hoaxer, on the other hand, may be more of a terrorist, in that hoaxers seek to disrupt and frighten. Table 21–1 lists differences between bombers and hoaxers.

Notification

After the call or, if possible, while the caller is still on the line, notification of key personnel must begin. Remember, in some cases there are only minutes until the time the caller stated the bomb will explode. Who should be notified? There must be internal as well as external notification.

Internal Notification

The process of internal notification is spelled out by the bomb threat emergency plan. Normally, the administrator, security director, plant manager, risk manager, director of nursing,

Table 21–1 Bombers and Hoaxers Compared

Trait	Bomber	Hoaxer
Has acquired knowledge of explosives	yes	no
Has acquired material	yes	no
Has constructed the device	yes	no
Has placed the device inside the facility	yes	no
Knows about where to place the bomb in the facility for maximum effect	yes	no
Will discuss the type of and reason for the bomb (is proud of the bomb)	yes	no

and public relations department are notified. Most facilities have a "calling tree" established for quick notification (each person who is called then calls two more people, and so on down the tree). Emergency calling trees must take into account off-hours, weekends, holidays, and vacations.

External Notification

Local law enforcement, the fire department, and emergency medical services must be notified. It is best if the bomb threat emergency plan has established a code to be used for this type of call. If not, then members of the media, who always monitor the police radio frequencies, will hurry to the facility and may impede the plan. In the bomb threat emergency plan, it should be established that only one law enforcement officer (hopefully a supervisor) will respond directly to the facility at a predetermined location. The fire department and emergency medical services should not respond directly to the facility but should stage themselves one or two blocks away. Because hoaxers like to see that their call has produced confusion and panic, a low-key approach is appropriate. This low-key approach also serves if the call happens to be real. If the caller is a legitimate bomber, then the minimal response will probably prompt the caller to call again. This time the caller will be more adamant and give more information to try to get the facility to evacuate.

Call Evaluation

In evaluating the call, the coordinator must consider some threat analysis factors.

- **Content of the threat message.** A real bomber will know the technology used, the precise location, how the bomb was placed, and when it will explode. In many cases, the bomber will volunteer this information to the operator.
- **Nature of target environment.** Are there any intra-facility tensions or controversies? Are there any social, political, or moral issues involved? Is there major construction at the site? Has there been a union strike, major layoff, or change in management?
- **Practicality of the threat.** Could the threat be carried out as described?
- **Timing of the threat.** Any particular events or activities planned at the time of the threat? Any significance—historic or otherwise—of the date? Does the threat come right at shift change (this could mean an employee placed the call)?
- **Responses available.** What type of response can be made within the given time frame?

- **Risk philosophy.** How much risk is the facility willing to accept? When should the facility be evacuated, a process with its own dangers?
- **Nature of area occupants.** Are the patients ambulatory? Are surgeries in progress? How many staff will be needed to assist the patients?

Based upon these factors, the coordinator, in consultation with law enforcement, can make a rational decision. Five levels of response (1 is highest level; 5 is lowest level) can be initiated.

1. immediate emergency evacuation
2. immediate general evacuation and search
3. general search, then evacuation
4. general search without evacuation
5. cursory search without evacuation

Special Circumstances

If the caller falls into one of the following three categories, the threat should be viewed as extremely high and the facility should respond accordingly.

1. **Panicked caller.** The caller may be the bomber or a second party. There will be panic in the voice. The party will usually apologize for placing the bomb or not being able to stop the bomber. Expressions of regret and panic such as "I couldn't make him stop! I'm sorry, I didn't mean for it to go this far, just get the people out!" are common. This type of panic will be much different than the peak emotion that the hoaxer has when placing the call. This call will be profoundly more urgent sounding.
2. **Persistent caller.** After calling the health care facility, the caller will contact another entity (e.g., police department, fire department, newspaper). These callers want to make sure that the facility takes the call seriously. They may also call the facility again if they do not feel that the facility is acting quickly enough to get the inhabitants out of the building.
3. **Caller with a mental disorder.** These callers are delusional. They may tell the operator that they are bombing the facility because it is a front for the Central Intelligence Agency or that voices made them take action against the devil.

THE SEARCH

The decision to search or not search the facility is contingent on a host of factors. In all instances, at least a cursory search should be made (unless the call is so urgent that immediate emergency evacuation is made). In most other cases, a routine search should be conducted.

Cursory Search

Search team members should be trained before a search is necessary. Team members should know the area they must search. They must also know not to turn any lights on or off, to stay in contact with the command center, and to use telephones—not radios—to let the command center know when they have cleared an area.

Several search teams are needed, and these teams should be established way in advance, before a search is necessary. One team should begin searching the outside of the facility and work inward. Other teams should be assigned different floors of the facility. They should search public areas first: restrooms, cafeterias, waiting rooms, elevators, and unlocked closets that the public could access. There should be enough search teams available that all areas can be searched and sealed off in less than seven minutes. Search teams should have the following equipment:

- flashlight
- gloves
- inspection mirror, for checking under and above objects
- wooden dowel, for moving objects out of reach
- socket screwdriver
- cutting pliers

Search Methods

The searchers should be instructed to search an area from the bottom to the top and use definite search methods. The two most common are the grid and spiral methods. In the grid approach, one person searches an area back and forth horizontally, while a partner searches the same area back and forth at a right angle, thus searching the area in a grid. The searchers will overlap each other, making for an effective search. In the spiral method, one searcher starts in the middle of the search area and searches in a spiral moving outward. The partner searches from the outside in a spiral moving inward. Again, the searchers will overlap. Once an area has been searched, it should be marked and secured.

Routine Search

In routine searches, the same manner of searching applies as in cursory searches. The main difference is that once the search teams have finished searching their areas, they will be assigned to other areas of the facility. They will supervise the search of individual departments, offices, and so on. They will need the assistance of the staff who work in the area. They are looking for anything out of the ordinary. The staff know their area and will be able to spot any unusual objects quickly.

> If staff members notice a strange object in their area, they should know not to touch the object in any manner. They should report their findings at once to the command center.

Even if an object is noted and reported, the search should continue. The suspected object may not be the bomb, or it may be one of several bombs. While waiting for the police bomb disposal unit, the search team should open external windows at the location of the bomb and close the door into the area. If time dictates, mattresses can be placed around the suspected object, but again, the object must not be touched.

Facility Response

For the most part, the facility should use the same emergency procedures for a bomb threat as for a fire. The facility should close all interior doors and keep patients in their rooms. The fire suppression system can be activated to close all smoke and fire doors to further isolate injury and damage if a blast occurs. All exterior windows may be opened in public areas to allow the blast energy to escape.

THE EVACUATION

Evacuation is difficult and dangerous and should be attempted only when it is clearly the best and only choice. In many cases, more injuries will result from trying to move some patients than from a bomb explosion. The facility should run several test evacuations to get an idea of how long a partial or full evacuation would take. Careful planning is the key to successful evacuation. If the evacuation is during inclement weather, where will the patients be staged for transportation? How will those evacuated be transported from the facility, and where will they go? In most locales, the emergency management systems have made these kinds of arrangements with other facilities. Be sure to check these arrangements and include them in the bomb threat emergency plan.

In most cases, if evacuation is deemed necessary, it will be partial. Patients, staff, and visitors should first be evacuated from the same level as the suspected bomb. If more evacuation is needed, decisions must be made based upon information from the fire department, plant engineering, and nursing services as to how quickly and safely further evacuations could occur.

KEY POINTS

- Planning is the key to managing a bomb threat call.
- Security and staff should be trained to analyze a call.
- Based on the analysis of the call, decision makers should be able to determine whether to evacuate the facility.
- Several different responses to bomb threats are possible, including several types of searches.

Chapter 22

Hostage Situations

CHAPTER OBJECTIVES

1. Know the different types of hostage takers and those most frequently involved in health care facility hostage crises.
2. Know how to handle a hostage situation.

INTRODUCTION

Glance at a morning paper or the evening news, and one will be reminded that violence is on the rise. Unfortunately, a health care facility is not immune to violence. Given the enormous number of health care facilities in the United States and the crises that take place inside their walls, it is not surprising that hostage situations occur in health care facilities.

When most people think of hostage incidents, they visualize political terrorists holding an ambassador or foreign diplomat captive. However, in a health care facility setting, politics are not the prime reason hostage incidents occur. In fact, of the 22 recorded hostage incidents in health care facilities, only one was directly related to politics (in Italy, a health care facility administrator was kidnapped to secure the release of political prisoners).

PROFILE OF A HOSTAGE TAKER

So why are there incidents of hostage taking in health care facilities? To fully understand many of the situations that have occurred, it is easiest to look at what type of individuals are involved. There are four main types of hostage takers in a health care facility setting:

1. the criminal or prisoner receiving treatment
2. someone who feels wronged by the health care system and wants to settle a score
3. a grieving person who is on the verge of losing a loved one
4. a mentally ill patient

Craig Perkins, Presbyterian HealthCare System, Charlotte, NC, contributed many of the guidelines contained in this chapter.

Most hostage takers from all four groups are males from 20 to 40 years old. Most will start out with an extremely high emotional level and progress downward to a more calm one. Most will experience mood shifts during the hostage incident, moving from excitement to calm, rage to fear, panic to rationalization. Mentally ill patients and criminal patients are the most likely to take hostages in a health care facility, so the next sections focus on them.

Mentally Ill Hostage Taker

The key to dealing with a mentally ill or emotionally disturbed hostage taker is simply realizing that the person is unbalanced, distraught, and possibly under the influence of drugs. It may be very difficult to communicate with this type of hostage taker. But some approaches are better than others.

- The hostage taker should be encouraged to vent frustrations. Many times, this type of individual simply wants someone to listen.
- People should show concern for the hostage taker by using the reflection or parroting technique. This technique involves "playing back" or emphasizing what the hostage taker has already said. Responses should be built from phrases such as "You are upset about," "If I heard you right," and "The problem, if I understand correctly, is." This technique tends to encourage communication and make hostage takers more willing to accept a solution.
- People should not argue with the hostage taker. Logic will not usually persuade someone who is mentally ill.
- People should stay focused on the hostage taker's main subject or concern without providing any solutions to the problem. They should be ready to distract the hostage taker if aggressive or violent behavior seems imminent.

Criminal Hostage Taker

Criminal hostage takers are unique since their situations and demands are clear. Their goals are more realistic and involve less planning on the part of the hostage taker.

Hostage situations involving criminals usually occur during a criminal act such as fleeing from treatment while under arrest or suddenly realizing that they will shortly be going to jail. In these cases the hostage taker's main objective is to obtain release and escape the police. Since criminals' demands are more specific, they are less likely to accept any compromises. A criminal hostage taker can be extremely dangerous.

If a criminal hostage situation occurs, staff members should take the following steps:

- They should contact security (who will contact the police) immediately. A uniform presence will help.
- Authorities should clearly state what can and cannot be done so the hostage taker will know what limits are being set.

- They should be businesslike and calm. A criminal hostage taker realizes that some deal will be made eventually and that proceeding in a businesslike manner may result in a better deal.

GENERAL RULES FOR RESPONDING TO A HOSTAGE SITUATION

The most important moments of a hostage incident occur 5 to 10 minutes after the start. In these critical minutes, the manner with which the incident will be handled is set. Staff members should take several steps during this period.

- They should secure the area, removing all people who are not involved in the incident without endangering their safety.
- They should call security—a step that can be forgotten in all the excitement. Security should then call the police.
- They should remain calm. A hostage taker will communicate better with someone who is calm.
- They should listen to the hostage taker's demands and assess the overall situation—the number of hostages, the hostage taker's behavior (e.g., affected by drugs, mentally disturbed), the weapons involved, and the location of the incident.
- They should not get directly involved unless directed to do so by security or the police. People tend to get caught up in the moment and feel the need to get involved, which can hinder negotiations.
- They should not make any deals with or promises to the hostage taker (they do not have the authority to do so) unless lives are in immediate danger. Anything promised to the hostage taker and not given may result in retaliation.

Hostage takers invariably select one person to act as a liaison with authorities or to complain to. Those placed in this role can take a few more steps to prevent further violence.

- They should listen intently to the hostage taker and express their concern. They should not say "I understand how you feel." This statement may anger a hostage taker who feels that no one can relate to his or her feelings.
- They should remain calm. Hostage takers may calm down as well in order to communicate.
- They should not show their true emotions (anger, despair, frustration) during the crisis because these tend to irritate the hostage taker.
- They should not lie to the hostage taker or promise something they know cannot be achieved.
- They should try to face the hostage taker at all times. Some hostage takers will stop thinking of someone as a person when face-to-face contact is broken. This increases the likelihood that the hostage taker will act violently.

TEN TIPS FOR THOSE TAKEN HOSTAGE

1. Do not lose hope. Avoid showing despair to the hostage taker.
2. Try to calm the hostage taker.
3. Do not speak unless spoken to by the hostage taker.
4. Do exactly as you are told and do not make suggestions.
5. Try to rest if possible but remain facing the hostage taker.
6. Request medical attention if you need it. Hostage takers do not want to have sick hostages.
7. Do not argue.
8. Be observant.
9. Expect noise and lights if a rescue attempt is made.
10. In case of a rescue, hit the floor and stay there.

Although most hostage incidents occur without warning, there are some signs that staff members can look for. When working in the critical areas, they should take note of any relatives or friends who seem to be having a physical or violent reaction to the death or dying state of a loved one. When dealing with a known drug user as a patient, staff members should realize that to obtain drugs, patients may act violently. Staff should listen for any complaints about the medical treatment of a patient by family members ("I know they did not do enough, and I'll make sure it doesn't happen again," "You didn't treat my mother like she should have been treated"). Dissatisfied, angry family members or friends may take action against the health care facility.

Plans are essential to hostage incident management. They help staff know how to recognize and deal with hostage situations. To prevent stressful situations and save lives, every facility should develop its own hostage incident management plan (see guidelines throughout this chapter as well as Appendix 22–A).

RESPONSIBILITIES OF SECURITY

Security officers' main objectives are to protect the scene and slow the process down. They should try to avoid making contact with the hostage taker. The presence of the uniform may escalate the situation. If there is no physical barrier between the hostage taker and the security officer, the security officer should wear a lab coat or other garment over the uniform. Security officers should not challenge or antagonize hostage takers.

The following sections discuss the duties of various personnel during a hostage crisis.

Security Desk Officer

After receiving a call about a hostage crisis, security desk officers should take the following steps:

- Have the supervisor go to the scene.

- Call the police at 911, informing them of the number of suspects and hostages, any demands that have been made, and the location of the incident. Also, the security desk officer should advise the police about which entrance to use, and, if necessary, which street routes to take so as not to be seen or heard by the hostage taker.
- Call the director of public safety/security and advise the director of the situation.
- Summon all security officers to the security office to await assignments.
- Keep phone lines clear.
- Alert all those on the security channel to keep radio traffic to a minimum.
- Dispatch an officer to meet the police and notify the officer on the scene when the police arrive. The officer who meets the police will escort the police to the hostage area, making certain to stay out of view of the actual hostage situation. This officer should then stand by at the scene and await further instructions.
- Stand by to receive and transmit information.
- Document all activity.

First Officer on the Scene (Supervisor)

After hearing the security desk officer's explanation of the hostage situation, the first officer on the scene should take the following steps:

- Go to the area. Avoid being seen by the hostage taker.
- Turn the security radio down as low as possible.
- Assess the situation, and advise the desk officer of the route that the police should take to the area.
- Set up a command post near the scene yet out of sight of the hostage taker.
- Contact the first person on the scene and any other person who has had contact with the hostage taker and have these people fill out a statement form.
- Always assume that a presumed hostage situation is real.
- Always assume that the hostage taker has a weapon and that it is functional, even if a weapon is not visible.
- Report any developments to the monitor surveillance tech, the security supervisor or security dispatcher.
- Calmly stand by and wait for the police.
- Assist the police in any and all tasks as requested.

Administrative Coordinator

During a hostage situation, the administrative coordinator should take the following steps:

- Ask the administrator on call to come to the security office.
- Ask the public information department to be prepared to handle press coverage if needed.
- Ask the plant engineering manager to come to the facility and be prepared to give information on the floor plans, heating, air conditioning, electrical systems, and so forth.
- Ask the switchboard manager to be prepared to make phone connections when needed.

- Meet security at the scene.
- If the hostage is a patient, gather as much information about his or her condition as possible (e.g., types of medication given and the time that the next dose is to be administered, physical and mental condition, type of life support system [advise security and police whether the patient can be removed from the machine]) as well as the physician's name and phone number.
- If the hostage is not a patient, gather as much information as possible about the hostage's identity and relationship to the hostage taker, if any.
- Keep other staff away from the scene and as calm as possible.
- Remain available to help police and security with any questions that may arise.
- Do not divulge any information to anyone other than security, police, and administration.

KEY POINTS

- Because health care facilities are stressful places, hostage situations may occur.
- There are basically four types of hostage takers associated with the health care environment.
- Planning and training are the keys to managing a hostage situation. Staff should be trained on what to do if a hostage situation occurs and if they are taken hostage.

Appendix 22–A

Hostage Incident Management Plan

PURPOSE:

The object of this plan is to provide guidance in the event a hostage incident occurs on hospital-owned or -leased property.

POLICY

- A hostage incident is a situation in which one person (the hostage taker) holds another person (the hostage) against his or her will by force, threat, or violence. Law enforcement officials, through negotiators at the scene, will attempt to obtain the release of the hostage or hostages.
- As soon as a hostage incident has been confirmed, the senior law enforcement officer present is in charge of controlling the incident.

PROCEDURE

- The first employee to identify a hostage situation should take the following steps:
  - Stay calm.
  - Focus on the individual, not the weapon.
  - Make no promises or commitments except that someone will come to help.
  - Step back.
  - Buy time.
  - Secure the immediate areas with the help of other employees by initiating OPERATION EVACUATION through the switchboard of the unit or floor where the incident is taking place. All patients, visitors, and employees should be evacuated.
  - With the assistance of other employees, immediately control access to the unit at elevators and stairwells.
  - Once relieved by security or law enforcement personnel, go to the boardroom for a debriefing.
    1. Note the number of hostages.
    2. Note the number of hostage takers.

3. Note weapons observed, descriptions, and number.
4. Note any threats or demands.

- Upon arrival at the scene of a hostage incident, security personnel should take the following steps:
  - Confirm the report of a hostage incident. If confirmed, contact the switchboard and have them notify the police department and
    1. the administrator on call
    2. the director of security
    3. the marketing department
    4. the materials management department
    5. the engineering/maintenance department
    6. the emergency department
  - Make arrangements through the switchboard to have the responding law enforcement officers meet at the campus entrance and escorted to the site of the incident.
  - Make arrangements to have the unit or floor involved locked out if accessed by an elevator. Contact maintenance for assistance.
  - Secure all access to the unit or floor by other means at all exits and entrances via stairwells or common hallways. **Only responding security and law enforcement personnel should be allowed on the scene.**
  - Call in all off-duty security personnel.
  - Post security, engineering, or environmental services personnel at all entrances to the facility. **All routine access is denied.**
  - Post staff at the entrance to the tactical operations center, which is the boardroom. Law enforcement operations will be initiated and conducted from here.
  - The director of security will respond to the boardroom tactical operations center.
  - Provide radio to the administration command post in the administration conference room and to the media command post in the education classroom.
- The administrative coordinator should take the following steps:
  - Activate the administration/command post in the administration conference room.
  - Send an administration representative to the boardroom to work with the senior law enforcement officer on the scene.
  - Assess need in conjunction with risk management for critical incident debrief, working also with psychological services.
- Marketing should provide a representative to staff the media command post in the education classroom.
- Engineering should take the following steps:
  - Provide representative to the boardroom.
  - Appoint a representative to bring all floor plans to the floor or unit involved in the incident, the floor above, the floor below, and the building overall.
- Materials Management should provide cellular phones for the media command post, administration conference room, and tactical operations center.
- Volunteer services should be prepared to evacuate the office area to be used by law enforcement personnel in support of the incident.

- Information services should provide telephone numbers of all telephones in the area of the unit or floor involved in the hostage incident.
- Risk management should assess need in conjunction with administration for critical incident debrief by psychological services.

REFERENCE

Joint Commission on Accreditation of Healthcare Organizations. Comprehensive Accreditation Manual for Hospitals. Standard EC 1.4, Effective 01/01/97. Joint Commission. Oakbrook Terrace, IL, 1996.

Chapter 23

Fire Prevention and Emergency Preparedness

James P. Finn

CHAPTER OBJECTIVES

1. Understand the purpose of emergency preparedness as prescribed by the Joint Commission on Accreditation of Healthcare Organizations (Joint Commission).
2. Know and understand how to organize an emergency preparedness plan.
3. Know the fire prevention training in health care facilities that is required by the Joint Commission and the National Fire Protection Association.
4. Know the Joint Commission standard for utility system failure.

INTRODUCTION

An emergency is an event that disrupts the normal operating procedures of a facility and requires that additional resources be called upon to maintain necessary levels of care. At one time, "disaster planning" and "emergency preparedness" were treated as synonyms. With the implementation of the Environment of Care standards by the Joint Commission on Accreditation of Healthcare Organizations (Joint Commission) in 1995, "emergency preparedness" took on a broader meaning. Emergency preparedness means that health care facilities understand, plan, and prepare for all potential situations that would disrupt normal operations. Prior to 1995, emergency preparedness referred to planning for a large influx of patients due to an external disaster.

Organizations need to determine what emergencies are most likely to occur and plan their response. For example, facilities in California will need to plan for a major earthquake, while facilities in the Midwest will have plans to deal with tornadoes. Most organizations have individual plans and procedures to deal with each type of event. It would be better if organizations had one plan or procedure to cover all emergencies.

This chapter examines policies and procedures associated with emergency preparedness.

DISASTER PLANNING

By now, every facility that is accredited by the Joint Commission has a written disaster plan. This plan is designed to give direction to facility employees in the event of a disaster— anything from an earthquake to a multivehicle accident. Disaster plans are activated for one reason: the influx of additional patients taxes the facilities' resources, so additional measures must be taken to handle the extra load. Disaster policies should cover

- activation of the plan
- general responsibilities
- medical staff responsibilities
- key locations
- deactivation of the plan

Activation of the Plan

It is important for everyone within the organization to know how and when the facility's disaster plan will be activated. It is common practice for each facility to use some type of overhead page, usually initiated by the facilities' PBX operators, to notify staff that the disaster plan has been activated. Once they hear the page, staff begin preparing. In many facilities, it is common for the potential number of victims expected to be included in the original page, if that number is known. When the number is given in the page, staff can prepare for the large influx of patients.

For example, imagine that a facility's code for disaster plan activation is "code yellow." A call comes in from a paramedic stating that 45 patients with various types of injuries will soon be arriving at the facility. The facility's PBX operators would include this number in the facility page, saying "code yellow—45."

Who will be responsible for activating the plan? Facilities must determine this in advance. Because of the additional resources that will be used when a disaster plan has been activated, it is only prudent that this activation decision be made by a person with the authority to initiate such expenditures. Typically, the facility's administrator on call makes the final decision. The administrator on call represents the facility's senior management and has the authority to quickly get things done, such as having the medical staff review which current patients may be discharged to free up beds in the facility.

The administrator on call will usually consult with the emergency department medical director and other key departments before making the determination to activate the plan (in some instances, the emergency department can handle the additional patient load without calling in additional staff because the injuries are not severe or the current emergency department patient census is low).

General Responsibilities

Every plan should spell out the responsibilities of every department, whether its role is small or large. The key departments should be listed at the front of the section on departmental responsibilities. Other departments should be listed alphabetically. The key players are those immediately involved with caring for the patients being brought in. In some of the best plans, different areas are designated to handle different types of patients. The emergency department may handle the most urgent cases, while adjacent areas handle the "walking wounded." This brings some order to the chaos and spreads the patient load as well as the additional staff over a larger area. Other departments are used to provide support services.

Here are some examples of what each department might be assigned to do.

- security: controlling access to the building and traffic
- public relations: handling media releases and dealing with media at the facility
- facility services and housekeeping: assisting with security, patient transports, and anything else that requires physical ability
- medical records: admitting additional patients
- clergy and guest relations staff: assisting with patients' family and death notification
- nursing units: helping physicians determine what other patients might be discharged to free up beds
- dietary: supplying snacks and beverages to the families of incoming wounded

It is very important that these assignments are made and departments understand what they are responsible for. Good planning makes disasters more manageable.

Medical Staff Responsibilities

The medical staff play an important part in the facilities disaster plan. Mechanisms need to be in place to call in additional physicians (especially surgeons and other specialists) to assist in caring for the influx of patients. The chief of staff should be responsible for coordinating the efforts of the medical staff, with plenty of assistance from the administrator on call. Depending on the number of casualties expected, additional physicians may be needed to perform triage. Attending physicians need to quickly assess which patients may be discharged to make room for possible admissions.

Key Locations

A facility's disaster plan should clearly refer to where in the facility various activities will take place. It is natural that the emergency department will be the first place that disaster victims are taken. But administrators should consider these additional questions.

- Where will we treat emergent patients?
- Where will we treat the "walking wounded"?
- Where will we contain the media so they have access to our public relations personnel but have no immediate access to the patients and patients' families?

- Where will we place family members of the patients? Is there a location that provides privacy and keeps them away from the media?
- If there are many fatalities, where will the bodies be kept? And where will next of kin be notified?

By being prepared, facilities will bring order to a chaotic situation.

Deactivation of the Plan

Just as it is important for one person to be responsible for activating the disaster plan, it is important that one person be responsible for canceling or deactivating the plan. In most instances, the administrator on call that activates the disaster response plan will be on hand to deactivate it. However, there may be times when that individual will need to be relieved by another senior manager simply because a facility remains under a disaster response for days rather than the typical few hours.

TYPES OF DISASTERS

There are two types of potential disasters facilities need to prepare for in their disaster plans: (1) internal disasters and (2) external disasters.

Internal Disasters

Internal disasters occur within a facility. The internal disasters faced most often by facilities are fire and loss of utilities.

Fire

Fire is the event most feared and most planned for by health care facilities. Because of organizations such as the National Fire Protection Administration (NFPA), the Joint Commission, and local fire departments, there are standards of practice and building codes that help keep facilities safer. The Joint Commission now requires all health care facilities it accredits to have a written management plan addressing life safety issues and including

- a completed Statement of Conditions document that helps an organization do a critical self-assessment of its current level of compliance and describe how to resolve any Life Safety Code deficiencies[1]
- an outline of the facility's process for protecting patients, personnel, visitors, and property
- procedures for identifying and maintaining all applicable required structural features of fire protection in accordance with the NFPA Life Safety Code[2]
- procedures for inspecting, testing, and maintaining fire alarm detection systems, automatic fire extinguishing systems, and portable fire extinguishers
- review of proposed acquisitions of bedding, window draperies, and other furnishing and decorations for fire safety
- life safety orientation and education program
- performance measures and annual evaluations of the life safety program[3]

It is very important to know, understand, and follow the Joint Commission guidelines. Nothing could be more important than performing all the required fire drills while genuinely critiquing the response of staff. One fire drill is required per shift per quarter. All elements of the system and all personnel located in areas housing or treating patients must be tested. If an organization is under interim life safety measures (ILSMs), it must perform twice as many fire drills. ILSMs are a series of 11 actions required to temporarily compensate for the significant hazards posed by existing Life Safety Code deficiencies or constructive activities.[4]

The Joint Commission allows organizations to randomly test staff performance instead of observing all areas if the following sites are included in the fire drill assessment:

- the smoke compartment in which the drill is initiated
- another smoke compartment on the same floor and immediately adjacent to the fire drill location (if one exists)
- another smoke compartment that is on a floor directly above or below the fire drill location (if one exists)
- an additional number of smoke compartments—20 percent of the total number of smoke compartments for the building (if the organization can prove satisfactory fire drill experience and has the approval of its safety committee, the amount of additional smoke compartments throughout the facility can be reduced to 10 percent of the total)[5]

Facilities need to critique how the fire alarm system and components of the life safety management plan functioned.

- Did the fire alarm strobes and chimes activate? Did they work properly?
- Did the fire alarm system component used in the drill (pull station, smoke detector) work properly?
- Did established smoke compartments close automatically? Was anything blocking the doors or keeping them from functioning as intended? Did the doors completely close and latch?
- Are hallways clear of obstructions to allow the transfer of people to other areas of refuge?
- Are all fire exit stairwells clear of obstructions to allow immediate access to egress traffic?
- Are all emergency exit lights functioning? Are there two exit lights visible from any location in the hallway?

Facilities should also critique staff knowledge and response.

- Did staff know where the nearest pull station was located?
- Did staff know what emergency telephone number to call to activate the fire response?
- Was anyone in immediate danger removed to an area of refuge?
- Was the fire properly contained?
- Did participating staff know where fire extinguishers were located?
- Did staff know where the shutoff valves are located for oxygen? Could they say when the oxygen valves were to be shut off?
- Could staff explain the process for evacuating patients? Do staff know the difference between horizontal and vertical evacuation and when each is used?

This is one situation whose outcome will be determined by what facility personnel learn and retain. There is a very high potential for injuries to patients, visitors, and staff and for damage to property and equipment if personnel do not know how to react properly and quickly. If an organization has decided that an emergency response team will respond to fire alarms, the team should also be critiqued during drill situations.

> There are emergency response teams, and then there are fire brigades. What is the difference? Fire brigade members must receive the same amount of training as someone in the local volunteer or municipal fire department. For this reason, facilities often call the groups that respond to fire alarms emergency response teams, not fire brigades.

Utility System Failures

Most health care facilities have backup systems for their backup systems. This is a great practice, but it can lull facilities into thinking they are covered for all potential outages. To be prudent, facilities should check, double-check, and triple-check their preparedness for utility outages. Is the facility prepared should the supply of water from a local utility provider be lost? How will the facility maintain supplies of fresh drinking water? How will the facility dispose of human waste when toilets cannot be flushed? How will the facility deal with infection control issues—in particular, hand washing? These are some of the issues associated with the loss of domestic water and sewer systems. But there are many other utilities, including electricity, telephone, and medical gases. Clearly, there is plenty to prepare for. As with life safety, the Joint Commission requires written utility management plans that do the following:

- promote a safe and comfortable environment of care
- assess and minimize the risk of utility failure
- ensure the operational reliability of all utilities
- establish criteria for the identification, evaluation, and inventory of critical operating components within the utility management program, addressing the impact of utility system failure on
  - life support systems
  - infection control systems
  - environmental support systems
  - equipment support systems
  - communication systems
- discuss requirements for the inspection, testing, and maintenance of critical operating systems
- cover development and maintenance of current operational plans for utility systems that help to ensure reliability, minimize risks, and reduce failures
- discuss investigation of utility system problems, failures, or errors and reporting incidents and corrective actions

- map the distribution of utility systems and labeling controls, for a partial or complete emergency shutdown
- establish an orientation and education program
- specify how performance measures and annual evaluations of the utilities management program will work
- cover emergency procedures for utility system disruptions or failures

External Disasters

For many years, health care facilities have been prepared to handle external disasters. Facilities used to believe that the Joint Commission's disaster planning or emergency preparedness standards addressed only external disasters; only recently have organizations realized internal disasters are involved as well.

> Every organization needs to assess the risks associated with doing business in its area. What acts of nature are most likely to affect the community? Tornado? Flood? Hurricane? Fire? Earthquake? Just as important, what nearby industries might affect the facility? A nuclear power plant? A manufacturing plant that houses or manufactures large quantities of hazardous chemicals? Are there major interstates or connecting highways where large accidents might result in an influx of many victims? Are these roads used to transport large quantities of hazardous materials? What kinds?

After assessing disaster-related risks in its area, an organization can start to develop one plan to prepare for the most probable emergencies, both internal and external.

KEY POINTS

- Emergency preparedness plans (disaster plans) should have five key parts.
  1. activation of the plan
  2. general responsibilities
  3. medical staff responsibilities
  4. key locations
  5. deactivation of the plan
- The Joint Commission requires that health care facilities have a written fire plan. The fire plan must contain education and mock fire drill components.
- The Joint Commission requires a plan for utility system failure.
- Emergency preparedness plans must cover both internal and external disasters.

REFERENCES

1. The Joint Commission on Accreditation of Healthcare Organizations, Comprehensive Accreditation Manual for Hospitals, Statement of Conditions (Oakbrook Terrace, IL: 1998), EC-8.

2. National Fire Protection Association, NFPA 101 Life Safety Code (1997), chapter 12 and 13.

3 The Joint Commission on Accreditation of Healthcare Organizations, Comprehensive Accreditation Manual for Hospitals, EC-13–EC-14.

4. Joint Commission, Comprehensive Accreditation Manual, EC-26.

5. Joint Commission, Comprehensive Accreditation Manual, EC-23.

Chapter 24

Gang Violence and Health Care Security

Rick J. Flinn

CHAPTER OBJECTIVES

1. Know the definition of a gang and the seven categories of gangs.
2. Describe the primary ways gang members interact with people in health care facilities.
3. Know some different gangs' colors and signs, and understand some gang language.
4. Know how to educate parents so that they may recognize if their child is in a gang.

INTRODUCTION

Despite some recent downward trends in the murder rate in the United States, violent crime continues to be an enormous concern for government, law enforcement, health care providers, and the community at large. In 1996, the nation's murder rate declined by 9 percent. Unfortunately, youth violence was on the rise. Actually, the Centers for Disease Control and Prevention reported that homicides among males between the ages of 14 and 25 were a genuine epidemic. If criminal activity is a barometer of social disorganization, what is happening with the nation's families and youth? Even more tragic, juvenile crime is predicted to increase by 114 percent in the next decade. One reason for this surge in youth crime and violence is the growth of organized gangs.[1,2]

In 1996, President Clinton recognized the issue as he spoke of key priorities for the nation during his 1996 State of the Union address. "The next step in our fight against crime is to take on the gangs, the way we once took on the mob," he said. Gang activity has reached nearly all of society. No longer are gangs in only inner cities and primarily engaged in misdemeanor crime. High-profile gang members are even idolized within the entertainment industry.

Gangs are organizations that have three or more people who use one shared organization name or identifying sign, symbol, or color and who individually or collectively engage in or have engaged in criminal activity. Key characteristics of a gang include

- formal organizational structure
- identifiable leadership

- identifiable territory
- regularly occurring interaction among members
- serious or violent behavior by members

Gangs have many things in common with legitimate organizations. Like many other organizations, gangs have a hierarchical structure. Specific responsibilities of each member are delineated, and members are accountable to their superiors. Performance is routinely evaluated, and leaders use a variety of techniques to ensure compliance. Leaders set goals and expect each gang member to participate. Group identity and loyalty are strong principles and serve as a solid foundation for interaction within the group. But there is one primary difference between gangs and legitimate businesses: the primary purpose of a gang is to commit crimes. Gangs' criminal acts can be divided into four major categories.

1. assault (with or without a deadly weapon)
2. robbery
3. manslaughter/homicide
4. the sale, distribution, and possession for sale of controlled substances

GANG DATA

Most Americans still believe that organized gangs are primarily located in large metropolitan areas. Clearly, the attitude of many is "it can't happen here or with my kids." Actually, criminal gangs are attracted to all communities throughout the country, either as areas to "lie low" or places to create new business. No geographical area is immune. In fact, towns with a population of 8,000 or less are prime targets, especially if there is easy access to a larger city for other business ventures.

Despite the absence of a precise reporting system for gang member activity, gangs are becoming more prevalent. There are over 5,000 identified gangs in the nation. Southern California has approximately 300 hard-core gangs with over 100,000 members. Overall, U.S. cities contain anywhere from 250,000 to 400,000 gang members. Nearly 700 cities routinely report gang activity, identifying over 47,000 gang-related incidents each year. And gangs handle over 25 percent of crack cocaine distribution. In 1992 alone, gangs made $150 billion from drug sales. Despite the limited tracking of gang-related crime, it is known that at least 10 to 30 percent of all homicides are gang related. Victims of gang violence are usually innocent bystanders or people who are not gang members. As a result of an increase in firearm availability and gun use among organized gangs, a bullet injures a child in this country every 92 minutes. Additionally, drive-by shootings, neighborhood feuds, and unlawful weapon discharges injure more non–gang members than rival gang members.[3]

Ninety percent of all gang members are juveniles. The average gang member is 16 or 17 years of age, with a typical age range from 12 to 25. The majority of gangs are concentrated in lower socioeconomic areas, yet the demographics show that migration is occurring. Nearly 80 percent of gang members are either African American or Hispanic.[4]

Most hard-core and affiliate gang members have reported that they do not expect to live past age 30. Members of these groups live for the moment and avoid long-term thinking. This mindset can be dangerous during criminal acts because it leads to fearlessness.

WHY DO YOUNG PEOPLE TURN TO GANGS?

The growth of gangs alarms most people. Many authorities wonder what attracts young people to these criminal organizations. Conditions in inner cities and some suburbs may be one factor. Many gang members have surfaced from neighborhoods plagued with overcrowding and unemployment, filled with high school dropouts and dysfunctional families, and lacking recreation and productive distraction. Unfortunately, gangs may offer young people some necessities that their families cannot. To some, gang membership may be the last resort. In general, the primary reasons for joining a gang are

- to get a greater sense of identity
- to gain recognition in the community
- to feel a sense of belonging
- to be disciplined
- to get some attention from others
- to acquire more money

The gang and its members become truly a surrogate family. Leaders are quite skilled in drawing in new members by promising money or drugs to, by intimidating, or by acknowledging vulnerable and impressionable teenagers. As one gang member put it, "A gangster's life is the life of a wanderer. A wanderer is a person with no safe place to return to. A safe place leads to success. When you leave home you can never return. To return is to be a coward. To play is to play to the end. We will live or die together. We will share the good things, and if there are bad things we will share those too." As this quotation suggests, members are generally loyal to their gangs, have no long-term aspirations, and do not consider the consequences of gang-related behavior.

Generally, most gangs fall into seven distinct categories:

- Crips
- Bloods
- Gangster Disciple Nation
- Vice Lords
- Latino affiliates
- Asian affiliates
- hate or bias groups

Examples of specific gangs in each category can be found in Exhibit 24–1. Regardless of affiliation, all gang members commit crimes and are capable of violence. They are territorial and can routinely be identified by their unique use of colors, graffiti, language, tattoos, hand signals, and general attire. Unfortunately, as certain gangs become better organized, signs and other identifiers become more obscure.

Gangs often extend into prisons. Rival gangs often feud in prison, and violence results.

Though organized gangs of women are fairly rare, over 100 organized gangs of women have been identified, with over 7,200 members. Typically, women align with other predominately male gangs.[4,5]

Exhibit 24–1 Categories of Gangs

Crips—originated in Los Angeles Kitchen Crip Gang 42 Crip Gang Rollin 80 West Coast Crip	**Latino affiliates** Mexican Mafia Latin Kings
Bloods—originated in Los Angeles West Side Pirus Inglewood Family Gangster Blood Stone Villain	**Asian affiliates** Natoma Scar Boys Saigon Cowboys
Gangster Disciple Nation Black Gangster Disciples Insane Gangster Disciples	**Hate or bias groups** Aryan Nation Ku Klux Klan White Supremacist
Vice Lords Conservative Vice Lords Insane Vice Lords	

GANGS AND HEALTH CARE FACILITIES

Because gang-related activity involves violence, health care institutions, especially emergency departments, are faced with managing the clinical issues associated with gang activity. And a gang member may choose to obtain routine health care at a particular facility. However the gang members and their victims arrive, the risks inherent in treating these patients create a huge challenge for all areas of health care facilities.

Several common conditions have been identified as the primary reasons gang members seek medical care.

- intentional injuries (i.e., blunt and penetrating injuries)
- assaults
- injuries associated with initiation rites
- sexually transmitted diseases
- illness induced by alcohol or other drug abuse
- unplanned pregnancy
- malnutrition[6]

Obviously, this patient population has legitimate needs, and health care providers must be prepared to deliver holistic care while ensuring a safe environment for other patients, visitors, and themselves. **When working with gang members, health care staff should consider the following points:**

- **Recognition of the gang member is of utmost importance.** Health care workers must become knowledgeable about local gangs and their common identifiers and get to know their slang (see Appendixes 24–A through 24–C). Staff must be on the lookout for the potential retaliation of rival gangs. Also, early identification helps to sort out members of rival gangs, in the case of multiple shootings. It is imperative to separate victims and

Exhibit 24–2 Early Warning Signs That Youths May Be Involved in Gangs

- Drug use/mood changes
- Decline in grades at school
- Truancy
- Change in friends
- Keeping late hours
- Withdrawing from family
- Change in clothing and jewelry
- Obsession with gangster rap music
- Many new possessions (e.g., very expensive stereos)

Exhibit 24–3 Clear Signs That Youths Are Involved in Gangs

- Having gang graffiti on walls, posters, or notebooks
- Wearing gang colors or apparel
- Having tattoos signifying gang affiliations
- Communicating using hand signals
- Disclosure of membership

Exhibit 24–4 Good Advice to Youths about Staying out of Gangs

- Do not associate or communicate with gang members.
- Do not attend gang parties or congregate at known gang hangouts.
- Do not wear gang-related apparel.
- Do not use gang slang.
- Do not use or imitate gang signs in public.

Exhibit 24–5 Tips for Parents and Youth Leaders Regarding Youth Involvement in Gangs

- Do not say it cannot happen.
- Demand that youths account for their time.
- Impress upon youths the importance of education and good grades.
- Spend quality time with youths.
- Listen to youths. Communicate with them about their concerns and fears.
- Get involved in youths' school activities.
- Establish rules, set limits, and be consistent, firm, and fair in punishment.
- Encourage good study habits.
- Respect youths' feelings and attitudes and help them develop good self-esteem.
- Ask questions when something seems wrong.
- Watch closely for negative influences.

continues

Exhibit 24–5 continued

- Get involved in community prevention and intervention programs. Urge others to become involved.
- Volunteer at the youth's school. Gangs are a community problem, and their influence does not stop at any particular boundary.
- Improve your own self-esteem so youths can model themselves after the most important role models—you.

---

families. Security coverage is paramount, at least initially, but often throughout the entire patient stay.

Early identification can be difficult sometimes because gang members may distort identifying information in an effort to maintain anonymity and avoid surveillance by law enforcement. Staff must be aware of the potential for the use of aliases, incomplete or false addresses, and false dates of birth. People who live outside California, especially members of the Bloods or the Crips, may use California phone numbers or addresses.

- **Each health care facility's security plan should include a process for managing victims of violence and a contingency plan for handling the unique risks associated with having a gang member as a patient.** Open dialogue with local law enforcement will assist in determining the risk to the institution and details regarding the characteristics of the specific gang. Health care officials can also assist law enforcement with tracking gang-related incidents—typically not a breech of patient confidentiality in that it is a criminal event. Clinicians may also be asked to participate in collection of evidence, such as bullet fragments and gang apparel. Evidence preservation is critical; the crime can be recreated if clothing and other items are kept intact.
- **Health care providers should assume an active role in the prevention of gang violence and crime.** Safety and security professionals must endorse a zero tolerance philosophy for gang-related activities among patients, visitors, and employees. The health care community, along with schools, families, social agencies, and others, can play a vital role in curbing gang activity. Graffiti must be immediately removed. Gang-related activity by employees must be restricted, in practice and in policy statements. Lastly, educational materials should be available for personnel and the general public. Information on the incidence of gang-related crime and violence, early warning signs that youths may be involved in gangs (Exhibits 24–2 and 24–3), and advice for youths, parents, and youth leaders (Exhibits 24–4 and 24–5) may prevent involvement in gangs or prepare parents to manage a gang-related crisis. Denial must be avoided at all costs.

CONCLUSION

Gang-related crime and violence have a direct impact on health care today. Security personnel and clinicians must work together to manage the clinical needs of gang members who fall victim to either illness or injury. The gang member's presence in the health care environment creates additional risks for personnel, yet early recognition and a comprehensive security response plan will assist in preventing acts of violence within the health care facility.

KEY POINTS

- Gangs are in small towns as well as large cities.
- There are seven distinct categories of gangs.
- Emergency departments and security officers must be trained in gang member identification and management.

REFERENCES

1. M. Rand, "Violence Related Injuries Treated in Hospital Emergency Department," *Bureau of Justice Special Report* (1997): 1–11.

2. S. Dobbin and S. Gatowski, "Statistics: The Juvenile Population in the U.S.," *www.ncjfcj/unr.edu* (1996):1–98.

3. G. Coward, *Gangs 2000* (California Department of Justice, Division of Law Enforcement and Bureau of Investigation: 1993) 1–5.

4. H. Kohl, *Background Facts: Gangs in America* (Committee on the Judiciary–United States Senate: 1995), 1.

5. American College of Emergency Physicians, *Emergency Department Violence: Prevention and Management* (ACEP Publications: 1997), 1–33.

6. S. Nawojczyk, *Street Gang Dynamics* (Nawojczyk Group, Inc.: 1994), 1–4.

Appendix 24–A

Street Gang Terminology

ace kool	best friend/backup
all is one	a term used by the Disciples
all is well	a term used by the Vice Lords
angel dust	PCP in crystal form
Audi 5000 G	goodbye/peace
babe	girl
banger	gang member or a person shooting in a drive-by
banging	gang activities/fighting or violence
base freak	girl who likes loud music, or dope fiend
base head	person hooked on cocaine
beam me up	person hooked on cocaine or looking for drugs
beemer	a BMW
bent	to get drunk or high
benzo	a Mercedes Benz
bet	the truth/I believe you
BG	baby gangster
big baller	a high roller/big-time drug dealer
bill	$100
bird	refers to kilo of cocaine
bitchin	something nice
BK	Blood Killer
BKA	Blood Killer always
BK rider	kills slobs
BK queen	fast food worker
Black Disciple	Black Disciple gang member note: not Black Gangster Disciple
blessed	initiated into the gang
blob	derogatory name for Blood gang member used by Crip gang members
Blood	Piru/non-Crip
blow chunks	vomit
bo	marijuana

315

bogey . . . . $100 piece of crack
bogie . . . . cop car
boned out . . . . quit/chickened out/left
book . . . . run/get away/leave
boo yaa . . . . sound of shotgun
bow . . . . marijuana
bowed out . . . . stoned/high on drugs or alcohol
boy . . . . heroin
B queen . . . . female Blood
brabs . . . . derogatory name for a Crip gang member used by Blood gang members
break . . . . run/get away
breakdown . . . . shotgun
brown paint . . . . heroin
bucket . . . . old, raggedy car
buck wild . . . . act crazy
bud . . . . marijuana
budded . . . . high
bullet . . . . one year in custody
bumper kit . . . . girl's butt
bumping titties . . . . fighting
bumpy face . . . . gin
B up . . . . take care
busted, popped a cap . . . . shot at someone
buster . . . . to go from a Crip set to a Blood set, or vice versa
busting . . . . involved in a violent act
button . . . . capsule of heroin or cocaine
BWPs . . . . bitches with problems
cabbage patch . . . . popular dance
check it out . . . . listen to what I have to say
chill out . . . . stop it/don't do that
china white . . . . Asian heroin
circle . . . . refers to ounces of cocaine
CK . . . . Crip Killer
CK ride . . . . drive-by shooting by a Blood gang
cluck . . . . cocaine smoker
clucker . . . . crack cocaine addict
colors . . . . item of clothing that identifies gang
colum . . . . Columbian marijuana
commercial . . . . Columbian marijuana
cookie monster . . . . Crenshaw Mafia gangsters
courting in . . . . initiation into the gang
courting out . . . . expulsion from the gang
C queen . . . . female Crip gang member

CR . . . . Colorado Rockies/Crips rule

crab. . . . . derogatory name for Crip gang member used by Blood gang members

crack queen. . . . . female crack addict who will perform illegal acts to obtain money to buy drugs

cragared down . . . . low-rider-type car

crank it . . . . turn up the music really loud

crumbs . . . . tiny pieces of rock cocaine

cuzz. . . . . another name for Crip

cuzzin . . . . cripping, gangstering

D. . . . . drugs

dead rag . . . . red rag/another Crip name for a Blood gang member

deft . . . . looking good

demonstration. . . . . gang fight

deuce. . . . . 22-caliber gun

deuce and a quarter. . . . . Buick 225 vehicle

dime speed . . . . 10-speed bicycle

dippin . . . . being nosey

dis . . . . no respect/disrespect

Disciple. . . . . Disciple gang member

Disciple queen . . . . Disciple gang's female sex object

dissen . . . . being disrespectful

do a ghost . . . . to leave/leave the scene

do a lick . . . . rob a store, armed robbery

dog . . . . a Crip

dork. . . . . nerd

donut. . . . . derogatory term for a Crip

double deuce. . . . . 22-caliber gun

down for mine . . . . ability to protect self

down with the set . . . . on the gang's own turf/mellow/fine/secure/OK

drag. . . . . hit off a cigarette

drag/mack/rush. . . . . ability to sweet-talk girls

dragon. . . . . bad breath

draped. . . . . a term used for a person wearing a lot of gold jewelry

dressed down . . . . wearing gang-related colors

drop a dime. . . . . snitch or tell on someone

dropping the flag . . . . leaving the gang

drove. . . . . get embarrassed

duckets . . . . money

dude . . . . male person

durag. . . . . handkerchief wrapped around head

dusted . . . . under the influence of PCP/crack

e ricket . . . . derogatory term for a Crip

eastly. . . . . very ugly person eight ball. . . . . ⅛ ounce of cocaine/40-ounce bottle of Old English 800 malt liquor

8-track. 2½ grams of cocaine

eleven-pointed pancake . . . . a Vice Lord who became a Disciple

ends. . . . . money

Esseys. . . . . Mexicans

everything is everything. . . . . it's all right

fag. . . . . homosexual

false flagging . . . . a deliberate gang misrepresentation in the form of a hand sign or slogan

federated. Crips' disrespect for the color red

firing on someone . . . . throwing a punch at someone or shooting at someone

forty . . . . 40-ounce bottle of beer

four five . . . . 45-caliber gun

5.0. . . . . 1988 Mustang

5-0. . . . . the police

500 . . . . BMW

fiend . . . . crack cocaine user

fifty. . . . . refers to $50 piece of crack

flip crip. . . . . a dope house that sells small amounts of drugs (usually no particular customers)

floatin . . . . driving fast

flue . . . . Blood members' name for blue

flue flag . . . . blue rag

fly . . . . good looking

flying your colors . . . . representing gang colors

freak . . . . good-looking girl

fresh . . . . good-looking/clean

frog. . . . . girl with low moral standards (jumps into anyone's car)

frontin. . . . . talking about someone, embarrassing them

fucc. . . . . fuck in Crip language

fugly . . . . extremely ugly

funk. . . . . bad smelling

G. . . . . gangster, homie

gaffled. . . . . cheated

gage . . . . shotgun

game. . . . . criminal activity

gangbanger . . . . gang member

gangbanging. . . . . gang activities

gangster . . . . gang member

gank . . . . cheat/steal/rob/sell imitation dope

gat. . . . . gun

g-down . . . . dress up
geed . . . . dressed nicely
geek . . . . someone who is loaded/high
geekin. . . . . crazy
get down . . . . fight
get jammed. . . . . to be accosted
get some gone. . . . . get out of my face
gettin the digits. . . . . getting a telephone number
ghost . . . . disappear
ghost it . . . . lose it
gig. . . . . gathering
girl . . . . cocaine
givin up the nappy dugout . . . . a girl that's intimate
glass house . . . . 1977–1978 Chevy
G-man. . . . . another name for Black Gangster Disciple
gone . . . . ugly
got it going on . . . . successful person or function
graveyard . . . . a drug house that has sold all its drugs and is out of drugs or was shut down by the police
G-ride (G-springs) . . . . gangster ride/stolen car
grob . . . . beer
hard-core. . . . . extreme
head hunter. . . . . term used for a female who performs sexual acts for cocaine
HIB. . . . . hair I bought/holding dope
high roller. drug dealer
holding down . . . . controlling turf or area
home boy . . . . fellow gang member
homes . . . . fellow gang member
homey. . . . . fellow gang member
hood . . . . neighborhood
hoodsta . . . . gangster
hook . . . . phony or imitation
hook me up. . . . . set up a deal
hook/trick . . . . phony or sissy
hoopty. . . . . car
hoo-rah . . . . loud talking
hound . . . . a good name for a Blood
hubba . . . . rock cocaine
hurl . . . . vomit
hustler. . . . . not into gangs—strictly out to make money or impress girls
hyped . . . . excited or anxious

ice . . . . crystal methamphetamine

ignorant fools . . . . derogatory remarks for Inglewood Family Gangster Bloods

illing . . . . making mental mistakes

in pocket . . . . a subject who has drugs ready to sell

in the mix . . . . involved in gang activities

jack . . . . rob

jacked-up . . . . beat up or assaulted

jammed . . . . confronted

jet . . . . run away

Jim Jones . . . . marijuana joint laced with cocaine and dipped in PCP

jimmy . . . . condom

jiving . . . . attempting to fool someone

joning . . . . talking about someone

juiced lifts . . . . hydraulics to raise and lower a car

jump on . . . . intimidation

jungle fever . . . . black and white together

key . . . . kilo of cocaine in powder form

kibbles and bits . . . . crumbs of cocaine

kicking back . . . . relaxing/killing time

kickin it . . . . taking it easy

kick you down . . . . give you something/set you up in drug trade

killa . . . . killer

kite . . . . a written letter

kite in the wind . . . . a letter in the mail

klucka . . . . dope fiend

knocked . . . . killed

knockin boots . . . . having sex

kool . . . . it's all right

laces . . . . chrome/spoke rims

lady . . . . girlfriend

lame . . . . boring

legit . . . . for real/proper

let's bail . . . . let's leave

lifts . . . . hydraulics to raise and lower a car

lil mallow . . . . friend

liquid juice/sherm/wack . . . . PCP

lit up . . . . shot at

lizard butt . . . . ugly girl

loc . . . . crazy/loco (Crips)

LOCs . . . . dark sunglasses

lok . . . . crazy/loco (Bloods)

lokes . . . . dark sunglasses

love . . . . rock cocaine

low budget . . . . cheap girl
ludes . . . . nickname for quaaludes
lynch mob . . . . a gang
mack/drag/rush . . . . ability to sweet-talk girls
mackin . . . . getting girls
main man . . . . best friend/backup
making bank . . . . making money, usually in illegal ways
man . . . . the police/anyone in charge
mark . . . . someone who wants to be a gang member
mission . . . . gang activity/contract hit
mobile . . . . proper/nice looking
molded/scratch . . . . embarrassed
money . . . . person with money
Monte C . . . . Monte Carlo vehicle
mud duck . . . . ugly girl
mushroom . . . . an innocent bystander shot in drive-by shooting
mut . . . . male slut
N/H . . . . neighborhood
N-hood . . . . term meaning "in their turf"
nice roller . . . . nice car
not . . . . don't think so
nut up . . . . angry/mad at somebody
O . . . . reference to 1 ounce of cocaine
O/G . . . . original gangster/old
old bird/old jude . . . . mother and father
old head . . . . older gangster (OGs)
on the pipe . . . . freebasing cocaine
on the strength . . . . based on the facts
187 . . . . penal code for murder in California
one time . . . . police in area/the police
OPP . . . . other people's property
packing . . . . gang member has a gun or big sexual organs
pacman . . . . cop
pad . . . . house
peace cut . . . . goodbye/see you later
peanut butter . . . . Crips' disrespect for Bloods
people . . . . Vice Lords, Latin Kings, etc., and their affiliates
pig . . . . police officer
pimped out . . . . well dressed
pipe head . . . . crack addict
piru . . . . another name for Blood
played out . . . . over/no longer used
player/hustler . . . . someone not into gangs—strictly out to make money
                                                         or impress girls

popped a cap/busted . . . . shot at someone
posse . . . . East Coast term for gang
possie . . . . group of friends
primo . . . . marijuana laced with cocaine
proper . . . . legal/not selling dope
prune . . . . derogatory name for a Grape Street Crip used by a Blood gang member
psyco . . . . crazy
puffer . . . . cocaine smoker
puggin . . . . a fighter/involved in a fight
punk out . . . . to chicken out
put em in check . . . . discipline someone
put in some work . . . . do a shooting
put that on the set . . . . to validate what you're saying is true
queen . . . . female member of a gang
rag . . . . color of gang handkerchief
raggin . . . . to complain
RAIDERS . . . . remember after I die everyone runs scared
raise . . . . leave
raisin . . . . derogatory name for a Grape Street Crip used by a Blood gang member
raspberry . . . . female who takes anything for sex
recruiting . . . . looking for good-looking girls
red eye . . . . hard stare
relative . . . . Bloods' term for homeboy
rickett . . . . derogatory name for a Crip gang member used by a Blood gang member
ride . . . . car
ride on/rode on . . . . go to another rival neighborhood in vehicles to attack other gangs
rig . . . . combination of hypodermic needle, bottle cap, and a string or nylon to tie off arm before injecting drugs
righteous . . . . a response that means true/yes
rip off . . . . steal/take
road dog . . . . close friend
robo cop . . . . popular dance
rock . . . . crystallized cocaine
Rockboys . . . . Cobrastones, Black P Stones
rock star . . . . cocaine prostitute
roll-em . . . . to assault and rob/robbery
roll em up . . . . arrested/forced out of scene
rollin . . . . doing well/having a nice car
rollin donut . . . . derogatory name for a Crip
rolling good . . . . selling drugs

rosco . . . . gun
ru (rooster) . . . . piru
rush . . . . ability to sweet-talk girls
safe house . . . . a house where large amounts of drugs and money are stored. Usually only a select number of members have access to house.
saggin . . . . jailhouse life/wearing pants real low/gangstering
Satin Disciples . . . . white Disciple gang members
scam . . . . to acquire illegitimately
scandalous . . . . deadbeat person/bad person
scank . . . . extremely ugly or disgusting
scratch/molded . . . . embarrassed
sell out . . . . to sell out your race
set . . . . specific gang/location of turf
shank . . . . jail term for homemade knife
sherm/wack/liquid juice . . . . PCP
shooter . . . . enforcer
shotcaller . . . . person in charge/gang leader
skeezer . . . . ugly girl
skins . . . . a female sexual organ
slangin keys . . . . selling dope
sling or slang . . . . deals or sells cocaine
slob . . . . derogatory nickname for Blood gang members used by the Crips
slob on the knob . . . . oral sex
smoke . . . . kill, shoot
smoker . . . . person who smokes cocaine
snake . . . . popular dance
snaps . . . . money
snoop . . . . derogatory term for a Blood gang member
snow bunny . . . . a white girl
space base . . . . PCP/rock cocaine
speed . . . . common name for LSD
speed ball . . . . combination of heroin and cocaine
springs . . . . vehicle
sprung . . . . a person addicted to cocaine
spue . . . . vomit
squad . . . . fight/argument
square . . . . cigarette
stall it out . . . . stop doing what you're doing
stank . . . . dirty girl
straight . . . . for real/serious
straight shooter . . . . metal pipe (usually a car antenna) that is used to smoke crack

strap . . . . a gun
strapped . . . . carrying a gun
strawberry. a term for a female who performs sexual acts for cocaine
sufferin need bufferin . . . . having problems
sup . . . . what's up/what's going on
take him out of the box. . . . . to kill a rival gang member
talking from the heart. . . . . making gang signs while beating on one's chest
talking head . . . . arguing, wanting to fight
talking smack . . . . aggressive talking/challenging
tango & cash. . . . . fentanyl
teenager . . . . $\frac{1}{16}$ ounce of cocaine
TG. . . . . tiny gangster
that's hard . . . . cool
through . . . . ugly
throw down. fight
thumper. . . . . gun
tore your drouse . . . . had a dispute
toss-up . . . . girl used for sex
to the curb. . . . . bad/bad position to be in
touring a gang. . . . . hang out with gang members without being in a gang
trey . . . . three
trey eight. . . . . 38-caliber gun
trick/hook . . . . phony or sissy
trip . . . . too much/something else
turkish. . . . . term used to describe heavy, ornamental gold necklace
or earrings
TWA. . . . . teenie weenie afro
twenty. . . . . $20 piece of crack
20 cents. . . . . $20 worth of cocaine
ugs . . . . Blood
under cover. plain gang car
up on it . . . . have knowledge of drug scene/in the know on the drug
scene/a person who's successful dealing drugs
uzi. . . . . any semiautomatic handgun
vamp. . . . . leave
vapors. . . . . fumes from freebased cocaine/to identify money-hun-
gry females
Vicki Lous . . . . derogatory name for Vice Lords
violation . . . . a breaking of a gang rule that results in a punishment
wack patient . . . . an individual who smokes PCP and is paranoid
wack/sherm/liquid juice . . . . PCP
wacky tobaccy . . . . marijuana
wad-up . . . . stoned/high on drugs or alcohol

water . . . . PCP
wave . . . . short, close-cut haircut
what it B like . . . . Blood gang member greeting
what it C like . . . . Crip gang member greeting
what's up . . . . what's going on
what's up G . . . . hello friend
what set you from? . . . . what gang are you a member of or do you claim to be from
whaz up . . . . hello
word . . . . ok/all right
yo! . . . . hey!
you played yourself . . . . you did yourself wrong

Appendix 24–B

Graffiti

One of the first indications that gangs are forming in a community is the graffiti placed on buildings, fences, and sidewalks. Graffiti usually appears on the rear and sides of buildings where it is less visible to the public. This is done because the gang is testing the community's reaction to the graffiti. If the community does not have a strong response to the graffiti, it will begin to appear on the front of buildings. When this happens, the gang is telling the community that it has control of that particular neighborhood. This is why it is important to remove or cover the graffiti as soon as it is seen. The community must try to keep the upper hand on the gang(s).

Many members of the public view graffiti as a childish prank. Gang members view graffiti as the neighborhood newspaper. Graffiti marks the gang's territory, announces gang leaders and sometimes provides clues to gang crimes. Graffiti is commonly used to eulogize fallen gang members.

If an officer observes gang graffiti in the community and this graffiti is crossed over, it is an indication that more than one gang is active in that area. It is also an indication that more than one gang is active in that area. It is also an indication that the two gangs are hostile and that violence is imminent.

Below are some examples of graffiti that might be seen in your area.

THIRTY-THREE CALI   33CALI

NINE-DUCE INGLEWOOD FAMILY GANGSTER BLOODS   92IFGB

BLACK GANGSTER DISCIPLES

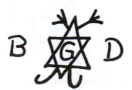

INSANE GANSTER
DISCIPLES

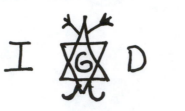

ROLLIN SIXTIES

CRIP KILLER

BLOOD KILLER

TWENTY-SEVEN MAC KILLER

REST IN PEACE

SIX-POINTED STAR OF DAVID SYMBOL USED
BY DISCIPLES

WHITE SUPREMIST GRAFFITI

CELTIC CROSS

SWASTIKA

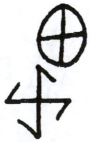

WHITE POWER

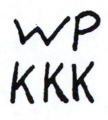

KU KLUX KLAN

All police officers should know how to read gang graffiti. Remember, gang graffiti can prove to be an excellent source of intelligence for law enforcement.

Appendix 24–C

Gang Affiliation Indicators

HAND SIGNALS

Hand signals are used by gangs to communicate with each other, to communicate gang affiliation and/or challenge rival gangs. The hand signals are made by forming letters, numbers, or symbols with the hands and fingers.

Gang members will also show disrespect to rival gangs by "throwing down" a rival gang's hand signals. In other words, gang members will take a rival gang's hand signals and turn them upside down to show disrespect. The "throwing down" of gang signs, if witnessed by the rival gang, is usually a prelude to violence.

Officers should not become too concerned with memorizing different hand signals; however, they should be generally familiar with their meaning(s).

TATTOOS

Tattoos are usually a strong indicator that a gang member is hard-core. If a gang member gets a gang tattoo, it could be an indication that the member is willing to display his or her gang membership to the police, friends, and family.

Gang members will usually tattoo a nickname on either the right or left arm., depending upon their affiliation with the Folks or Peoples Nation. Tattoos will also consist of the gang's initials, such as "62ECC" for Six Deuce East Coast Crips or "OG" for Organized Gangster Disciples, or Original Gangster.

Tattoos are also worn to honor slain gang members. These tattoos usually consist of the letters "RIP" with the deceased gang member's nickname. Another way of eulogizing a deceased gang member is with the teardrop tattoo or by wearing a gold tooth with the outline of a teardrop.

CLOTHING

The following information details current ways in which gang members are using popular sports and other clothing to represent individual gang affiliations. It should be noted that the wearing of this clothing does not always signify gang affiliation.

Atlanta Braves	Braves products are worn by gangs that are aligned with the Peoples Nation (e.g., Vice Lords and Bloods). The A signifies almighty.
British Knights	These gym shoes are worn by Crips for the logo "B-K," which signifies Blood killers.
Burger King	Logo initials "B-K" signify Blood killers.
Chicago Bulls	The color combination red and black represents the Bloods, Vice Lords, Latin Counts, Mickey Cobras/Cobra Stones, and Black P Stone Nation gangs. The letters B-U-L-L-S, signify boy your look like stone.
Cincinnati Reds	Reds products are worn by 4-corner Street Hustlers Vice Lords gang.
Colorado Rockies	Rockies products are commonly worn by Crip gang members. The logo "C-R" signifies Crips rule.
Columbia Knights	These gym shoes are worn by Bloods for the logo "C-K," which signifies Crip killers.
Converse	These gym shoes are worn by gangs that are aligned with the Peoples Nation (e.g., Vice Lords and Bloods). Worn for the five-pointed star.
Dallas Cowboys	Cowboys products are worn by gangs affiliated with the Peoples Nation for the five-pointed star.
Duke	Duke clothing is worn by gangs affiliated with the Folks Nation (e.g., Disciples and Crips). The letters D-U-K-E signify Disciples utilizing knowledge everyday.
Georgetown Hoyas	The colors are black and blue. The letters H-O-Y-A-S signify Hoover's on your ass. The G stands for gangster. Commonly worn by the Disciple gang members.
Kansas City Royals	The colors are black and blue. The letters "K-C" signify Kitchen Crips, a gang based out of Los Angeles, California, with a subset in St. Louis, Missouri. 87 Kitchen Crip gangsters.
Raiders jacket	Because of its popularity with entertainers and rap artists, this jacket is very popular with both black and white youth. It is the jacket of choice of the Gangster Disciples and Crips. The team's letters R-A-I-D-E-R-S signify remember after I die everybody runs scared.
Kings jackets	A Kings jacket has the same color combination as a Raiders jacket. It also is a jacket of choice of the Gangster Disciples and the Latin Kings.

LA Dodgers	The color combination is blue and white. This is the preferred clothing of the Disciples. D stands for Disciples.
Magic jacket	The color combination is blue and black. This jacket is popular with Crips and Gangster Disciples.
San Diego Padres	The initials S D stand for six deuce, as in Six Deuce East Coast Crips.
White Sox	The color combination is black and white. White Sox clothing is preferred by the Gangster Disciples and some Crips.
UNLV	The colors are red and black. U-N-L-V spelled backward stands for Vice Lord Nation United.

Chapter 25

Workplace Violence in the Health Care Environment

CHAPTER OBJECTIVES

1. Understand the need for a policy concerning violence in the health care workplace.
2. Understand the legal aspects of maintaining a safe and secure facility.
3. Review the Occupational Safety and Health Administration guidelines to help prevent violence in the workplace.
3. Know how to recognize potentially violent employees and potentially volatile situations.
4. Learn the various components of workplace violence prevention.

INTRODUCTION

There is no doubt that health care facilities, once a safe haven, are experiencing an alarming increase in violence. Health care staff face a more violent workplace than they once did.

Bureau of Labor Statistics data reveal that, among all types of workers, health care workers have the highest incident of assault injuries. Violence in health care facilities is so pervasive that the Occupational Safety and Health Administration (OSHA) has published guidelines to help prevent violence in the health care setting.

Not only are health care workers subject to death and injury, but patients and those visiting the facilities have been the victims of violence. These victims usually file lawsuits claiming negligent security against the facility. Claims against health care facilities for negligent security and premises liability are among the fastest-growing types of litigation today.

There are also employee lawsuits. In many instances, facilities are finding that the courts are permitting employees to go beyond the limitations of workers' compensation and to file lawsuits against their employers when they are victims of workplace violence.

With these two types of lawsuits becoming more prevalent, a brief discussion of the legal aspects of health care facility security is in order. The following discussion is not to be considered legal advice. Readers should always consult with their facilities' legal departments about premises liability and negligent security.

NEGLIGENCE

The cornerstone of most of these lawsuits is a breach of duty, commonly called negligence. To understand what negligence is, it is necessary to understand the basic definition of a tort.

> When a tort occurs, party A (being a person or legal entity) owes a duty to party B (another person or legal entity) and breaches that duty by act or omission and proximately causes damages (injury) to party B.

In these facility security cases, both the facility and the person committing the violence are party A. The employee or a third-party visitor is party B. The duty is the legal requirement, based upon community and industry standards, to provide a reasonably safe environment for working and visiting. In this discussion, "duty" means "adherence to a standard of care." This standard of care is established by a review of the facility, the area surrounding the facility, incidents of security threats in other facilities in the community, and the national industry standards for similar facilities in similar settings. This review must be made by an expert in the field of security, preferably health care security. The findings of the review are presented in court in the form of an expert witness opinion.

The breach of the duty would be the claim of inadequate security or the failure to act on information that could have prevented the violent act. Consideration of this breach is based upon the fact that the facility does not meet the standard of care as established by the opinion of the expert witnesses and other facts in the case. The breach of duty means that party A did not fulfill the duty of reasonableness. In other words, based upon community and industry standards, party A did not act in a reasonable manner to prevent the violent act. Obviously, both parties in the case will have expert witnesses who may disagree on the standard of care or duty.

In most employee injury cases, workers' compensation is the only recourse for recovery for the employee. However, if the employee can show that the employer had actual knowledge (notice) of something or should have known (constructive notice) something that could have led to anticipating the violent act and preventing it from occurring, the employee may be able to claim that the employer was grossly negligent and proceed with the lawsuit outside of the confines of workers' compensation.

The damages are the physical and emotional injuries the employee or third party received due to the violent act. These damages consider the lost wages, medical bills, and pain and suffering resulting from the event. In many of the lawsuits that have been filed by employees, the employees claim emotional damages in the form of post-traumatic stress. The employees usually claim that they are so emotionally handicapped by the event that they are totally disabled and cannot work in a similar setting again.

It should be pointed out that the facility's insurance carrier will usually pay for the defense and compensatory damages in these cases. But punitive damages awarded by the court are not usually covered by insurance. Punitive damages in the hundreds of thousands and even millions of dollars are not uncommon in these cases. This is especially true for facilities in which there have been several violent events.

OSHA GUIDELINES

While the OSHA guidelines are not to be considered regulations, failure to adhere to these guidelines may lead to sanctions for not maintaining a safe and healthy workplace. These guidelines, which appear in Appendix 25–A, address only the violent acts that patients may commit against staff. The guidelines have four basic components.

1. management commitment and employee involvement
2. work site analysis
3. hazard prevention and control
4. safety and health training

Management Commitment and Employee Involvement

Both management commitment and employee involvement are essential to keeping health care facilities safe. Top managers must show their support and concern for worker safety. They can do so by providing a written policy that expressly prohibits any workplace violence and providing funding for educational programs to fully inform and train staff on this issue. In response, employees must give management sufficient feedback on the zero-based policy (i.e., no violence is acceptable) and accept the fact that they can make a difference in the workplace by promptly reporting events that have or are likely to happen.

Work Site Analysis

Work site analysis is a step-by-step review of the facility and the likely areas where violence has or probably could occur. This analysis should be conducted either by a security professional or by a threat assessment team. It should include analyzing and tracking records, monitoring trends, analyzing incidents, screening surveys, and analyzing workplace security.

Hazard Prevention and Control

Once workplace hazards are identified, the next step is to design measures through engineering design or administrative and work practices to prevent or control these hazards. If violence does occur, how a facility responds can help prevent future incidents.

Safety and Health Training

Training and education ensure that all staff are aware of potential security hazards and how to protect themselves and their coworkers through established policies and procedures. Everyone must learn to practice "universal precautions for violence": violence should be expected but can be avoided or mitigated through preparation.

WORKPLACE VIOLENCE

As stated above, the OSHA guidelines address only patient-to-staff violence. They do not cover the full definition of workplace violence used by security professionals today: Any incident at the workplace that results in physical or psychological injury to someone, damage to property, including graffiti, or loss of productivity.

As this definition shows, workplace violence can take many forms. In addition to the possibility of injury from patients, health care staff must be alert to other threats. Who knows when a disgruntled employee may return to the workplace and commit unthinkable acts? What about the possibility of a family member causing a life-threatening injury to a supervisor in retaliation for the supervisor's reprimanding the family member's loved one? The following sections discuss factors that may make workplace violence more likely at health care facilities.

Downsizing

Probably every health care facility and medical clinic has downsized within the past five years. The fear of losing one's job increases stress, as does being asked to "do more with less." Any staff member will probably say that the overall quality of care the patient is receiving has diminished in recent years. Where there were once only 4 to 6 patients for every nurse, reduced staffing levels mean that some nurses may have to tend to 8 to 10 patients. In many cases, facilities require that a family member stay with the patient at all times to help in rendering care and to monitor the patient. Lower budgets and smaller staffs increase stress for the staff and for the patient's family.

Stressful Emergency Departments

Lacking health insurance, more and more families today use the local emergency department as their family physicians. This causes a higher patient load at the same time that budget cuts are reducing staff rosters. In addition, the prevalence of gang-related violence and domestic violence—both of which land their victims in the emergency department—is increasing. With more patients, fewer staff, worried families and friends anxiously awaiting news about patients, and rival gangs following victims to emergency departments, is it a wonder that violent acts occur in emergency departments?

Some facilities use patient representatives to inform family members of patients' status, thus reducing anxiety and violence. These long waits are more tolerable if information is provided regularly.

Drug and Alcohol Abuse and Domestic Violence

Health care staff are not immune to the normal societal ills. Currently, 1 in 10 adults in the United States has a substance abuse problem. This causes an enormous amount of stress and possible family violence.

All family issues, from substance abuse to domestic violence, can easily spill over into the workplace. A facility must determine, in advance, its position on exposing other staff and patients to domestic violence. A corporate statement must discuss whether a staff member will be allowed to stay on duty if he or she thinks there is a good possibility that a family member will come to the facility to commit a violent act.

The Facility Environment

No one except staff wants to be at a health care facility. No one wants to be sick or injured or to have a loved one who is sick or injured. Fear of being in the health care facility, of losing a loved one, and of financial ruin are very real. People handle these fears in different ways. For some, violent acts are spontaneous events. Others may become violent after they decide that their loved one's death was the facility's fault.

PREVENTING VIOLENCE IN THE HEALTH CARE FACILITY

Written Corporate Policy and Procedure

A comprehensive corporate policy stating that the corporation has zero tolerance for violence must be drafted, distributed, and discussed. The policy should address not only physical assaults but also verbal threats and damage to property. Exhibit 25–1 shows a sample policy.[1]

Employees should be required to report incidents. A method of reporting anonymously should be established so that employees will feel comfortable making reports. The policy must clearly state that there will be no reprisals against anyone for making such a report.

Exhibit 25–1 Sample Policy Regarding Workplace Violence in the Health Care Facilities

---

Purpose

The hospital system is committed to providing each employee a work environment that is safe and secure and free of prejudice, harassment, threats, intimidation, and violence.

Policy

In order to protect employees, their belongings, and hospital property, as well as maintain an orderly working environment and prevent disclosure of confidential hospital information, the following security measures are necessary, and all employees must abide by them.

- Each applicant for employment will undergo a pre-employment background investigation and a criminal records check, consistent with his or her position. The exact criteria will be determined by the director of human resources.
- This policy, when implemented, requires the participation of all employees. Attendance at related educational sessions will be mandatory.
- No friends or relatives of an employee will be permitted on hospital premises without the approval of that employee's supervisor.
- The hospital reserves the right to conduct searches of persons and their personal belongings whenever it is deemed necessary. This includes employee vehicles. An employee's consent to searches is required as a condition of employment. An employee's refusal to give consent will result in immediate discharge. For the purposes of protection and security, the hospital utilizes electronic surveillance on its facilities. All employees are required to wear their identification badges at all times while on hospital property.

The following rules have been established to define and protect the rights and property of City Hospital System and its employees. It is the policy of the hospital to prosecute employees who

---

continues

Exhibit 25–1 continued

commit criminal offenses against the hospital or its employees. The following actions are subject to disciplinary action up to and including termination:

- distribution of non-work-related written or printed material
- using hospital vehicles, copying machines, or other materials or equipment for unauthorized personal use
- defacing hospital identification badges or name tags, or using duplicated or altered badges, name tags, or parking decals for unauthorized purposes
- horseplay, dangerous practical joking, and other unsafe conduct
- insubordination or uncooperative conduct, including refusing to follow a supervisor's requests, instructions, or orders
- posting, defacing, or removing notices or signs, or writing on bulletin boards or company property, unless authorized to do so
- unauthorized entry into or exit from hospital premises at points other than those established as normal areas of entry and exit for employees. This includes leaving points of entry or exit to the hospital or its facilities and/or its offices unlocked or in any way unsecure when it is the employee's responsibility to secure same. This is not limited to the employee's work area. This includes the practice of propping open doors to gain access back into an office and/or facility.
- stealing or damaging any hospital property
- falsifying or omitting pertinent facts on any hospital-required reports or documentation
- engaging in illegal, immoral, or indecent conduct on company premises or off premises while on hospital business
- bringing onto hospital property, including hospital-owned or -leased parking areas, any firearm, knife, explosive material, toxic agent, or any other weapon or device intended to be used as a tool of violence
- threatening, intimidating, coercing, harassing (including verbal, physical, and visual sexual harassment), or interfering with fellow employees on hospital premises or creating discord or lack of harmony. Harassment includes
  - verbal harassment such as name calling, derogatory comments or slurs based on sex or other criteria
  - physical harassment, such as assault, impeding or blocking movement, or any physical interference with normal work or movement when directed at an individual
  - visual forms of harassment, such as displaying derogatory posters, cartoons, or drawings that are offensive
  - requests for sexual favors or unwanted sexual advances
  - any other conduct that unreasonably interferes with an employee's performance of his or her job or that creates an intimidating, hostile, or offensive work environment
- use of abusive or threatening language toward another employee, a supervisor, or any other person on company premises
- unauthorized opening of or tampering with locks, unauthorized duplication of keys issued by the hospital, or unauthorized entry to restricted or locked areas, unauthorized loaning of keys to nonemployees or employees not issued the same keys, or unauthorized release of keypad entry information to nonemployees or employees not authorized to know that information

continues

Exhibit 25–1 continued

- unauthorized entrance to hospital premises or unauthorized areas during nonscheduled work hours
- inducing another employee to violate hospital policies
- violation of other hospital policies regulating employee business conduct
- using, possessing, selling, giving away, or being under the influence of prohibited or controlled substances (unless prescribed by a licensed physician and approved by the employee's supervisor) or intoxicants while on hospital time and property. Alcoholic beverages may be served at appropriate hospital-sponsored functions with administration approval.

Procedure

- Any violations of this policy are to be reported to the employee's supervisor for investigation and action.
- When appropriate, the supervisor or manager may confer with the director of human resources with the assistance of the director of security for further action and investigation.
- Violations of this policy that are sustained as a result of an investigation will result in disciplinary action up to and including termination.

This policy should also discuss the corporation's various methods for assisting employees who find themselves in potentially violent situations. It is important to have an employee assistance program whose leaders work closely with the security department.

The policy should state that those who breach the policy will be disciplined up to and including termination. In addition, the policy should note that in certain circumstances law enforcement will be brought in and the perpetrator will be prosecuted.

This policy must be conveyed in writing and in employee forums to all employees (see Appendix 25–B). Everyone in the organization must be advised of and acknowledge understanding of the policy.

Supervisor and Staff Training

The facility should conduct training sessions concerning the workplace violence policy. These training sessions should be conducted on various days and shifts to reach all employees.

Separate sessions should be held for general employees and for supervisors. Obviously, some information will apply to all employees, while some will be aimed at supervisors in particular. Having separate sessions will minimize training time and allow more focused question-and-answer sessions. Ideally, these training sessions should be mandatory and videotaped so that they may be watched by new hires and employees just promoted to supervisors. The following sections will assist the facility in developing the various training sessions.

DEALING WITH PATIENTS IN THE PREASSAULTIVE STAGE*

Staff should be trained to implement and utilize common sense interventions for any patient assessed as being in the preassaultive phase. The following therapeutic interventions are geared toward decreasing the patient's stress level.

- Approach the patient with caution (not fear). The patient will respect the fact that staff have recognized that he or she may lose control and are taking appropriate action by treating the patient and the situation with respectful caution.
- Avoid startling the patient. Approach the patient from the front and do not begin speaking until you have first made eye contact. Gauge your actions by the patient's responses. Do not address the patient when he or she cannot see you or you are out of the patient's view.
- Avoid provocation whenever possible.
- Be aware of your facial expression. Strive for a neutral expression that does not convey judgment, fear, anxiety, or disgust. Avoid smiling when communicating with a paranoid patient, who may misinterpret your expression (i.e., the patient may think you are laughing at or mocking him or her or that you view him or her with contempt).
- Keep your tone of voice calm and speak normally. Avoid yelling, rapid speech, escalating pitch, and any terminology that the patient might not understand. Use vernacular in situations where it is appropriate. Street language may also be therapeutic, depending on the patient and conditions and circumstances. This decision is a matter of judgment.
- Do not use profanity and rude gestures in response to a patient's usage of such tactics. Do not show shock in response to the language or the gestures. The patient is expressing himself or herself in the only way possible at that particular time. Sometimes patients will curse and use rude gestures in an attempt to frighten you, get you to keep your distance, or keep you at emotional arm's length. Sometimes the patient behaves in that manner because that reflects his or her personality. In any case, try to decipher what the patient's behaviors signify without being judgmental.
- Use open-ended questions that provide openings for the disturbed patient to verbalize feelings (e.g., "How are you feeling now?"). Remember, although what you say is important, how you say it is even more important, because the patient will respond to a gentle but assertive tone.
- Avoid promises. Never make promises that the next shift will have to honor. If staff on the next shift's workload or unit activities prohibit them from honoring the promise you made, that might be viewed as a provocation by the already disturbed patient, and the staff will find themselves confronted with a hostile, untrusting, preassaultive patient.
- Avoid using "okay" at the end of your sentences because this term implies choices when none may exist, and its usage could be confusing and ambiguous to patients, some of whom may already have considerable difficulty processing the stimuli in their environment.

---

*Adapted from Carol A. Distasio, "Violence in Health Care: Institutional Strategies To Cope with the Phenomenon," *Health Care Supervisor*, Vol. 12:4, © 1994, Aspen Publishers, Inc.

- Avoid challenges. Do not confront the patient. Nobody wins in a confrontation with a violent patient. Keep your goal (i.e., to calm the patient) in mind constantly.
- Be aware of your posture. Avoid threatening or closed communication positions (e.g., arms folded or crossed over your chest). Strive for neutral, nonthreatening positions. Listen attentively when the patient speaks, and let your posture show your interest.
- Remove anything that may be used as a weapon by the patient from your person (e.g., scissors, stethoscope). Wearing dangly pierced earrings is not a good idea when working in a psychiatric unit or in situations involving potential violence.
- Know where the nearest exit is, and do not permit any obstacles to come between you and that exit in any interaction with a patient who is in the preassaultive stage.
- Avoid vulnerable positions (e.g., do not lean over the patient's chair or bed, do not "get in the patient's face"). Again, let your actions be governed by common sense.
- Do not turn your back on any patient in the preassaultive stage under any circumstances. The patient may think your turning your back expresses a lack of respect, which is a provocation. Moreover, when you turn your back you communicate a disregard for the patient's feelings and send all the wrong messages to the patient: "I'm not afraid of you. See, I turn my back on you." "You're not a threat to me" (denial). "You can't hurt me, I'm the physician" (or other staff member).
- Equally important, all staff must take responsibility for personal safety, and denial of the very real risks that exist with any emotionally disturbed preassaultive patient is not prudent or therapeutic. Besides, it will do nothing to decrease your personal risks. On the contrary, in all probability, it will increase those risks.
- Organize all supplies (and only those supplies) needed to provide a treatment before entering a patient's room, ask permission to enter the room, explain the purpose of the visit, and ask permission to perform the treatment—all before proceeding over to the patient. Keep the patient's room free of items that may be used as weapons as much as possible.
- Use paper meal trays and plastic utensils for very disturbed patients, when indicated, and encourage the patient to eat in his or her room or other quiet area, where stimuli are reduced or can be more readily controlled.
- Stand in the doorway when awakening a sleeping patient, and call the patient's name until he or she awakens. Do not shake or yell at the patient, and keep your distance until the patient is fully awake and aware of his or her surroundings. Do not awaken the patient using the intercom at the nurses' station because the patient may be startled awake by a voice but will have no person in his or her room with whom he or she can have eye contact and talk directly. Using the intercom with a sleeping patient who is experiencing auditory hallucinations or paranoid delusions may exacerbate psychiatric symptoms—not to mention increase anxiety and provoke anger in the patient.
- Strive for early cue recognition and early interventions. This approach affords you the best chance of avoiding progression to the violent stage.
- Show empathy for the patient's plight but communicate very clearly that you expect the patient to maintain self-control. It is very frightening to some patients to feel that they are going to lose control. Reassure the patient that staff will help assist with self-control if he or she cannot maintain it. The patient needs to know that staff will retain control of the situation.

- Attempt to distract the patient and redirect attention. Encourage time-outs for patients whose stress levels are escalating.
- Be assertive. Be firm but compassionate. Remember, the patient is a troubled human being who is experiencing emotional and psychological disturbances that may be more frightening for the patient than they are for the staff. Act at all times with respect and concern for the patient.
- Ask family or significant others to assist with the patient's care, if appropriate, and invite them to participate or contribute to the patient care planning process. The patient should also be invited to participate in the plan of care.
- Use verbal skills to defuse situations whenever possible.

OFFENDER PROFILE

Though all different kinds of people have the potential to become violent in a workplace, a certain profile of the typical offender has emerged.

- The person is a male.
- He is in his thirties or forties.
- He is white.
- He is a socially isolated loner who does not have a support system.
- He owns guns and displays a fascination with weapons.
- He has a long history of frustration and failure.
- He blames others for his failures.
- He cannot handle defeat or rejection.
- His identity is tied to his work.
- He has demonstrated emotional or mental instability in the past.
- He is intimidating and defiant, or he blatantly violates organization procedures.
- He has made threats against the organization or an individual.
- He has a history of violence. He has made threats or acted out violently before.
- He is often from a battered home filled with violent conflict.
- Often, one of his parents abused alcohol or other substances.
- He is suicidal.
- He has experienced some precipitating event, such as being fired or getting divorced.
- He has gone from job to job during his lifetime.
- He is chronically disgruntled.
- He takes criticism poorly.

IDENTIFYING A VIOLENT PATIENT OR VISITOR

Contrary to popular belief, people do not just "go off." They always display signs of increasing stress and agitation. Staff should summon help quickly if someone in the work environment displays any of the following signs.

- talks and complains loudly, uses profanity, and makes sexual comments
- makes unnecessary demands for services

- says that he or she is going to lose control
- paces about the waiting room in a very agitated manner
- starts to focus his or her attention on or stares at one person
- appears very tense and angry
- challenges authority
- appears to be drunk or under the influence of drugs
- has a history of previous violence

DEALING WITH A PERSON WHO APPEARS TO BE BECOMING VIOLENT

Planning is the key to surviving a potentially violent episode. Each facility should plan and prepare written policies and provide training for staff who may have to cope with potentially violent persons. Staff should learn at least the following strategies:

- Do not argue with or provoke the hostile person.
- Some eye contact may be okay, but avoid staring at the person. It could be interpreted as confrontational.
- Be honest about the situation and explain the reason for any delays if delays are causing the agitation.
- Make comments only about the person's behavior and not about him or her personally.
- Do not violate the person's space. Keep at least two to three arm's lengths away from the hostile person, and do not allow yourself to be backed into a corner. Leave room for your escape if necessary.
- Talk to the person in a firm tone, making sentences short and direct.
- Listen to and acknowledge your concern for the person's anger. Do not accept the blame for any of the accusations made. Never say "I understand."
- Try to separate the person from others. Move him or her into another room if possible.
- Check for weapons. Look for the possibility of a weapon, either on the person or a potential weapon in the area (i.e., a lamp, chair, etc.).
- Make no heroic attempts to subdue or control the patient.
- Do not lie to the patient.
- Get help! Call the warning code or similar emergency code to alert security and health care facility staff to a threat. The code should trigger a rapid response from trained personnel in the health care facility to report to the area.

If violence occurs, take the following steps:

- Call facility security and/or the police at 911.
- Do not attempt to subdue the person yourself.
- Give the patient drugs if he or she demands them.
- Keep other patients away from the incident.

After all episodes of violence are over, reflect on and talk about what could be done better the next time. Report episodes of verbal and physical abuse to the department manager, security, human resources, and/or administration.

CONCLUSION

The subject of workplace violence is a very important one for health care facility security. A facility must not only address the regulatory and legal demands associated with workplace violence but also ensure that visitors, patients, and staff feel and are secure. Health care facilities must once again become a safe harbor and protect society's most fragile members.

KEY POINTS

- Lawsuits for negligent security are becoming more common.
- OSHA has passed standards for preventing violence in health care facilities.
- Stress in today's health care facilities increases the likelihood of violence.
- Facilities must have a written policy concerning workplace violence.
- Staff must be trained in recognizing potentially violent employees and visitors.

REFERENCE

1. Joint Commission on Accreditation of Healthcare Organizations; Comprehensive Accreditation Manual for Hospitals; Standard EC 1.4, Effective 1/1/97; Joint Commission; Oakbrook Terrace, IL; 1996.

SUGGESTED READING

Occupational Safety and Health Administration, Guidelines for Preventing Violence for Healthcare and Social Service Workers; Document 3148; U.S. Department of Labor; 1996.

Appendix 25–A

OSHA #3148: Guidelines for Preventing Workplace Violence for Health Care and Social Services Workers*

EXTENT OF PROBLEM

Statistics from the Bureau of Labor Statistics indicate that more assaults take place in the health care and social service industries than in any other industry. One statistic shows that in 1993 health care and social service workers sustained more assault injuries than all other workers (BLS, 1993). The settings for nearly two-thirds of the nonfatal assaults included nursing homes, hospitals, and institutions rendering in-patient care and other social services (Toscano and Weber, 1995).

According to a number of studies, assault on health professionals is not a phenomenon born in recent years. In the period between 1980 and 1990, 106 health care workers were killed while performing their jobs (Goodman et al., 1994). This number was comprised of 27 pharmacists, 26 physicians, 18 registered nurses, 17 nurses' aides, and 18 health care workers in other areas. This same study found that 69 registered nurses were killed on the job between 1983 and 1989. In nursing homes and personal care facilities, homicide was the main cause of traumatic occupational death among employees.

The rate of assault per one hundred employees among health care staff at a psychiatric hospital was far above the rate of injuries found in other industries. The nursing staff at a psychiatric hospital experienced 16 assaults per 100 employees per year (Carmel and Hunter, 1989), while only 8.3 out of every 100 full-time workers in all industries and 14.2 out of every 100 full-time construction workers sustained injuries of all types (BLS, 1991). After being injured on the job, 43% of 121 psychiatric hospital workers who sustained 134 injuries missed work, and 13% of them missed more than three weeks.

While the occurrence of violence in the health care and social service industries is of great concern simply due to the threat it poses to workers' physical safety, even more disturbing are underlying issues such as under reporting and health care workers' attitudes toward on-the-job violence. Some incidents of workplace violence are not reported, and many health care workers see violence and assault as everyday job-related risks. Several reasons for under reporting and the belief that assault must be accepted may be identified, and they include an absence of institutional reporting policies, worker opinions that reporting incidents will prove

---

*Source: Occupational Safety and Health Administration, Guidelines for Preventing Violence for Healthcare and Social Service Workers; Document 3148, U.S. Department of Labor; 1996.

to be futile in the end, or worker worries that a report of assault will reflect negatively on the worker's job performance.

RISK FACTORS

The rate of assault among health care and social service workers continues rising due to the following:

- The increased presence of guns and other weapons in the health care and social service setting.
- The trend among the police and the criminal justice system of using hospitals to detain criminals and severely disturbed, violent persons.
- The growing number of mentally disturbed individuals who are released without the assurance that they will be monitored in the future, which is added to the fact that they now also have the ability to decline medication and hospitalization, unless they may do harm to themselves or others.
- The likelihood that a hospital, clinic, or pharmacy will become a target for robbery due to the presence of money or drugs.
- Certain conditions and situations such as the unmonitored movement of people through the institution, the increasing presence of gang members, alcoholics, drug addicts, trauma patients, upset family members, the frustration created by long emergency room waits in patients who expect medical attention.
- The inadequate staffing levels experienced especially during busy times such as at meal times and during visiting hours.
- Situations such as examinations and treatment which place the worker in a one-on-one situation with the patient.
- The unavailability of assistance and the inability to obtain assistance using communication devices or alarm systems, which are especially serious in remote and high-crime areas.
- The staff's unfamiliarity with the characteristics of assaultive behavior and escalating hostility.
- Dark parking areas.

OVERVIEW OF GUIDELINES

In January 1989, OSHA made available general recommendations to employers on how to ensure safety in the workplace. OSHA subsequently published violence prevention guidelines, and these guidelines take the generic recommendation one step further by offering a list of the most important risk factors and ways to minimize their effects.

OSHA's objective is to ensure that workers are no longer faced with dangerous situations by adopting certain routines and by acquiring security devices such as an alarm system.

The guidelines set forth by OSHA apply to a wide range of health care and social service workers employed in a variety of settings. The workers include physicians, registered nurses, pharmacists, nurse practitioners, physicians' assistants, nurses' aides, therapists, technicians, public health nurses, home health care workers, social/welfare workers, and emergency medical care personnel. Also affected are auxiliary workers such as secretaries and clergy.

The employee environment may be a psychiatric facility, a hospital emergency department, a community mental health clinic, a drug abuse treatment clinic, a pharmacy, a community care facility, or a long-term care facility.

VIOLENCE PREVENTION PROGRAM ELEMENTS

Four essential factors which are required for a successful safety and health program are in fact also necessary in preventing workplace violence, (1) management commitment and employee involvement, (2) worksite analysis, (3) hazard prevention and control, and (4) safety and health training.

Management Commitment and Employee Involvement

In order to sustain a working safety and health program, it is vital that management and the employees work together. One can opt to use committees or teams, but, if so, one must ensure compliance with the applicable provisions of the National Labor Relations Act.

When management and top officials are clearly involved, the occurrence of workplace violence will be dealt with in a positive manner. Management commitment should include the following:

- A visible consideration for the workers' emotional and physical well-being.
- A fair balance between concern for the workers' safety and the patient's safety.
- A clear division of duties among management, supervisors, and employees so that each does his part in preventing workplace violence.
- A method by which managers, supervisors, and employees can be held responsible for their actions.
- A medical and psychological program designed to treat employees who have been the victim of assault or who have seen an assault take place.
- A serious consideration of safety and health committees' recommendations.

By making sure that employees are involved in the effort to promote workplace safety more ideas on how to improve and execute safety measures are obtained.

Employee involvement has to have the following:

- A strict compliance with existing workplace violence prevention program measures.
- The expression of concerns and ideas pertaining to safety and security in the workplace.
- The fast and honest reporting of absolutely all violent incidents.
- Active involvement in committees which concern workplace safety.
- Receiving training on safety and security issues, such as on how to recognize escalating hostile behavior, assaultive behavior, or criminal intent and how to deal with each of these issues.

Written Program

A comprehensive safety and security policy needs to be written out, though the level of complexity of the program should reflect the size and complexity of the organization. The most important function of a safety policy is to set forth concrete goals that are realistic given the size of the institution and that can be changed to fit any given situation.

Once a safety policy is devised, it should be made available to all employees, and all workers must be made aware of the date of effectiveness. Every workplace violence prevention program should do at least the following:

- Communicate to managers, supervisors, co-workers, clients, patients, and visitors the fact that no violence, threatening, or otherwise hostile behavior will be tolerated in the workplace.
- Guarantee employees the right to report violent incidents without negative repercussions and ensure that no negative actions are taken against any worker who is the victim of workplace violence.
- Motivate employees to report all occasions of violence and how they think risk factors might be minimized. Keep written records of all incidents for the purpose of measuring perceived risk and effectiveness of safety measures.
- Set forth a plan of action for creating a safe work environment, which includes working together with safety experts such as law enforcement representatives and others who might be able to point out important risk factors and how to minimize their effects.
- Place people who have had or will be having training on how to create a safe workplace in the health and social service industries in positions of authority in the program. Budget an appropriate amount of resources for safety training.
- Reiterate to the employee that management is dedicated to creating a worker-supportive environment which values employee safety and health and patient or client satisfaction equally.
- Set up a company briefing as part of the initial effort to address such issues as preserving safety, supporting affected employees, and facilitating recovery.

Worksite Analysis

An essential component of creating a safe work environment is examining the physical setting and identifying existing or potential hazards for workplace violence. This process includes determining if certain practices create risks or if certain locations are especially dangerous.

A group referred to as the "Threat Assessment Team," "Patient Assault Team," similar task force, or a coordinator should be in charge of determining where the risks for violence lie and how violent incidents might be avoided. This same group should then also be responsible for putting the workplace violence prevention program into practice. Senior management, operations, employee assistance, security, occupational safety and health, legal, and human resources staff should be present on the team.

By examining records such as workers' compensation claims and illness and injury records, the team or coordinator may notice that assaults recur in similar situations. In that case, anything which can be done to ameliorate the situation should promptly be done.

Worksite analysis programs should involve reviewing workers' records, examining each violent incident with attention to the development of patterns, considering workers' suggestions and complaints, and assessing the workplace's general security.

Records Analysis and Tracking

This particular component of a workplace violence prevention program requires analyzing medical, safety, workers' compensation, and insurance records to review occasions of violence in the workplace. It may be noted that violence is more likely to occur in specific locations or in certain departments or units, and individuals with certain job titles and tasks may also be more susceptible. In addition, some violence may be associated with a time of day. By keeping track of such factors and reviewing their role in each violent incident, it is possible to determine a baseline from which to assess the safety measures' success.

Monitoring Trends and Analyzing Incidents

Contacting similar local businesses, trade associations, and community and civic groups is one way to learn about their experiences with workplace violence and to help identify trends. Use several years of data, if possible, to trace trends of injuries and incidents of actual or potential workplace violence.

Screening Surveys

One important screening tool is to give employees a questionnaire or survey to get their ideas on the potential for violent incidents and to identify or confirm the need for improved security measures. Detailed baseline screening surveys can help pinpoint tasks that put employees at risk. Periodic surveys—conducted at least annually or whenever operations change or incidents of workplace violence occur—help identify new or previously unnoticed risk factors and deficiencies or failures in work practices, procedures, or controls. Also the surveys help assess the effects of changes in the work processes. The periodic review process should also include feedback and follow-up.

Independent reviewers, such as safety and health professionals, law enforcement or security specialists, insurance safety auditors, and other qualified persons may offer advice to strengthen programs. These experts also can provide fresh perspectives to improve a violence prevention program.

Workplace Security Analysis

The team or coordinator should periodically inspect the workplace and evaluate employee tasks to identify hazards, conditions, operations, and situations that could lead to violence.

To find areas requiring future evaluation, the team or coordinator should do the following:

- Analyze incidents, including the characteristics of assailants and victims, an account of what happened before and during the incident, and the relevant details of the situation and its outcome. When possible, obtain police reports and recommendations.
- Identify jobs or locations with the greatest risk of violence as well as processes and procedures that put employees at risk of assault, including how often and when.
- Note high-risk factors such as types of clients or patients (e.g., psychiatric conditions or patients disoriented by drugs, alcohol, or stress); physical risk factors of the building;

isolated locations/job activities; lighting problems; lack of phones and other communication devices; areas of easy, unsecured access; and areas with previous security problems.

- Evaluate the effectiveness of existing security measures, including engineering control measures. Determine if risk factors have been reduced or eliminated, and take appropriate action.

HAZARD PREVENTION AND CONTROL

After hazards of violence are identified through the systematic worksite analysis, the next step is to design measures through engineering or administrative and work practices to prevent or control these hazards. If violence does occur, post-incident response can be an important tool in preventing future incidents.

Engineering Controls and Workplace Adaptation

Engineering controls, for example, remove the hazard from the workplace or create a barrier between the worker and the hazard. There are several measures that can effectively prevent or control workplace hazards, such as those actions presented in the following paragraphs. The selection of any measure, of course, should be based upon the hazards identified in the workplace security analysis of each facility.

Assess any plans for new construction or physical changes to the facility or workplace to eliminate or reduce hazards.

Install and regularly maintain alarm systems and other security devices, panic buttons, hand-held alarms or noise devices, cellular phones, and private channel radios where risk is apparent or may be anticipated, and arrange for a reliable response system when an alarm is triggered.

Provide metal detectors—installed or hand-held, where appropriate—to identify guns, knives, or other weapons, according to the recommendations of security consultants.

Use a closed-circuit video recording for high-risk areas on a 24-hour basis. Public safety is a greater concern than privacy in these situations.

Place curved mirrors in hallway intersections or concealed areas.

Enclose nurses' stations, and install deep service counters or bullet-resistant, shatter-proof glass in reception areas, triage, admitting, or client service rooms.

Provide employee "safe rooms" for use during emergencies.

Establish "time-out" or seclusion areas with high ceilings without grids for patients acting out and establish separate rooms for criminal patients.

Provide client or patient waiting rooms designed to maximize comfort and minimize stress.

Ensure that counseling or patient care rooms have two exits.

Limit access to staff counseling rooms and treatment rooms controlled by using locked doors.

Arrange furniture to prevent entrapment of staff. In interview rooms or crisis treatment areas, furniture should be minimal, lightweight, without sharp corners or edges, and/or affixed to the floor. Limit the number of pictures, vases, ashtrays, or other items that can be used as weapons.

Provide lockable and secure bathrooms for staff members separate from patient, client, and visitor facilities.

Lock all unused doors to limit access, in accordance with local fire orders.

Install bright, effective lighting indoors and outdoors.

Replace burned-out lights, broken windows, and locks.

Keep automobiles, if used in the field, well-maintained. Always lock automobiles.

Administrative and Work Practice Controls

Administrative and work practice controls affect the way jobs or tasks are performed. The following examples illustrate how changes in work practices and administrative procedures can help prevent violent incidents.

State clearly to patients, clients, and employees that violence is not permitted nor tolerated.

Establish liaison with local police and state prosecutors. Report all incidents of violence. Provide police with physical layouts of facilities to expedite investigations.

Require employees to report all assaults or threats to a supervisor or manager (e.g., can be confidential interview).

Keep log books and reports of such incidents to help in determining any necessary actions to prevent further occurrences.

Advise and assist employees, if needed, of company procedures for requesting police assistance or filing charges when assaulted.

Provide management support during emergencies. Respond promptly to all complaints.

Set up a trained response team to respond to emergencies.

Use properly trained security officers, when necessary, to deal with aggressive behavior. Follow with written security procedures.

Ensure adequate and properly trained staff for restraining patients or clients.

Provide sensitive and timely information to persons waiting in line or in waiting rooms. Adopt measures to decrease waiting time.

Ensure adequate and qualified staff coverage at all times. Times of greatest risk occur during patient transfers, emergency responses, meal times, and at night. Locales with the greatest risk include admission units and crisis or acute care units. Other risks include admission of patients with a history of violent behavior or gang activity.

Institute a sign-in procedure with passes for visitors, especially in a newborn nursery or pediatric department.

Enforce visitor hours and procedures.

Establish a list of "restricted visitors" for patients with a history of violence. Copies should be available at security checkpoints, nurses' stations, and visitor sign-in areas. Review and revise visitor check systems, when necessary.

Limit information given to outsiders on hospitalized victims of violence.

Supervise the movement of psychiatric clients and patients throughout the facility.

Control access to facilities other than waiting rooms, particularly drug storage or pharmacy areas.

Prohibit employees from working alone in emergency areas or walk-in clinics, particularly at night or when assistance is unavailable. Employees should never enter seclusion rooms alone.

Establish policies and procedures for secured areas, and emergency evacuations, and for monitoring high-risk patients at night (e.g., open versus locked seclusion).

Ascertain the behavioral history of new and transferred patients to learn about any past violent or assaultive behaviors.

Establish a system—such as chart tags, log books, or verbal census reports—to identify patients and clients with assaultive behavior problems, keeping in mind patient confidentiality and worker safety issues. Update as needed.

Treat and/or interview aggressive or agitated clients in relatively open areas that still maintain privacy and confidentiality (e.g., rooms with removable partitions).

Use case management conferences with co-workers and supervisors to discuss ways to effectively treat potentially violent patients.

Prepare contingency plans to treat clients who are "acting out" or making verbal or physical attacks or threats.

Consider using certified employee assistance professionals (CEAPs) or in-house social service or occupational health service staff to help defuse patient or client anger.

Transfer assaultive clients to "acute care units," "criminal units," or other more restrictive settings.

Make sure that nurses and/or physicians are not alone when performing intimate physical examinations of patients.

Discourage employees from wearing jewelry to help prevent possible strangulation in confrontational situations.

Community workers should carry only required identification and money.

Periodically survey the facility to remove tools or possessions left by visitors or maintenance staff which could be used inappropriately by patients.

Provide staff with identification badges, preferably without last names, to readily verify employment.

Discourage employees from carrying keys, pens, or other items that could be used as weapons.

Provide staff members with security escorts to parking areas in evening or late hours. Parking areas should be highly visible, well-lighted, and safely accessible to the building.

Use the "buddy system," especially when personal safety may be threatened. Encourage home health care providers, social service workers, and others to avoid threatening situations. Staff should exercise extra care in elevators, stairwells, and unfamiliar residences; immediately leave premises if there is a hazardous situation; or request police escort if needed.

Develop policies and procedures covering home health care providers, such as contracts on how visits will be conducted, the presence of others in the home during the visits, and the refusal to provide services in a clearly hazardous situation.

Establish a daily work plan for field staff to keep a designated contact person informed about workers' whereabouts throughout the workday. If an employee does not report in, the contact person should follow-up.

Conduct a comprehensive post-incident evaluation, including psychological as well as medical treatment, for employees who have been subjected to abusive behavior.

Post-Incident Response

Post-incident response and evaluation are essential to an effective violence prevention program. All workplace violence programs should provide comprehensive treatment for victimized employees and employees who may be traumatized by witnessing a workplace violence incident. Injured staff should receive prompt treatment and psychological evaluation whenever an assault takes place, regardless of severity. Transportation of the injured to medical care should be provided if care is not available on-site.

Victims of workplace violence suffer a variety of consequences in addition to their actual physical injuries. These include short- and long-term psychological trauma, fear of returning to work, changes in relationships with co-workers and family, feelings of incompetence, guilt, powerlessness, and fear of criticism by supervisors or managers. Consequently, a strong follow-up program for these employees will not only help them to deal with these problems but also help prepare them to confront or prevent future incidents of violence (Flannery, 1991, 1993, 1995).

There are several types of assistance that can be incorporated into the post-incident response. For example, trauma-crisis counseling, critical incident stress debriefing, or employee assistance programs may be provided to assist victims. Certified employee assistance professionals, psychologists, psychiatrists, clinical nurse specialists, or social workers could provide this counseling, or the employer can refer staff victims to an outside specialist. In addition, an employee counseling service, peer counseling, or support groups may be established.

In any case, counselors must be well trained and have a good understanding of the issues and consequences of assaults and other aggressive, violent behavior. Appropriate and promptly rendered post-incident debriefings and counseling reduce acute psychological trauma and general stress levels among victims and witnesses. In addition, such counseling educates staff about workplace violence and positively influences workplace and organizational cultural norms to reduce trauma associated with future incidents.

TRAINING AND EDUCATION

Training and education ensure that all staff are aware of potential security hazards and how to protect themselves and their co-workers through established policies and procedures.

All Employees

Every employee should understand the concept of "Universal Precautions for Violence," i.e., that violence should be expected but can be avoided or mitigated through preparation. Staff should be instructed to limit physical interventions in workplace altercations whenever possible, unless there are adequate numbers of staff or emergency response teams and security personnel available. Frequent training also can improve the likelihood of avoiding assault (Carmel and Hunter, 1990).

Appendix 25–B

Sample Employee Handbook
Discussion of Workplace Violence

The safety and security of City Health System personnel, patients, and visitors are of vital importance. Therefore, workplace violence will not be tolerated. Any employee who commits an act of violence at work against a person or property will be immediately dismissed and, where appropriate, the matter will be referred for prosecution by legal authority. In addition, any employee who fails to comply with designated security protocols or fails to use security devices will be subject to disciplinary action, including immediate discharge.

Workplace violence is conduct in the workplace against employers and employees committed by persons who either have an employment-related connection with the establishment or are outsiders. This conduct may involve (1) physical acts against persons or employer property or (2) verbal threats of profanation, or vicious statements that are meant to harm or cause a hostile environment, or (3) written threats, profanation, vicious cartoons or notes, and other written conduct of intense distortion that is meant to threaten or create a hostile environment, or (4) visual acts that are threatening or intended to convey injury or hostility.

DETAILED POLICY

Workplace violence can and must be prevented. Achieving that goal requires the combined efforts of all employees, supervisors, and managers. Anything less than total commitment to the elimination of workplace violence is not enough—the hospital intends to see that violence is stopped, and all employees must do their part to achieve this result.

All employees are entitled to perform their work, regardless of location, whether on the employer's premises or elsewhere, free from violence. A nonviolent workplace assurance procedure has been implemented which includes a procedure for employees to follow should a violent act or threat occur. All employees are expected to know these procedures. In addition, all employees are expected to report any suspicions they have about any potential acts of violence. All such reports shall be fully investigated. No reprisals will be taken against any employee who makes such a report. Any employee who takes any reprisal, regardless of the magnitude of the reprisal, against a person who reports an act of violence or a suspicion of violence, shall be subject to immediate discipline, including discharge.

All employees will receive training concerning their roles and responsibilities in maintaining a nonviolent workplace. Additionally, audits will be conducted periodically to ensure that this policy is being followed. Any instance of failure to follow the provisions of this policy will be considered in such decisions as pay increases, promotions, and career development.

All employees are expected to comply with this policy, but management personnel must assume extraordinary responsibility to ensure that both the spirit and intent of the policy are met. In addition, managers are responsible for both the (1) prevention and (2) stopping of harassment and forms of violence. Due to the pernicious nature of harassment, managers will be held to a higher standard of responsibility in both preventing and stopping it.

A management response team has been established and is directed by the security director at each facility. The management response team is responsible for tracking and reviewing past incidents of violence, reviewing policies to ensure readiness to respond to incidents of violence, conducting training of hospital staff, and establishing a liaison with local law enforcement and emergency services.

PROCEDURES

1. Pre-employment screening of applicants will be conducted in an attempt to minimize the likelihood of hiring an individual with violent propensities.
2. Employees will be educated so that they can recognize and understand violence and how it can be prevented.
3. Employee education will focus on assisting employees in understanding themselves, including their attitudes, motivations, and decision-making styles so that they will not resort to violence.
4. Security protocols will be developed by each facility, and employees will be made aware of these protocols.
5. Supervisors and managers will ensure that all employees use designated security devices.
6. All employees will be encouraged to report any persons who may commit or have committed a violent act.
7. All employees shall report immediately any acts or threats of violence to the security department, their supervisors, or management response team members.

Chapter 26

Investigating Patient Abuse Claims

CHAPTER OBJECTIVES

1. Understand the definition of abuse.
2. Know most states' requirements concerning reporting and investigation of abuse claims.
3. Know the basic questions to ask in an investigation of patient or resident abuse.
4. Understand how to use photographs and take statements in an investigation.

INTRODUCTION

It is no secret that health care facilities and nursing homes are facing more scrutiny than ever before. Allegations of abuse are at an all-time high. Newspapers and television news broadcasts feature many stories on nursing home abuse. In 1998, President Clinton signed a bill calling for more inspections and more severe sanctions for nursing homes where abuse occurs.

At the same time, the government has reduced the funding for nursing home care. Managed care has caused many health care facilities to purchase nursing homes so they can move their patients into a less costly environment. Nursing homes that become part of a health care facility find themselves with the advantage of having a security department to call upon to investigate alleged abuse claims.

Lower funding means lower wages at nursing homes, which means more difficulty attracting and retaining high-quality staff. Where does this leave patients and residents? Residents are often not given timely, adequate care or are victims of an employee's frustration. Is it any wonder that allegations of abuse are at an all-time high?

> As many security professionals know, abuse claims often come down to one person's word against another's: a patient says there was abuse, but a staff member says there was not. Part of the problem in these cases is a difference of opinion over the definition of abuse. This chapter defines abuse as the willful infliction of physical pain, injury, or mental anguish; unreasonable confinement; or the willful deprivation by a caretaker of services that are necessary to maintain mental and physical health.

Unfortunately, people often consider allegations true until an investigation proves otherwise. Until this proof comes, the reputations of the staff member and the facility are in question.

So, upon hearing of an allegation of abuse, what should facility leaders do? Where must the abuse be reported? What happens if the abuse is proven to have taken place? To answer these questions, this chapter will review a typical state law addressing abuse in nursing homes. Differences among states' laws in this area tend to be minor.

REPORTING REQUIREMENTS

The facility is required to report any injury of unknown origin, or any allegation of abuse, to its licensing body and to the department of social services or adult protective services (in some states, the department of health and human resources) within 24 hours of learning of the allegation or injury. If the allegations appear to involve a criminal act, they must also be reported to the local police.

After the initial reporting, the facility has five working days to complete an investigation of the allegation. Again, the five-day investigation period starts at the time the facility becomes aware of an injury of unknown origin or allegation of abuse. The facility should record everything learned during the investigation. This includes a chronological list of events surrounding the alleged incident or injury of unknown origin; statements from the victim, witnesses, and alleged perpetrator; and all pertinent documents (e.g., patient charts, physician orders, lab tests, nursing notes).

Based upon the findings, investigators must decide if the allegation is substantiated or unsubstantiated. Their decision must be reported in writing. Most states have a standardized reporting form (see Exhibit 26–1). If the allegation is substantiated, the facility must state what action it has taken against the perpetrator.

INVESTIGATIONS

Investigations into allegations of abuse or injuries of unknown origin should proceed as follows:

- Seek medical care for the injured person (if applicable).
- Prepare a report.
  - Establish the who, what, when, where, and how.
  - Interview the person making the allegation.
  - Determine if there are any witnesses. Locate the witnesses and the suspect.
  - Gather statements and other documentation and photograph the injury.
- Complete the investigation.
  - Determine if the allegations are substantiated or unsubstantiated.
  - Report the findings within five days. Explain the actions taken against the perpetrator.

Based upon the information furnished, the licensing body may elect to open an independent investigation. For this reason, it is vital that facilities conduct their investigation in a timely, professional manner. Unfortunately, most facilities lose credibility due to the lack of professionalism in their investigation. They usually have a manila folder and just drop state-

Exhibit 26–1 Sample Reporting Form

NURSE AIDE AND HEALTH CARE PERSONNEL REPORTING GUIDELINE

I. FACILITY INFORMATION

a) Facility/Agency Name: _____ b) Facility Type: _____

c) Street: _____ City: _____ State: _____ Zip: _____

d) Facility/Agency License #: _____ e) Provider # (If certified): _____ f) County: _____

g) Facility/Agency Contact Person: _____ h) Phone #: (_____) _____

II. ALLEGED PERPETRATOR INFORMATION:

a) Full Name: _____ Title: _____

b) Phone #: (___) _____ c) Date of Hire: _____ d) SS #: _____ e) Date of Birth: _____

f) Last Known Complete Address: _____

City: _____ Sate: _____ Zip: _____

III. ALLEGATION TYPE: (Circle all that apply.)

1. Resident abuse   5. Fraud against resident
2. Resident neglect   6. Fraud against facility
3. Diversion of resident drugs   7. Misappropriation of facility property
4. Diversion of facility drugs   8. Misappropriation of resident property

IV. RESIDENT INFORMATION:

a) Resident's Name: _____ b) Room #: _____ c) Age: _____

d) Address (if different from facility's): _____ City: _____ Sate: _____ Zip: _____

e) Other Information: _____ f) Phone #: (___) _____

g) Interviewable: ____ Yes ____ No • h) Mental Status: _____

i) Mental and Physical Limitations: _____

V. RESIDENT'S LEVEL OF CARE: (Circle one.)

1. Adult care   2. Home care   3. Acute care
4. Nursing home   5. Hospice   6. Adult care resident in a nursing home

7. Other _____

VI. SPECIFIC ALLEGATION: (Attach additional sheets if needed.)

a) Date and Time of Occurrence: _____
b) Exact Location of Incident: _____
c) Physical Injury: _____ No _____ Yes (Describe injury in detail) _____

d) Resident's Emotional Response to Incident: _____
e) Allegation: (Include details) _____

f) Other Comments: _____

continues

Exhibit 26–1 continued

VII. WITNESS(es):_____ No _____ Yes _____ Number (Include resident victim if resident is a witness. Provide last known complete address, area code, and phone number. Indicate witness' relationship to resident victim and alleged perpetrator.)

a) (1) Name: _____ b) Title/Relationship: _____ c) Phone: (___) _____

d) Street:_____ City and State:_____ Zip: _____

a) (2) Name: _____ b) Title/Relationship: _____ c) Phone: (___) _____

d) Street:_____ City and State:_____ Zip: _____

a) (3) Name: _____ b) Title/Relationship: _____ c) Phone: (___) _____

d) Street:_____ City and State:_____ Zip: _____

(LIST ADDITIONAL WITNESSES ON THE BACK)

VIII. ACTION TAKEN BY FACILITY: (Fill in all blanks that apply.)

a) Allegation Substantiated by Facility? _____ No _____ Yes • b) Date Investigation Completed:_____

c) Person Who Conducted Facility Investigation and That Person's Title: _____

d) Was Incident Reported to Local DSS? ___ No ___ Yes • e) Date Reported: _____ f) County: _____

g) On-Site Visit? _____ No _____ Yes • h) Date of On-Site Visit:_____ i) Name: _____

j) Adult Home Specialist? _____ No _____ Yes • k) Adult Protective Services? _____ No _____ Yes

l) Reported to Police?: _____ No _____ Yes • m) Date Reported: _____ n) Date Investigated: _____

o) Name of Police Dept.: _____ p) Phone #: (___) _____

q) Name of Investigator: _____ r) Title: _____

s) Charged? _____ No _____ Yes • t) Specific Charges: _____

u) Alleged Perpetrator's Employment Terminated? _____ No _____ Yes • v) Date: _____

w) Other Action: _____

IX. COPIES OF THE FOLLOWING ARE ATTACHED TO REPORT: (Please check all boxes that apply.)

a) ☐ Statement from resident

b) ☐ Resident diagnoses

c) ☐ Statement from alleged perpetrator

d) ☐ Statement(s) from witness(es)

e) ☐ Time cards for alleged perpetrator and witness(es) for date of allegation

f) ☐ Assignment sheet(s) for alleged perpetrator and witness(es) for date of allegation

g) ☐ Documentation of alleged perpetrator's orientation and/or training related to allegation

h) ☐ Prior disciplinary actions/problems for alleged perpetrator

i) ☐ Plan of care, care plan, treatment plan, etc.

j) ☐ Pertinent medical record documents supporting allegation (e.g., medication administration record, physician orders, nursing notes, social assessments, emergency room reports, X-rays)

k) ☐ Controlled drug reconciliation record

l) ☐ Police report

m) ☐ List of other agencies also notified

n) ☐ Any other supporting or pertinent documents (specify): _____

_____

_____

_____

o)_____   p)_____

(Printed name and title of person preparing report)   (Signature of person preparing report)   (Date)

ments, reports, and other documents into the file without thinking about presentation. It is not uncommon to see statements written on the back of documents and telephone numbers written on napkins.

Exhibit 26–2 Some Questions To Consider in an Abuse Investigation

Who
- was the victim?
- are the victim's family members?
- discovered the abuse?
- made the report?
- was the supervisor on duty at the time of the alleged abuse?
- was working in the area at that time?
- saw or heard something of importance?
- was the last person to see the victim before the alleged abuse took place?
- was the victim's primary caregiver at the time of the alleged abuse?
- contacted administration?
- was the victim's physician?
- was the staff member who treated the injuries of the victim?
- was the primary investigator on the case?
- assisted the primary investigator?
- is the primary suspect in the alleged abuse?
- hired the primary suspect (check to see if reference and criminal record checks were completed)?

What
- was the alleged abuse?
- was the extent of the abuse?
- actions were taken by the supervisor?
- happened (in chronological order)?
- did the reporting person see, hear, and do?
- did the primary caregiver say about the alleged abuse?
- are the job functions of the primary suspect in the case?
- did other witnesses see, hear, and do?
- evidence was obtained?
- photographs were taken?
- statements were taken?
- physical evidence of abuse was present?
- outside agencies have been contacted?
- medical treatment did the victim need as a result of the alleged abuse?
- changes in the victim's behavior have been noted?

continues

Exhibit 26–2 continued

- did the outside agencies say and do as a result of your notification?
- did the victim say happened?
- did the victim do as a result of the alleged abuse?
- could have caused the abuse (e.g., assault, fall, self-infliction, blunt object pressure)?
- did the primary suspect say about the alleged abuse?

When

- did the alleged abuse take place?
- was it discovered?
- was it reported to a supervisor?
- was it reported to administration?
- was the last time the victim was seen before the alleged abuse?
- were outside agencies contacted?
- were family members contacted?
- were the statements of the witnesses taken?
- were the photographs of the victim and crime scene taken?
- did the primary suspect start working at the facility?

How

- was the alleged abuse discovered?
- was the alleged abuse reported?
- was the alleged abuse committed?
- did the abuser get into the facility, room, etc.?
- did the victim say the alleged abuse occurred?

Where

- did the alleged abuse take place?
- did the person who discovered the abuse first see the victim?
- was the person who discovered the abuse prior to seeing the victim?
- was the reporting person when he or she learned of the abuse?
- was the supervisor when he or she learned of the abuse?
- was the victim last seen before the alleged abuse took place?
- were the witnesses at the time of the alleged abuse?
- was each staff member at the time of the alleged abuse?
- were the photographs of the victim taken?
- was the victim taken for medical treatment?
- did the primary suspect work prior to working at your facility?

Staff at most facilities do not know what questions to ask and how to take written statements. Exhibit 26–2 lists some important questions to ask—the who, what, when, where, and how. The why will be established after the perpetrator is named.

Taking a statement entails more than handing someone a piece of paper and saying "tell me what you know about the alleged incident." First, all statements should be taken on the same type of form (see Exhibit 26–3). Most statement forms should contain a section that identifies the person giving the statement, including name, age, date of birth, and address.

Exhibit 26–3 Statement Form

Case Type _____ Case Number _____ Page _____ of _____
Statement of _____ Age _____ Date of Birth _____
Address _____ Phone _____
Connection with case (circle one):   witness   suspect   victim
Place Statement Taken _____ Date _____ Time _____

_____
_____
_____
_____
_____
_____
_____
_____
_____
_____
_____
_____
_____
_____
_____
_____
_____

I certify by my signature that the above statement is true to the best of my knowledge. No threats, promises, or inducements have been made in regards to this statement.

Witnesses _____   Signed _____
_____   Address _____

                                        Date _____ Time _____

There should also be a section that notes the place where the statement was taken and the date and time it was taken. At the bottom of the statement, there should be a place for the person giving the statement as well as two witnesses to sign.

Before taking a statement, the investigator should spend a few minutes conducting an interview. They should ask basic questions (e.g., Where were you at 8:00 P.M.? What first drew your attention to the patient?). They should not ask too many questions because their questions might give away information about the investigation. After a brief interview, the investigator should ask the person to write out a statement. If the person is unable to write, the investigator may write the statement for the person. However, the statement must contain the person's exact words, not the investigator's summary. After the statement is completed, the investigator should read the statement back to the statement giver, then ask for any corrections or additions. If there are none, the statement giver should sign the statement. The investigator conducting the interview as well as another staff member should sign as witnesses. The second staff member can testify that the investigator read the exact statement to the statement giver before signing took place.

Photographs

Photographs can document the extent of injury at a specific point in time. But photographs may be subpoenaed by opposing parties in lawsuits. Therefore, facility leaders should confer with the facility's attorney before establishing a policy on the use of photographs in an abuse investigation.

After seeking advise from counsel and establishing a policy concerning the use of photographs, facility leaders should *never* stray from the policy. If the policy is sometimes adhered to and sometimes not adhered to, a good opposing attorney will argue that the variance is part of a cover-up.

Camera Type

When possible, facilities should use both a camera that produces photographs instantly and a 35mm camera. Using the instant camera ensures that there is at least some photographic documentation. But there are problems with instant cameras: colors may be distorted by the use of a flash, and it is almost impossible to enlarge the photographs.

The 35mm camera offers a wider range of film speeds. Films of 400 speed or higher eliminate the need for a flash. If the camera user is not proficient in photography, a flash can "wash out" colors and not accurately show the injury. In addition, flashes can disturb patients.

What To Photograph and When

Investigators should be sure to photograph everything that is related to the case. If a patient is found lying on the floor with a broken hip, the entire room needs to be photographed. Measure and record the distances from each piece of furniture to where the patient was lying.

The photographs should be taken as soon as possible after the alleged incident or unexplained injury. The photographs should accurately depict what can be seen with the naked eye. Investigators should photograph the injury up close and at a distance, showing the entire body. A photograph should be taken showing a ruler or marked piece of tape beside an abrasion or "skin tear" to show its length.

Documentation of Photographs

Certain information about each photograph should be recorded in a photo log.

- photographer's name
- date, time, and place taken
- make and model of camera
- brand and speed of film used
- name of person photographed
- distance from the photographer to the subject

- lighting source
- description of photograph (e.g., "injured area")

KEY POINTS

- Though there are official definitions of the term, abuse may be almost any action that a patient or resident considers abusive.
- All health care facilities must report actual or alleged patient abuse.
- Facilities must investigate each allegation thoroughly.
- The investigation should cover who, what, when, where, and how.
- Specific guidelines should be followed for taking statements and photographs.

Chapter 27

VIP and Executive Protection

CHAPTER OBJECTIVES

1. Know the standard set by the Joint Commission on Accreditation of Healthcare Organizations for VIP protection.
2. Know how to define the terms "executive protection" and "VIP protection."
3. Know how to establish a VIP protection plan in a health care setting.
4. Know why an executive protection plan is necessary in a health care setting.
5. Understand the basic components of an executive protection plan.

INTRODUCTION

The Joint Commission on Accreditation of Healthcare Organizations, under EC1.4 - I-3 (1999), requires that facilities have an established plan for "handling of situations involving VIPs or the media." What makes a person a VIP? For the purposes of this chapter, VIPs are people who, by virtue of their public status, either can cause a disturbance to facility operation or be in danger while on the property. A facility's list of VIPs may include politicians, entertainers, businesspeople, criminals, and average people caught up in unusual situations.

What is executive protection, and how does it work in a health care facility? For the purposes of this chapter, an executive protection plan, unlike a VIP protection plan, is ongoing and protects a principal. Facility executives may need protection for everything from a kidnapping to such risks as personal and professional embarrassment, poor health, or interrupted travel. The objective is to provide a reasonable degree of protection while still allowing the principal to carry on with his or her normal life.

SECURITY WITH DIFFERENT TYPES OF VIPS

Security directors have much to think about when planning for VIP visits. For instance, it is best if facilities designate certain inpatient rooms as VIP rooms. These rooms should be in an area where access can be easily controlled and have adjacent rooms available for VIP staff.

> Security must be advised about when and where press briefings will occur. The media should be given controlled access to information. It should be made very clear to the media that any attempt to directly contact the patient or interfere with patient care will result in all members of the media being ejected from the property. Likewise, public relations should work with the media and supply timely and accurate nonconfidential information.

VIPs visiting health care facilities tend to fall into one of four categories.

1. government leaders
2. businesspeople
3. entertainers
4. criminals

Security directors should remember that VIPs often bring their own security detail. In these cases, the security director oversees communication about the VIP more than protection of the VIP. The type of VIP visiting the facility may dictate the role security plays. Exhibit 27–1 provides a sample VIP protection policy.

Government Leaders

Most international, national, or state leaders will probably have their own security detail. If the VIP is coming to the facility for a business function (e.g., a ground breaking), security will probably provide escorts throughout the facility and property. If the VIP is a patient, security may communicate with the medical staff about the VIP's security needs and help handle the media. It is important that security explain to the medical staff that it is essential to limit the number of outside people that have access to the VIP and the length of time they spend with the VIP.

> If the president, vice president, or members of their immediate families are coming to visit the facility, or if the facility is considered the primary health care facility during one of these people's visits to the area, Secret Service advance team members will contact the facility, explain their security needs, and gather information about the facility.

Businesspeople

Many high-profile businesspeople and captains of industry will also have their own security detail. But some high-profile businesspeople will not, and they may not feel that protection is necessary. If this is the case, security should meet with the VIP's advance or media relations representative and agree upon the degree of protection the VIP will accept. At the

Exhibit 27–1 Sample VIP Protection Policy

Policy

This policy provides guidelines for handling VIP visits.

Purpose

The purpose of this policy is to help facility staff provide a reasonably safe and secure environment of care for VIPs.

Procedure

VIPs fall into four basic categories.

1. government leaders
2. businesspeople
3. entertainers
4. criminals

Government Leaders

- Leaders of other nations will probably have a dignitary-style escort from the State Department, Secret Service, military, or another government agency. Other politicians may have security with them as well.
- Security should notify the head nurse as soon as possible that a VIP will be present.
- Facility staff must limit the number of the VIP's visitors and the length of their visits.
- Staff should be prepared to handle members of the media and direct them to the proper authorities.
- Staff should cooperate and coordinate with the VIP's protective detail.

Businesspeople

- Businesspeople and captains of industry may arrive with their own private protective detail.
- Security should notify the head nurse as soon as possible that a VIP will be present.
- Businesspeople may not want VIP-type treatment.
- Staff should cooperate and coordinate with the VIP's protective detail.
- Staff should be prepared to handle the media.

Entertainers

- Entertainers may arrive with their own private protective detail.
- Security should notify the head nurse as soon as possible that a VIP will be present.
- Staff must limit the number of the VIP's visitors and the length of their visits.
- Staff should be prepared to handle members of the media and direct them to the proper authorities.
- Staff should be prepared to handle fans of the celebrity.
- Staff should cooperate and coordinate with the VIP's protective detail.

Criminals

- Criminals will be in the custody of the state detention officers.
- Staff must limit the number of the VIP's visitors and the length of their visits.
- Staff should be prepared to handle members of the media and direct them to the proper authorities.
- Staff should cooperate with detention officers.

very minimum, security should have personnel on hand during the entire visit to respond to any incidents.

As is the case with other VIPs, the level of security for VIP businesspeople will vary depending on the nature of their visit (e.g., for inpatient stay, for brief ceremony).

Entertainers

Entertainers may attend ground-breaking ceremonies or visit patients during the holidays. In these situations, the VIPs will have their own security detail, and the locations and times they visit certain areas will already be set.

If entertainers are patients, security may be required to take a more active role. The VIP may not have enough security to provide coverage 24 hours a day, 7 days a week.

Medical staff should be reminded to limit the number of persons who may come into contact with the VIP. They may encounter eager fans, both inside and outside the facility, trying to see the entertainer.

Criminals

Suspects in high-profile cases will often be brought to health care facilities for treatment or evaluation. They will be accompanied by law enforcement officials who are required to stay with the suspects at all times. The security director should help the medical staff understand the concerns and requirements of the law enforcement officials. It is extremely important that the number of persons who come in contact with a prisoner patient be limited and that back hallways and service elevators be used when moving the patient. It is a good policy to consider all prisoner patients dangerous and an escape risk.

EXECUTIVE PROTECTION

The security director should determine the level of protection that should be provided to various facility leaders. Most people no longer think of health care facilities as primarily places of healing. Facilities are now seen as businesses, often part of much larger organizations, which means that facility leaders need as much protection as any other CEOs.

In addition, stress is high in health care facilities. Patients and visitors are under stress from illness, fear, or pain. Staff are constantly being asked to do more with less. A facility leader may face an angry family member whose loved one has just died or employee who has just been laid off after many years of loyal service. What can a security director do to protect corporate executives in these situations?

First, security directors must determine what types of threats could arise. In most cases, health care facility executives are not threatened because of their political beliefs or because someone wants ransom payments. Facility executives tend to face threats from spontaneous events, such as confrontations with upset employees or family members. But these spontaneous confrontations can escalate into hostage situations or kidnappings quickly. Therefore, security directors should not rule out the need for a crisis response plan. A crisis response plan will be necessary if the executive or a member of his or her family is kidnapped.

Crisis Response Plan

The first step in assembling a crisis response plan is to gather information about the principal, including

- a recent photograph and physical description
- place of birth
- date of birth
- health profile
- name of personal physician
- vehicles (including motorcycles and boats) and their license or tag numbers
- addresses and floor plans (including gas and electrical shutoffs) of homes
- recent photographs of family members and physical descriptions of them
- names and addresses of places executive or family members frequent (e.g., schools, churches, clubs)
- location of banking records and credit cards
- attorney's name and address

Once the basic information is gathered, a "what if" meeting should be held with the executive, chief financial officer, senior vice president, corporate attorney, director of public relations, director of security, director of plant operations, and either local, state, or federal law enforcement representatives. Many facilities elect to have the director of security chair this meeting because security directors have an ongoing relationship with law enforcement.

Meeting participants should decide who will be contacted if an event occurs and what role they will play in the crisis response plan. The chief financial officer should determine how much money could be made available quickly in a crisis. The director of public relations must understand that absolutely no information about the event should be released to the media unless authorized by law enforcement. And if an event occurs at the facility, the director of plant operations will need quick access to floor plans, electrical and telephone system prints, air flow shutoffs, and other facility information.

How can security directors help prevent these crises? Because most principal protection crises occur spontaneously, access control can be the key. Administrative offices should be located on a nonpublic floor. Controlled access into and out of the executive area must be maintained. In addition, security must be notified ahead of time if there is a potentially volatile situation (e.g., a potentially violent employee has been terminated or an unforeseen patient death has upset family members).

CONCLUSION

Whether protecting facility executives or VIPs just visiting the premises, security directors will succeed only if they plan ahead.

KEY POINTS

- The Joint Commission on Accreditation of Healthcare Organizations requires health care facilities to have a plan for VIP visits.
- There are basically four types of VIP patients.
- Health care executives need an executive protection plan.
- There are precise steps in designing VIP and executive protection plans.

Chapter 28

Parking and Security

CHAPTER OBJECTIVES

1. Know who the customers of a health care facility's parking areas are.
2. Evaluate the different systems of paying for parking.
3. Understand the security measures needed in various parking structures.
4. Know the components of and how to assemble a parking control program.

INTRODUCTION

Parking issues cause problems in many medical facilities. Patients want and need to park close to the facility. Visitors want easy access between the parking area and medical facility. They also want free or very low cost parking. Physicians want primarily quick access from the parking area into the facility. Volunteers like to have a designated space for parking. Employees want a safe, easily accessed parking area that always has plenty of empty parking spaces so they do not have to waste time driving around looking for a space. Administrators want a parking program that affords them special parking and does not generate complaints about the number of spaces, the proximity to the facility, and the safety of the area.

A few facilities may have managed to meet all these needs, but in most facilities, parking has and always will be a problem. There are two basic rules in health care parking: (1) there is never enough, and (2) what parking is available will be reduced due to construction. As facilities grow, they must plan for changing parking needs. Usually, most available land goes to the new construction, not for parking.

Exhibit 28–1 contains some questions that facility directors should ask themselves as they plan parking structures. Exhibit 28–2 contains a policy listing many of the parking-related decisions that one facility in Charlotte, North Carolina, made.

SPECIALLY DESIGNATED PARKING

Facilities need to decide in advance who, if anyone, needs specially designated parking. Decisions should be based on need, not desire. This decision should be fairly easy. The pa-

Exhibit 28–1 Questions To Consider While Planning Parking Areas

---

Style and Design

- Should there be just one entrance on the first level, or should there be multiple entrances to the parking facility?
- Where should the facility be located? The needs of patients and patrons should be considered first, then the needs of employees and others who may use the facility.
- What kind of signage will be used? The best signs are direct and simple. Signs should offer directions on where to park, how to pay, and how to enter and exit.
- Will the facility conform to state and local laws governing design? Will it meet Environmental Protection Agency and Americans with Disabilities Act guidelines?
- Where will security cameras, screamer alarms, and help buttons be located?
- What will parking regulations be? How will they be enforced? Giving warnings, issuing tickets, and towing cars are all options.
- How will employees register to park?

Payment Method

- Will drivers pay on foot before they return to their cars, or will they pay as they exit in their cars?
- How will the facility keep the cashiers accountable for the money they handle?
- What kinds of supplies (e.g., tickets, machine tape, tokens, stamps) will be needed for the payment method?

Staffing

- What personnel will need to be hired to run the parking structure? Parking attendants will need to serve as cashiers as well as give directions and assist with other parking functions. Because cashiers will be handling money, their backgrounds should be thoroughly checked.
- Is it worth the time and expense to have valet parking? What will the costs of staffing and supplies be? What extra insurance will be needed? Is there an area big enough for valets to park the cars?
- What department will oversee parking personnel?
- Will staff wear uniforms?

Other Topics

- Will shuttle service to and from the parking structure be necessary?
- What kind of lighting systems will be used in the structure?
- How will equipment in the structure be repaired? Will there be a service contract with a vendor, or will there be individual service calls?

---

tient is always the one who needs special treatment the most. Patient parking should be as close to the facility as possible, clearly marked, and with easy access and egress. The number of spaces needed is determined by the mix of services offered at the facility. If the facility is a physician's office, the parking spaces should turn over approximately every 45 to 55 minutes. If the facility is for one-day surgery, the turnover time may be 4 to 6 hours. For the emergency department, the turnover may be 2 to 3 hours. Many health care facilities are using valet parking for patients coming to the emergency and maternity departments. This valet parking reduces the need for parking close to the facility and will make patients happy. The last thing these patients want to be worried about is parking.

Exhibit 28–2 Sample Parking Policy

Policy

Because the automobile is the dominant form of transportation in Charlotte, City Health System is dedicated to providing safe, convenient parking for patients, visitors, employees, students, volunteers, physicians, physician's office staff, clergy, and others who use the facilities. The facility makes the following regulations to ensure efficient, cost-effective use of available parking lots and decks.

Parking Assignments

- Parking deck B (1,430 spaces)
  -Visitors: levels 1–4
  -Physicians: level G with overflow to levels 2–4
  -Physicians' office staff: level G with overflow to levels 2–4
  -Clergy: level G with overflow to levels 2–4
  -Day shift employees: levels 5–7
  -Night shift employees: level 5
  -Volunteers: levels 1–4
- Parking deck E (848 spaces)
  -Day shift employees: levels A, C, and D
  -Students: levels C and D
  -Evening shift: level B with overflow to level C
  -Overflow patients from cancer center and emergency department: level B
- Cole lot (187): day shift parking for health system employees and medical center tenants
- 1600 East Fifth Street lot (78 spaces)
  -Employees whose office is on Fifth Street and tenants of the building
  -Visitors to the building
- Medical center lot (48 spaces)
  -Patients of physicians in the medical center
  -Commercial tenant parking
- Medical tower deck (760 spaces): patients and visitors using the medical tower and outpatient surgery center as well as tenants who lease offices in the building and their employees
- The A lot (20 spaces): restricted, with security-controlled access, to patients with disabilities, outpatient surgery patients, endoscopy patients, and other high-turnover patient and visitor traffic
- Emergency department/cancer center lot
  -emergency department patients and their families
  -cancer center patients
  -maternity department patients
- Other areas:
  -16 spaces in front of child development center: reserved for child dropoff and pickup
  -spaces along service entrance off 5th Street will be used for service and delivery vehicles only

Valet Parking

Valet parking is available to maternity patients and other patients who need special assistance because of their condition (e.g., patients who are older, patients with small children).

continues

Exhibit 28–2 continued

Physicians responding to emergencies in the emergency department, surgery, delivery room, and other departments may have their cars valet parked by the emergency department attendant. The operating room may use the spaces marked in the ambulance drive area.

Parking Cards

Parking will be controlled through the following mechanisms:
- Employees: time/identification cards issued by the personnel department
- Students: identification cards issued by the personnel department
- Physicians: parking cards issued by the medical staff coordinator
- Physicians' office nurses: parking cards issued by the nursing office
- Clergy: parking cards issued by the chaplain's office
- Volunteers: access codes given to the department daily

Paid Parking

Except for people belonging to those groups listed in the "Parking Cards" section above and other people named by the administration, everyone will pay for parking.

- Parking charges for the B deck will be $1.00 per day. Visitors or patients who park more than once in a day will not have to pay again for that day. To avoid duplicate charges, visitors and patients must save their exit codes after paying the initial $1.00. The parking deck cashier will give the visitor or patient a new exit code for free parking after having been shown the exit code from earlier in the day.
- Parking charges for the A deck will be $3.50 for the first hour and $1.00 per half-hour thereafter. There is no maximum charge. Parking is free with a parking gate ticket stamped by the tenant.

Violations by Employees and Towing Procedures

- First violation: A public safety officer will issue a citation describing the violation. A copy of the citation will be left on the front windshield of the employee's vehicle.
- Second violation: A public safety officer will issue a citation describing the violation. A copy of the citation will be left on the front windshield of the employee's vehicle. A copy of the citation will also be sent to the employee's supervisor listing the number of citations and the reason they were issued.
- Third violation: The employee's auto will be towed at the owner's expense. No notice will be given before towing.
- An employee can receive a citation for any violation of the parking policy dealing with employees (e.g., a vehicle has no displayed parking sticker, is parking in a restricted area of the deck, or is taking up two spaces or otherwise improperly parked).
- Each violation will be added to the employee's record of citations to be kept by the public safety office. Any additional violations after the initial towing will result in more towings.
- Cars parked in areas marked "towing enforced" will be towed regardless of the number of previous violations.

Procedures for Security Assistance to Motorists

Security officers shall provide assistance to motorists who encounter difficulty while on health system property.

continues

Exhibit 28–2 continued

- Visitors reporting automotive trouble on corporate property should be directed to the security department.
- Security officers may use the equipment available to them to open locked cars, jump a dead battery, or inflate tires.
- Security officers may not change tires or perform mechanical services. If these services are required, the security officer should offer to contact a service station or relative of the driver.

Authorized by: _____

President and CEO

Date _____

Second, facilities need to decide whose desire, not need, for special parking should be accommodated. Those who will be making frequent trips into and out of the facility should be accommodated if possible. Physicians usually visit a health care facility in the early morning, late afternoon, and early evening. Spaces set aside for physicians can usually be used for other groups at other times.

Volunteers really do need assistance in parking. They are giving the health care facility a precious gift—their time. In most cases, volunteers are senior citizens. While still active, they will appreciate being allowed to park close to the facility. Facilities should work with the head of volunteers to determine the number of spaces needed. In most cases, volunteers are at the health care facility between 9:30 A.M. and 2:30 P.M. While this is prime time in the parking lot, volunteers may need only a few predetermined spaces. Some health care facilities that offer valet parking at the emergency department offer to valet park volunteers if the volunteer spaces are full.

Visitor parking normally peaks between the hours of 5:30 P.M. and 8:30 P.M., Monday through Friday, and from 1:00 P.M. to 4:00 P.M. on the weekends. Visitor parking spaces tend to turn over every 1 or 1.5 hours. Again, the key concern of visitors is easy access to the parking area. The parking supervisor should travel all the main roads leading up to the health care facility. Are there adequate signs showing the way to the visitor parking area? Are there signs helping drivers unfamiliar with the facility?

One health care facility had a long drive that dead ended at the front of the health care facility. There was always a traffic jam at the front of the facility, mostly from visitors asking where to park. The traffic was so bad that the health care facility hired off-duty police to direct the traffic. The parking deck for visitor parking was located on the left side of the long drive. In front of the deck was a small 24-inch by 30-inch sign that directed visitors to park in the deck. When a consultant reviewed the problem, it was easily corrected. The consultant recommended that a larger sign be placed on the right side of the road, facing the oncoming traffic. The traffic jam at the front of the health care facility quickly ended. Now the approaching drivers could see the sign and understand that they needed to turn into the deck.

The facility should also review the number of parking spaces available for people with disabilities. Most building codes require that 5 percent to 10 percent of the total number of parking spaces be designated for people with disabilities. For a health care facility, these percentages are far too low. Most professionals in the industry believe that 12 percent to 15 percent is more reasonable. In addition to vehicles marked with a handicapped tag, the health care facility has patients who need special parking when they come to the health care facility for radiation or chemotherapy because their treatments leave them physically weak. These patients need a designated parking area.

FEES AND PAYMENT SYSTEMS

Next, facilities must decide whether to charge visitors for parking. If they decide to charge for parking, then they must decide on the rate of parking fees and how they will be paid.

Most health care facilities charge for visitor parking. If the visitor is the primary family member for the patient, many health care facilities offer the visitor free parking after seven days.

Fees will depend on the location of the facility. Most urban health care facilities charge the usual city parking fees. If they offered lower rates, many city workers would simply park at the health care facility and take a bus downtown. The amount to charge for parking must also be determined by the method of collection. If cashiers are used, then the wage and benefit for the cashiers must be incorporated into the parking fee. **There are two basic methods of payment for parking.**

- **Flat rate.** In the flat rate system, visitors park as long as they like for one price. The driver pays either a cashier or a money machine on the way into or on the way out of the parking area.
- **Variable length.** In the variable length system, parking is charged by the half-hour or hour. Some health care facilities with limited visitor parking spaces charge premium prices for parking during peak visitor time. Their goal is to get some visitors to visit in off-peak hours. In a variable pay system, drivers receive a parking ticket when they drive into the lot. When they leave, they pay an attendant for the time they parked.

There are several types of variable pay systems. In some systems, drivers are asked to be sure to take their parking tickets with them into the facility. On the way out, they stop by the cashier before going to their vehicles. The cashier determines the length of time the driver has parked, charges accordingly, and gives the driver an exit code. This exit code is similar to the codes used at service station car washes. In this "pay on foot" parking system, vehicles do not idle for long periods of time at a cashier's booth. This can be critical for the facility if the area around the facility has an emission problem. In some areas, the Environmental Protection Agency closely monitors "stack" time. A similar pay on foot system lets the driver insert the ticket into a reader, and the reader determines the parking fee. The driver pays the reader and then receives an exit code. In both systems, the exit code is only valid for a set amount of time, usually 15 minutes. This keeps drivers from paying for parking as they arrive rather than as they leave.

PARKING AREA DESIGN

Several lot designs are available for facilities. Some facilities may elect to have open, surface lot parking. While surface lots are relatively inexpensive to build and use, they tie up valuable land space. In most urban locations, surface lots are simply not an option. Moreover, surface lots have many security problems. Anyone can simply walk into the lot, break into a vehicle or rob a visitor, and run away. It is simply very difficult to control walk-on or walk-through traffic on a surface lot. The lot should have "no trespassing" or "no loitering" signs. In addition, closed-circuit television (CCTV) and security patrols should cover the lot. If the lot has a cashier's booth, excess cash should be pulled from the booth as needed to keep the cash exposure low. Many facilities that use surface lot cashier booths, especially away from the main campus, do suffer robbery attempts.

Parking decks can solve many parking problems. More spaces can be built using less land. And while building parking decks is not cheap, the use of prefabricated building systems has improved the per space cost. But most visitors do not like parking decks. They have a hard time finding their vehicle when they return, and they feel unsafe on the decks. While most people in urban settings are used to decks, people who live in suburban or rural settings usually are not.

To make people more comfortable with parking decks, security directors must make sure that the directional signs leading up to deck entrances are readable and understandable. They should ask various visitors if the signage is sufficient. Remember, the signs must be adequate for the visitor, not the parking director. Bright lights will make people feel safer, as discussed in the "Security" section below.

EMPLOYEE PARKING

Handling employee parking can be both the easiest and the most difficult aspect of structuring a parking program for a health care facility. The first order of business is to establish how many employee vehicles will be on the property at any one time. All employees who will be parking on campus should be required to register their vehicles. In most cases, human resources can handle the registration process and then forward the completed form to security or parking. The registration form (see Exhibit 28–3) should ask employees to list the year, make, model, color, and license tag number of all the vehicles that they might drive to work. The registration form should have a place where employees can note the shift they will be working if the employee works rotating shifts on a regular basis. Once their vehicles are registered, employees should receive parking decals and be told to place them on the prescribed area of their vehicle.

The registration forms should then be forwarded to the parking director, who should enter the names on all three shifts in the database. After all names have been entered, the database should be separated by work shift to determine the maximum number of employee vehicles that could be on the property at any one time. Calculations of the needed spaces should also take into consideration that most shifts overlap. The parking director must plan for the fact that for approximately 45 minutes to 1 hour at the beginning and the end of the shift, two shifts' worth of vehicles will be on the property.

Exhibit 28–3 Sample Parking Registration Form for Employees

Parking Registration Form
(Please print.)

Last Name	First Name	Middle Initial

The number on the front of your badge is your employee identification number. In order to register your vehicles, it is mandatory that you provide your employee identification number. Employee # _____ or Driver's license number (only if not an employee) _____ Please register all vehicles you may drive to work:

	Year	Make	Model	Color	Tag #	State	Sticker #
Car 1							
Car 2							
Car 3							
Car 4							
Car 5							

What shift(s) do you work? _____

Employee signature _____   Date: _____

- Any changes in the above information must be reported to the public safety department.
- If you drive a temporary car (e.g., rental car) to work, please call public safety with the above information so you will not be ticketed.

The public safety department welcomes you and appreciates your cooperation with the vehicle registration program.

Most facilities try to let the third shift park as close to the building as possible to decrease the chance of a crime occurring. Parking directors should also take into account the fact that the second shift always leaves after dark and the first shift arrives before dawn in the winter months.

Security should maintain a strong physical presence in the employee parking areas during shift change times. For this reason, many security departments have their shift changes either a half-hour before or a half-hour after those of health care facility departments. A facility can place CCTV and intercoms throughout the employee parking areas, but nothing makes an employee feel safer than seeing a well-trained, physically fit officer in the parking lot. The officer should be either in an elevated security booth or standing outside a security vehicle with the overhead emergency lights on. High visibility is the key.

Some facilities have utilized card access to allow only the designated employees into and out of their parking lot. This system can be very effective. Using this parking lot card access system with the facility access/egress identification system can be cost-effective and add to the security of the campus.

Some facilities attempt to mix employees and visitors in one common deck. This is normally not a good idea because there are large numbers of employee vehicles entering or exiting the deck at certain times of day. This volume of moving traffic can make a visitor unfamiliar with the facility very uncomfortable. It is also very difficult to regulate where the employees park in the deck. Employees are just like everyone else: they want the closest parking space possible. If the parking is unregulated, most of the closest parking spaces will be taken by staff, and the patients and visitors will be left to park on the upper levels of the deck.

One system that seems to control employee parking works in the following manner. The employee enters the parking deck through a designated set of parking gates. Located at the gates is a card reader. The reader not only permits the employee access to the deck but starts a tracking mechanism. The employee must proceed to the employee parking area (called a nesting area) on one of the upper levels of the deck. To enter the nesting area, the employee activates another card reader. The employee is then free to park anywhere in the designated spaces. When leaving, the reverse is done. The employee swipes the card to exit the nesting area, then swipes to use the designated exit gates. If employees do not complete the card access and egress loop, their cards will not allow them to exit via the employee gates. They then must go to a cashier area and pay the "lost ticket" price for parking.

If an employee tries to circumvent the system by going to the nesting area, then turning around and leaving to park in a lower area, the computer will recognize the short time duration and "hold" the vehicle in the nesting area. Likewise, when employees leave the nesting area, they have a preset time to exit the deck, or their exit will be blocked.

INFRACTIONS

The facility must have a well-structured, well-enforced parking program. Most facilities have some form of vehicle ticketing program. Some are very strict, charging employees parking fines; others have little credibility because they are not enforced. Some facilities allow an employee a certain number of tickets per year. (Exhibit 28–4 shows a parking courtesy reminder, and Exhibit 28–5 shows a sample employee parking citation.) Employees who exceed the number lose the privilege of parking in the employee areas and must pay regular visitor prices to park in the visitor area. Some facilities will not allow employees to park anywhere on the property for 30 days if they exceed the allotted parking tickets. Most facilities allow parking citations to be automatically deleted from an employee's parking record after a set time. Most facilities hold citations for 90 days and start the cumulative process over again. Some do, however, demand that parking infractions such as parking in a fire zone or blocking the path of emergency vehicles always stay on the employee's parking record.

Exhibit 28–4 Parking Courtesy Reminder

NAME:_____

DEPARTMENT:_____   EXTENSION: _____

HOSPITAL PERMIT #:_____   COLOR: _____

MAKE: _____   MODEL: _____

TIME:_____   STATE/LICENSE: _____

LOCATION: _____

The following parking regulations have been violated:

	PATIENT/VISITOR		HANDICAPPED
	RESERVED AREA		LOADING ZONE
	PROHIBITED AREA		DRIVEWAY/RAMP
	ASSIGNED AREA		CARELESS
	FIRE ZONE/PLUG		NO PERMIT

OTHER: _____

_____

_____

_____

_____

_____

_____

_____

☐

VISITOR: PLEASE ASSIST US BY PARKING PROPERLY.

NO RESPONSE IS NECESSARY._____

☐

EMPLOYEE: PLEASE ASSIST US BY PARKING PROPERLY AND COMPLYING WITH
HOSPITAL PARKING POLICY. PLEASE CONTACT SECURITY IF YOU HAVE ANY
QUESTIONS. THIS DOCUMENT IS A WARNING CITATION. NO RESPONSE IS NEC-
ESSARY._____

OFFICER:_____   DATE: _____

A discussion of parking procedures would not be complete without a mention of towing
vehicles. It is unfortunate, but some visitors and staff will park in areas clearly marked "towing enforced." Before a vehicle is towed, an attempt should be made to contact the owner of
the vehicle and give that person a chance to move to a designated parking area. If the vehicle
is not moved, or if contact cannot be made with the owner, security should take a photo of the
vehicle, clearly showing that the vehicle is parked in a tow-away zone. The photo should also

Exhibit 28–5 Sample Employee Parking Ticket

City Health System
**Employee
Parking Citation**

       DATE   TIME   LOCATION

AUTO MAKE   COLOR   TAG   STICKER NO.

REGISTERED TO: _____ DEPT. _____

_____ PARKED IN NO PARKING ZONE

_____ PARKED IN RESTRICTED AREA

_____ PARKED IN FIRE LANE

_____ STICKER NOT DISPLAYED OR IMPROPERLY DISPLAYED

_____ IMPROPERLY PARKED:

_____

_____ OTHER:

_____

A COPY OF THIS CITATION WILL BE SENT TO YOUR SUPERVISOR. UPON IS-
SUANCE OF A THIRD VIOLATION, THIS AUTO WILL BE TOWED FROM THE PROP-
ERTY, IF YOU HAVE ANY QUESTIONS, PLEASE CONTACT PUBLIC SAFETY.

                            OFFICER BADGE NO.

try to capture full views of the vehicle, noting any damaged areas. Once all documentation is made, the vehicle should be towed. Unfortunately, most facilities must set examples to maintain an orderly parking program.

SECURITY

Parking directors should make sure parking areas are clean and brightly lit. While most security and lighting consultants suggest that the acceptable lighting standard for a deck is five-foot candles, the parking director may want to double the lighting. Increasing lighting is one of the best ways to deter crime and improve the appearance of a deck. The brighter the deck, the less fear and crime.

Signs that say "no loitering," "no trespassing," or "lock your vehicle" make people feel safer and reduce crime. Signs should tell visitors when an area is monitored by CCTV.

Facilities should always have someone monitoring a camera in a parking area. The person monitoring the camera can call for a security officer to respond if there is an emergency.

Often, drivers cannot remember where they parked their vehicles in parking decks. They may wander the lot, upset, confused, and not aware of people who may be nearby. This type of behavior can make them an easy target for a criminal. To help people remember the locations of their cars, some parking decks have color coded the levels of the deck. Some have even placed numbered ticket stamps at the elevator entrance so drivers can stamp the back of their ticket.

Parking decks have elevators, and with elevators come other security issues. Most experts agree that glass-backed elevators and fire stairwells are the safest. In addition, employee elevators can have card reader access into the elevator lobby. Not only is this a security feature, but it allows employees easy and full access to elevators during shift change time.

Some health care facilities have utilized integrated security systems to their fullest potential. In one facility, each level of the parking decks had enough cameras to fully cover the level, including the elevators. In addition, located throughout each level of the deck were audible intercom alarms. If people needed nonemergency assistance, they looked for the large blue sign, blue light, or column. At that location was a call box that would put them in contact with security via an intercom. If the people were in distress and shouted, or if any other noise above the set decibel level was noted, the intercom would automatically open and security could hear everything in the area. At the same time, the same level of the parking deck would appear on a large monitor in the command room, and the VCR would start to record the level. A special "tone" would activate on the security officers' radio to alert them to the possibility of a problem in the parking deck.

This system, while elaborate, can significantly improve security and people's comfort at the facility. It can also serve in unexpected ways. One December, a young woman on the way to visit a sick relative was in a parking deck. Her son, approximately two years old and acting like a "terrible two," accompanied her. Several times the youngster set the audible alarm off by screaming and yelling. The person monitoring the cameras noted the obvious distress of the young mother but did not speak over the intercom. When the mother and son entered the elevator, the youngster again began to shout and misbehave. His shouting opened the intercom alarm in the elevator, and the interior of the elevator was visible on the camera. Deciding that the young mother needed some help, the security officer said in a deep, rich voice, "Young man, this is Santa. You'd better behave—remember, Christmas is coming!" You can imagine the son's amazement. As the mother and son exited the elevator, the son now acting very much the gentleman, the relieved mother spotted one of the security cameras, went up to it, and gave a big "okay" sign to the camera. You cannot beat public relations like that.

Because parking attendants will handle cash, it is helpful to have a system of checks in place. Cashiers should each have their own drawers and be accountable for the cash that comes into and goes out of these drawers. Supervisory personnel should audit the parking garages at least four times a week. Exhibit 28–6 contains a parking cashier daily balance form, and Exhibit 28–7 contains a sample audit procedure form. Supervisors should compile weekly garage statistics (Exhibit 28–8) to track weekly cash flow and note year-to-date statistics for the parking area.

Parking lot attendants and security officers will sometimes find themselves helping patients, visitors, and employees with problems other than lost tickets and stolen purses. If there is an automobile accident, for instance, the security department will need to complete a motor vehicle accident form like the one found in Exhibit 28–9. If visitors lock themselves out of their cars and ask security officers for help in opening the cars, the officers should first have the drivers complete a release form like the one found in Exhibit 28–10.

KEY POINTS

- Parking affects customer service in a health care facility.
- The facility should conduct a thorough assessment to decide whether to charge for parking and, if so, what to charge and what payment method to use.
- Parking decks and lots have a high potential for crime.
- Several groups need their own designated parking areas.
- Staff should register their vehicle with parking or security.

Exhibit 28–6 Parking Cashier Daily Balance Form

Date: _____ Day: _____	Date: _____ Day: _____
Lane #01 Shift: _____	Lane #02 Shift: _____
Gross: $ _____	Gross: $ _____
Neg. Validation: _____	Neg. Validation: _____
Net: $ _____	Net: $ _____
Present Cash: $ _____	Present Cash: $ _____
(−)Starting Cash: $ _____	(−)Starting Cash: $ _____
Net Amount Accountable: $ _____	Net Amount Accountable: $ _____
Lane Is (+) _____	Lane Is (+) _____
(−) _____	(−) _____
Even _____	Even _____
Cashier Name/s _____	Cashier Name/s _____
_____	_____
Verified By: _____	Verified By: _____
Amount Deposited: $ _____	Amount Deposited: $ _____
Receipt from Business Office:	Receipt from Business Office:
_____	_____
Notes:	Notes:

Exhibit 28–7 Parking Garage Audit Procedure

---

1. The parking garage will be audited by supervisory personnel a minimum of four times weekly (random times/days): day shift both during week and on weekends, and evening shift both during week and on weekends.
2. Supervisory personnel will arrive unannounced to security booth and collect all stamped tickets, all cash in drawer minus bank, and (X) out register tape and note amount.
3. Supervisory personnel will fill out form below and, if necessary, research and explain discrepancies. Forms must be completed.

PARKING GARAGE AUDIT FORM

Officer on duty:_____   Date: _____   Time: _____

Supervisor: _____   Shift: _____

Denomination of Tickets: $1.00 $2.00 $3.00 $4.00   Nonrevenue

Quantity					Total ____

Total cash in drawer minus bank: _____

(X) out amount on register tape: _____

Explanation of discrepancy (if any): _____

_____

_____

_____

Signature of supervisor: _____

Signature of parking garage officer: _____

Courtesy of St. Joseph's Hospital and Medical Center, Paterson, New Jersey.

Exhibit 28–8 Weekly Garage Statistics

Week Beginning _____   Week Ending _____

Day	Actual	Overage	Short	Nonrevenue Tickets	ID	Paid Tickets
Monday	$	$	$			
Tuesday	$	$	$			
Wednesday	$	$	$			
Thursday	$	$	$			
Friday	$	$	$			
Saturday	$	$	$			
Sunday	$	$	$			
TOTALS	$	$	$			

YEAR-TO-DATE TOTALS

Total Receipts	Cars Entered	Cars Exited	ID Card Exits	Nonrevenue Exits	Paid Exits
$					

Signature _____

Exhibit 28–9 Security Department Motor Vehicle Accident Report

Case: _____   Date: _____

Hospital Vehicle Involved? Yes: ( )   No: ( )

Hospital Property Damaged? Yes: ( )   No: ( ) _____

Police Department Investigating?   Yes: ( )   No: ( )

Department: _____ Officer:_____ Badge #:_____

Citations Issued: Yes: ( )   No: ( )   Unknown: ( ) _____

Date/Time of Accident: _____

Location of Accident: _____

Reported By:_____ Date/Time: _____

Pictures Taken? Yes: ( )   No: ( ) _____

Weather Conditions: _____ Visibility: _____

Light Conditions:_____ Road Conditions: _____

Vehicle #1.

A. REGISTERED OWNER OF VEHICLE

Name:_____ Home Telephone: _____

Address: _____

Insurance Company: _____

Policy #: _____ Agent: _____

B. Driver

Name: _____ State/Driver's License #: _____

Address: _____

Home Telephone #:_____ Business Telephone #: _____

Business Address: _____

Was Driver Injured? Yes: ( )   No: ( )

Transported to Medical Facility? Yes: ( )   No: ( )

Name of Medical Facility: _____

C. Vehicle:

Year:_____ Make: _____ Model: _____

Color: _____ State/License #: _____

D. Passengers? Yes: ( )   SEE BACK OF REPORT   No: ( )

Injured? Yes: ( )   SEE BACK OF REPORT   No: ( )

Exhibit 28–10 Release of Liability for Courtesy Services

Type of Service:

    Auto Unlock _____   Tire Inflate _____   Battery Boost _____

    Other (describe) _____

Vehicle:

    Make _____ Model_____ Year _____ Tag # _____

I, the owner/custodian of the above vehicle, do hereby release and discharge the employees and agents of _____ Medical Center from any civil or criminal actions that may arise from the performance of the above courtesy service. I understand that these services can cause damage to the vehicle, even if performed in a proper manner and that I warrant that I am releasing any claim for damages.

Signed this _____ of _____, _____.

_____   _____   _____

Owner/Custodian   **Driver's License #**   **Medical Center Representative**

Chapter 29

Managed Care

CHAPTER OBJECTIVES

1. Understand the part managed care has played in the evolution of health care.
2. Know key managed care terms.

INTRODUCTION

The health care business is unlike most others. For instance, a health care facility cannot set up shop beside another facility unless it proves to the state that there is a real need for the duplication of services. Retail stores and other businesses, by contrast, are free to open beside their competitors' stores. Also, customers of health care cannot always pay for what they purchase. Can you imagine someone going to the local tire store, demanding that new tires be put on a vehicle, and then not paying for the tires? But if people come to the emergency department, under federal law, they must be allowed to see a physician. And if the patients cannot pay the bill? The facility may refer the accounts to a collection agency and perhaps eventually take the patients to court and receive a judgment for the amount of the service. But if the patients are truly indigent, how will they pay?

Health care is undergoing rapid change. Owing partly to the growth of managed care, health care is now as much about doing business as it is about caring for patients. Managed care organizations attempt to control the cost of health care, not necessarily provide better health care.

The concept of managed care derives from the Medicare diagnosis-related group (DRG) concept of the early 1980s. Under the DRG guidelines, Medicare would pay a health care facility based upon national averages for a particular illness or condition. If the facility could treat the patient in the allotted time for the allotted amount, the facility made some profit. In most cases, Medicare paid somewhere between 60 percent and 66 percent of the facility's normal charges. Today's managed care contracts are written with even deeper discounts.

Security professionals today should have a basic understanding of managed care. This chapter will help to provide that knowledge. The sections below give an overview of managed care, defining many key managed care terms. Exhibit 29–1 lists other important terms used in managed care.

Exhibit 29–1 Other Key Managed Care Terms

ALOS—average length of stay; calculated as the average number of patient days of hospitalization for each admission, expressed as an average of the population within the plan for a given period of time

ambulatory care—health care services that are rendered on an outpatient basis, or to patients who are not confined overnight in a health care institution; outpatient care; may be provided within a doctor's office, medical clinic, acute care hospital, or free-standing ambulatory surgery center

basic health services—benefits that all federally qualified HMOs must offer, defined under subpart A, 417.104(a), of the Federal HMO Regulations to include at least physician services, outpatient services to include diagnostics, inpatient services, instructions on how to secure emergency care in and out of the service area, 20 outpatient visits per enrollee per year, home health, and preventive services

capitation—a prospective reimbursement based on the historical cost and expected use of health care services for the average member. In exchange for providing a defined set of health care services for members, providers receive a monthly capitation rate (which usually varies depending on the age and sex of the individual) for each member enrolled in their practice.

COBRA—Consolidated Omnibus Budget Reconciliation Act of 1985; a federal law requiring every hospital that participates in Medicare and has an emergency room to treat any patient in an emergency condition or active labor, whether or not covered by Medicare and regardless of ability to pay. COBRA also requires employers to provide continuation benefits to specified workers and families who have previously had benefits that have been terminated.

continuum of care—a spectrum of health care options, ranging from limited care needs through tertiary care, that has become the focus for an IDS to provide the appropriate expertise for the patient without providing a more expensive setting than necessary. An integrated delivery network can take full advantage of the continuum by ensuring good communication throughout the patient episode and by using step-down, long-term care, rehab, subacute, or assisted living center features as soon as they can be used.

DRG—diagnosis-related group; a Yale University–derived system of classification for 383 inpatient hospital services based on principal diagnosis, secondary diagnosis, surgical procedures, age, sex, and presence of complications; used as a financing mechanism to reimburse hospitals and selected other providers for services rendered; used to describe patient mix in hospitals and to determine hospital reimbursement policy.

emergency services—an important definition that determines whether care will be reimbursed; may involve care within a plan or may address those services that are essentially out-of-area emergencies. HCFA defines emergency services as covered inpatient or outpatient services that are furnished by an appropriate source other than the HMO or competitive medical plan (CMP) for care needed immediately because of injury or sudden illness, when such care cannot be delayed for the time required to reach the HMO or CMP provider or authorized alternative

continues

Exhibit 29–1 continued

without risk of permanent damage to the patient's health, and when transfer to an HMO or CMP source is also precluded because of risk or unreasonable distance given the nature of the medical condition. Many believe that a standard definition of emergency service should be developed at the state or federal level.

   fee splitting—an unethical "kickback" practice of a physician, surgeon, or consultant returning part of the professional fee back to the referring physician for making the referral; practically ruled out under the relationships of managed care in which the PCP is at risk or sharing risk with specialists

   gatekeeper—a physician who directs and coordinates the care of a member in a managed care plan. The gatekeeper is responsible for authorizing referrals to specialists and hospitalizations.

   hospital alliance—a voluntary formation or collaborative grouping of two or more hospitals as a system or network (or other looser alliances) for the purpose of competing with the strengthened negotiating position of one entity in dealing with one or more health plans for managed care contracts, and possibly reducing costs through shared services or group purchasing. Some say that loose affiliations will not bring the strongest advantages possible, but others say that the need for tightly integrated structures should be determined solely by whether they are needed to compete effectively.

   member—an individual enrolled in or covered by a managed care plan

   provider—a physician or other health care practitioner who delivers health care services to individuals in a managed care plan

   purchaser—a public or private entity or organization that buys health coverage for workers, dependents, retirees, or other beneficiaries

   Source: Adapted from R. Rognehaugh, *The Managed Health Care Dictionary,* second edition, © 1998, Aspen Publishers, Inc.

OVERVIEW OF MANAGED CARE*

Managed Care Organizations (MCOs)

According to the American Association of Health Plans (AAHP), MCOs are entities that offer a health maintenance organization (HMO), preferred provider organization (PPO), or point of sale (POS) plan, or any combination of these. They can be owned by national managed care firms, physician groups, hospitals, commercial health insurers, Blue Cross and Blue Shield plans, community cooperatives, private investors, or other organizations. The following summaries provide information on the structure of various MCO models.

HMOs

HMOs offer comprehensive health care services to members for a fixed monthly fee by contracting with or employing hospitals, physicians, and other health care professionals to

---

* This section was adapted from W. Knight, What Is Managed Care? *Managed Care: What It Is and How It Works,* pp. 20–43, © 1998, Aspen Publishers, Inc.

provide medical care to enrollees. Half of the HMOs in operation today are owned by national managed care firms, and the remainder are divided among Blue Cross and Blue Shield and independent ownership. Roughly 10 to 12 percent of the nation's HMOs are owned by providers, including physician groups and hospitals. These provider-sponsored HMOs enroll more than five million people.

Historically, HMOs have differed from other managed care plans in many ways, including provider payments, benefits, and plan structure; however, as the market demands greater adaptability, HMOs are taking on characteristics of other managed care models. For example, HMOs have developed products with more flexibility for obtaining care from providers outside their own network of providers. **Although the differences between HMO models are fading, there remain four basic models.**

1. **Staff model.** Physicians and other health care providers are salaried employees and provide care exclusively to individuals enrolled in the HMO. Care is usually delivered at clinics owned by the HMO.
2. **Group model.** The HMO contracts on an exclusive basis with a large physician practice to provide comprehensive benefits to the HMO's enrollees. While the HMO and the physician practice appear to be the same organization, they are distinct entities.
3. **Independent practice association (IPA) model.** The HMO contracts with physicians or groups of independent physicians (known as IPAs) to provide care to HMO members in the physicians' own offices. These physicians are usually organized as solo practitioners or small group practices and see patients other than those enrolled in the HMO.
4. **Network model.** The HMO contracts with several larger multispecialty groups or IPAs, not individual physicians or small practices, who also see patients not enrolled in the HMO. An HMO that uses several contracting methods is often called a network-model HMO.

PPOs

PPOs are networks of hospitals, physicians, and other health care professionals that provide medical care to individuals for a negotiated fee. PPOs are often sold as an option (also known as a rider) to a traditional insurance plan. In contrast with HMOs, PPOs do not assume the financial risk of arranging for health care benefits; risk is often assumed by the sponsoring organizations, such as an insurance company, third-party administrator, or self-insured employer. Consequently, PPOs do not perform many of the functions customary for HMOs and other risk-bearing MCOs, such as underwriting, utilization management, and quality assurance. Since the sponsoring organization determines what benefits are covered in the plan, PPOs are not in a position of making treatment decisions or denying claims; therefore, they have limited member service functions. Through a PPO, a sponsoring organization offers its beneficiaries access to a broad array of health care providers at discounted fees. Clients can also purchase utilization management services, such as case management and utilization review, as stand-alone products or to complement the PPO network offerings. While exact numbers on PPO enrollment are difficult to ascertain, the AAHP estimates that over 91 million people are covered through a PPO.

Provider-Sponsored Organizations (PSOs)

PSOs are managed care organizations that are owned or controlled by health care providers. While many of the original HMOs were (and still are) provider controlled, PSO is a recent term used to describe the emerging provider organizations that form for the purposes of directly contracting with purchasers to deliver care to beneficiaries. Unlike IPAs and other provider groups, PSOs are structured to assume the insurance risk of providing medical care to a set group of patients. As a result, many PSOs are licensed HMOs. PSOs are formed by IPAs, physician–hospital organizations (PHOs), integrated delivery systems (IDSs), and the like—sometimes as joint ventures with large provider organizations or MCOs.

IDSs

IDSs are groups of hospitals, physicians, and other health care professionals and facilities that provide the full spectrum of health care services under one legal structure. Because of their ability to assume risk directly from the purchaser, IDSs can function both as a participating provider in a managed care network and as a direct competitor of plans. In fact, many IDSs that are formed by academic medical centers or larger hospitals compete directly with other managed care plans. IDSs tend to own the hospitals and facilities in the system and employ the affiliated physicians, although some IDSs are joint ventures created to gain greater leverage in highly penetrated managed care markets.

PHOs

A PHO is a legal entity formed by a hospital and physicians to contract with managed care plans and employers. PHOs are composed of one or more hospitals and their medical staff, and other community physicians and health care professionals who become members or shareholders of the PHO. The majority of PHOs are separate business entities, not hospital divisions.

The PHO assumes responsibility for the contracting, administrative, and marketing functions of its members. PHOs enter into full- or partial-risk arrangements with MCOs. Most PHOs were formed by hospitals in response to the growing dominance of managed care plans in their market and are still perceived as hospital controlled, even though the majority of them have equitable hospital and physician ownership and board representation. In 1995, 67 percent of PHOs surveyed indicated that they were equally owned by physicians and hospitals.

Administrative Organizations

Rather than provide all of the administrative functions necessary to deliver patient care, some MCOs and provider groups work in conjunction with third-party administrators (TPAs) and other administrative organizations and intermediaries. The following sections discuss some of these administrative organizations.

TPAs

Typically, a TPA provides claims processing, enrollment, and other administrative functions for self-funded employers, PPOs, and small or emerging MCOs. Some TPAs assume broader responsibilities, such as utilization review, actuarial analysis, and network development. Most do not assume insurance risk, however.

PPO Intermediaries

PPO intermediaries negotiate and manage managed care contracts on behalf of individual physicians. These organizations can represent a handful of or numerous providers, in multiple or single specialties, and in wide or confined geographic areas. They also vary in their scope of services offered. Some PPO intermediaries assume all responsibility for building and managing PPO networks, in turn leasing them to insurance companies or self-funded employers. Others contract on behalf of a small group of physicians within a single country.

Managed Care versus Traditional Insurance

To understand the essence of managed care, it is often useful to contrast it to traditional insurance programs. Although this may seem meaningless given the permeation of managed care features into most traditional insurance plans, such a comparison engenders a good comprehension of managed care.

From a financial perspective, health care is a transaction between two or more parties involving a medical treatment: one who seeks it (patient), one who provides it (health care professional), and one who pays for it (insurer and employer). Sometimes more than one role is occupied by the same entity or individual. For example, the person who pays for a medical procedure on his or her own is seeking and paying for medical care. Other times, multiple organizations will fulfill a single role, as with the employer and insurer who share the cost of health coverage.

Managed care introduces a new role to the equation: one who arranges for medical care. Network-based MCOs will arrange for health care professionals to deliver medical care within certain cost and utilization parameters. Some MCOs employ health care professionals to provide care, as well. As such, managed care plans are positioned to provide, arrange, and pay for medical care, depending on their organizational structure. Traditional health insurance companies, on the other hand, pay for only the health care services incurred by individuals.

Total Patient Health

A managed care system differs from traditional indemnity insurance in many ways, most significantly in how it regards the individuals for whom it is contractually obligated to provide medical care. Unlike indemnity insurance policies, which pay the medical bills of patients who develop particular illnesses or medical conditions, a managed care plan has responsibility for providing the full spectrum of medical care to individuals enrolled in the plan. This includes medical services that

- keep patients in good health (e.g., annual physical exams)
- detect illnesses or conditions (e.g., cancer screenings)
- treat acute illnesses (e.g., hospitalizations, surgical procedures)
- minimize complications from chronic ailments (e.g., home care, medical equipment)

Managed care, then, regards each individual as a total patient and not the sum of individual body parts that need repair on occasion. This perspective is fundamentally different from that of traditional insurers, which take no ownership for a person's health status. By agreeing to provide a broad range of health care services to an enrollee for a fixed fee, a managed care plan, one could argue, has implicitly accepted the challenge to keep that person healthy. Conversely, one can assert (as many opponents of managed care do) that accepting a fixed fee for a patient encourages MCOs to enroll only the healthiest individuals and to deny necessary medical care to members to keep costs down.

A managed care plan will provide a continuum of care adapted to the particular health needs of patients and designed to maintain or improve patient health. Such an approach necessitates processes and functions not required in traditional insurance plans, including health education literature, wellness programs, and disease management programs.

Benefit Coverage

Generally, traditional insurance plans cover basic medical and surgical procedures and hospitalizations, while MCOs cover the full range of health care services, including preventive care services, physician visits, hospitalizations, home care, and various outpatient treatments and services. There is usually greater patient cost sharing in traditional plans in the form of higher co-insurance amounts. MCOs require deductibles and co-insurance for certain procedures or products, particularly those with high utilization. The majority of them charge patients a small fee per visit, or copayment, for most services.

Access to Health Professionals

The most common way people differentiate managed care from traditional insurance is the mechanism for seeing health care professionals. Managed care plans create "networks" of health care professionals they direct members to use. Complete or maximum payment for medical services is predicated on the member using these providers. Depending on the type of managed care product, the plan may require the member to see his or her designated primary care provider (PCP; also called a gatekeeper) to obtain authorization from the plan before receiving specialty care. With many MCOs, the member typically needs to receive authorization for hospitalizations, outpatient procedures, and diagnostic services. The frequency of services or treatments may be limited to a certain number of visits or days. While most traditional insurance plans have incorporated medical management techniques of managed care (e.g., precertification for hospitalizations), they usually allow unrestricted access to specialty care providers.

Provider Payment

In a traditional insurance arrangement, health care professionals are paid a certain fee for each procedure they perform (i.e., fee for service). This fee-for-service payment mechanism creates incentives for physicians to perform services for financial gain, not necessarily because the procedures may be effective or appropriate in treating a patient. As a result, total health care expenditures continue to escalate without a clear sense of improved patient care. The payment policies of managed care plans are designed to make providers more accountable for the services they perform. This is done by limiting the frequency of unnecessary medical procedures, reducing the per unit cost of services, compensating physicians for total treatments or cases, or prepaying physicians for the partial or total medical care of a patient (i.e., capitation). While capitation is not the only way MCOs pay physicians, it is the one payment mechanism that is most closely associated with managed care, particularly managed care's negative attributes. Many insist that capitation payment systems encourage physicians to withhold necessary medical care solely for profit and to eschew patients who consume more health care resources.

Population-Based Health Management

Because individuals are enrolled in the managed care plan, MCOs have the opportunity to understand the unique medical experiences of each patient. Using computers and other information systems, MCOs can collect patient information from medical records, claims, enrollment data, patient surveys, and other sources to develop programs to treat and manage patient care. Such information includes past and current medical conditions and illnesses, historical use of specific health care services, and lifestyle behaviors that affect the health of individual patients and within specific categories, such as gender and age. The collection and analysis of this information enables the MCOs to first identify the prevalent risk factors and incidence of diseases among their membership and then develop target programs to best care for their membership. Population-based health care management, as this is called, is an element of health care management unique to managed care, although such initiatives are still in their infancy.

The Future of Managed Care

It is difficult to define managed care given its continuous modification and contradictory perceptions of it. Because managed care is shaped by fluid market forces, its structure and focus change frequently and swiftly, sometimes faster than one can absorb. Such rapid mutations do not permit easy comprehension. Moreover, the various perceptions of managed care mold the understanding of it among its key audiences. Consequently, clear definitions of managed care are elusive and are outdated almost as soon as they are formulated. Continuous change in the managed care market is inevitable as purchasers, consumers, providers, and others grapple with how best to deliver quality health care with finite economic resources.

KEY POINTS

- Managed care has dramatically changed the health care industry.
- There are many forms of managed care organizations, including HMOs, PPOs, POSs, PSOs, IDSs, and PHOs.

Chapter 30

Medicaid and Medicare Fraud

John Thomas Readling

CHAPTER OBJECTIVES

1. Understand the magnitude of Medicare and Medicaid fraud and abuse.
2. Know how to define health care fraud and abuse.
3. Know the federal laws (criminal and civil) pertinent to health care fraud.
4. Understand some complex health care fraud schemes.
5. Know what agencies are the primary investigators of health care fraud.

INTRODUCTION

Health care fraud and abuse are complex problems involving hundreds of millions of dollars. Because of the complexities of billing and payment methods and the fluid nature of crime related to health care, those charged with fraud and abuse investigation have a monumental task. This chapter will discuss the scope of the health care fraud problem, summarize the basic laws involved, and provide an overview of some of the more common schemes employed to fraudulently obtain huge amounts of money.

During fiscal year 1997, national health care expenditures exceeded $1 trillion dollars, or approximately 13.5 percent of the gross domestic product—about one-seventh of the U.S. economy. Of this total amount, approximately 14.6 percent was attributed to the Medicaid program, 19.6 percent to the Medicare program, and 12.2 percent to other public programs.[1] With so much money involved, it is easy to see why organized criminal enterprises have targeted this field. Both simplistic and sophisticated schemes have been devised to illegally obtain millions of dollars of government funds.

The General Accounting Office recently estimated that fraud and abuse account for approximately 10 percent of health care costs, a figure that many believe is very conservative.[2] (It is difficult to establish a precise figure.) If this 10 percent figure is accurate, fraud and abuse accounted for $100 billion dollars nationwide in 1997 alone.

The per capita spending in the United States measured approximately $4,000 in 1997.[3] Again, if this 10 percent figure is accurate, every person in the United States was the victim of a $400 larceny.

Fraud and abuse drain the nation's resources, and everyone wants to stop them. State and federal law enforcement have become more vigilant about fraud and abuse, and yet they continue. Politicians have made speeches about fraud and abuse, and yet they continue. New laws have been enacted, yet the fraud and abuse continue. If so many people know about health care fraud and abuse and are so concerned, how is it that fraud and abuse continue?

To greedy thieves, the government is an "easy mark"; any people with knowledge of the system can simply take as much as they can and the government has made it easy for them to do so. In fact, if they are sophisticated in their approach, the government will even assist them with their billings. These thieves often see the fraud as almost a victimless crime. To them, the government is a large, nameless, and faceless bureaucracy.

Unscrupulous health care providers commit fraud because they either believe the government does not pay them what they are worth or they are out to maximize profits through fraudulent manipulation of the system. Whatever the rationalization, the health care providers who commit these acts are just white-collar criminals who have chosen to use health care funds as their target.

The solution to the fraud and abuse problem is as complex as the bureaucracy that oversees the health care expenditures. The payment systems established for Medicare and Medicaid seem to be rooted in two basic premises: (1) claims should be processed as promptly as possible, and (2) health care providers are honest. While a vast majority of health care providers are honest, this assumption of honesty makes the system an easy target for those who are not. In addition, many more government employees are involved in funds disbursement than in the detection and investigation of health care fraud and abuse.

Consider the hundreds of thousands of claims submitted for payment. Most claims are processed by companies hired by the government to function as claim processing centers. These companies are usually paid on a per claim basis. The more claims they handle and the faster they handle them, the more profitable these companies are. Most of these firms do have some basic edit functions in their automated processing systems. These often include cross-references on provider numbers and recipient numbers and other edits relating to the claims. If an electronic claim passes through the initial company edits, the claim is automatically paid.

Those involved in health care fraud often take the time to learn proper submission techniques, ask for help with claim submission, and determine what type and what amount of claims either would be denied or would generate suspicion on the part of program integrity personnel or fraud investigators. By keeping their claims below certain thresholds, perpetrators of some fraudulent schemes can remain active for years and receive funds regularly.

There are more sophisticated computer programs designed by fraud investigators to serve as "edits and audits" that are designed to identify potentially fraudulent claims before the claims are paid. These programs, if utilized, do tend to slow the payment process. The slowing of the payment process is not welcomed by the companies who handle the claims, those who disburse the funds, and the health care providers who must wait longer for payment. In fact, it is argued by some that it is cheaper to pay the fraudulent claims than it is to slow the process, identify the criminals, and either stop the illegal payment before it goes out or prosecute and recoup funds after payment has been made.

Because of the emphasis on payments, most health care fraud investigations in this country are "pay and chase." The funds are first paid to fraudulent health care providers and then, if the investigators are able to identify criminal activity, they initiate an investigation and attempt to prosecute the individuals and recover the fraudulently obtained funds. But there are few fraud investigators and many frauds perpetrated on the system. The likelihood of detection and prosecution is low.

The CBS program *60 Minutes* recently aired a segment on health care fraud and abuse. An accountant had discovered that two sets of books were being maintained by Columbia/HCA, one of the largest health care providers in the country. The accountant provided the government with evidence that suggested that cost figures presented to the government, on which certain payments are based, had been inflated. The U.S. Department of Justice initiated an investigation, and the government may attempt to recover as much as $1 billion from Columbia/HCA. Not only is the amount of the alleged fraud staggering, but the fact is that until the allegations were made by a private citizen, the government did not even know the fraud was going on!

WHAT IS HEALTH CARE FRAUD?

Simply stated, health care fraud is obtaining health care funds the provider is not legally entitled to. Malcolm K. Sparrow defines criminal fraud as requiring "a deliberate misrepresentation or deception, leading to some kind of improper pecuniary advantage."[4(p.50)] In most cases, the fraud requires that the health care provider make, or cause to be made, a false statement of a material fact in a direct application for payment or in documentation of cost reporting.

As discussed later in this chapter, some types of fraud are so blatant that the criminal intent of the provider is clear. Some of these types of fraud would include billing for services that were not rendered, billing for expensive equipment or tests when more inexpensive equipment or tests were actually provided, and billing for brand-name drugs when generic products were actually used.

Other types of fraud and abuse are not so obvious. Imagine, for example, that a home health agency provides a willing physician with the names of people who do not really need home health care. The physician signs a paper saying that the people do need health care. The home health agency then provides some form of home health care to the people and is paid for its service by government funds. The physician gets a kickback from the agency.

Identifying this type of fraud is somewhat difficult because it involves questioning a physician's judgment. If there are recipients who are clearly not entitled to receive home health services, challenging the judgment of the physician is easier. When cases are not so clear, other health care professionals must be willing to step in and question a colleague's decision. In most cases, health care professionals do not want their own decisions scrutinized and therefore do not feel comfortable scrutinizing the decisions of others. In addition, the line between deliberate fraud and poor judgment is fuzzy. For all these reasons, these types of cases are often difficult to detect, prove, and prosecute.

CRIMINAL STATUTES

There are numerous criminal and civil laws being utilized in the war against health care fraud and abuse. This text will focus on the most prevalent federal statutes. Because of the great number of different statutes enacted by states and the fact that many state statutes mirror the federal statutes, no discussion of state law will be attempted.

Making or Causing To Be Made False Statements or Representations

Title 42, Section 1320a-7b, of the United States Code is considered one of the definitive laws for criminal penalties relating to Medicare and Medicaid fraud. The law, appearing under the Public Health and Welfare laws, is specific in targeting acts involving federal health care programs. Within the statute, the term "federal health care program" is defined as any health care benefit funded in whole or in part by the U.S. government or any state health care plan, which includes the state Medicaid programs. Part (a) of the statute states that a person who does one of the following acts is guilty of a felony.

(1) knowingly and willfully makes or causes to be made any false statement or representation of a material fact in any application for any benefit or payment under a Federal health care program . . .

(2) at any time knowingly and willfully makes or causes to be made any false statement or representation of a material fact for use in determining rights to such benefit or payment,

(3) having knowledge of the occurrence of any event affecting (A) his initial or continued right to any such benefit or payment, or (B) the initial or continued right to any such benefit or payment of any other individual in whose behalf he has applied for or is receiving such benefit or payment, conceals or fails to disclose such event with an intent fraudulently to secure such benefit or payment either in greater amount or quantity than is due or when no such benefit or payment is authorized,

(4) having made application to receive any such benefit or payment for the use and benefit of another and having received it, knowingly and willfully converts such benefit or payment or any part thereof to a use other than for the use and benefit of such other person,

(5) presents or causes to be presented a claim for a physician's service for which payment may be made under a Federal health care program and knows that the individual who furnished the service was not licensed as a physician, or

(6) for a fee knowingly and willfully counsels or assists an individual to dispose of assets (including by any transfer in trust) in order for the individual to become eligible for medical assistance under a State plan . . . if disposing of the assets results in the imposition of a period of ineligibility for such assistance.[5]

Violation of the provisions noted above by an individual is a felony. Upon conviction the individual may be fined up to $25,000, or imprisoned for not more than five years, or both. Misdemeanor provisions are also included in the statute for those individuals acting on behalf of another.

Only the first five of the parts of the statute listed above deal directly with the health care provider. It is important to note that the statute goes beyond the concept of criminal penalties for services not rendered. Item (1) above notes that any claim that contains a false statement or representation of a material fact can have action taken against it. *Black's Law Dictionary* defines a "material fact" as "one which constitutes substantially the consideration of the contract, or without which it would not have been made."[6(p.1128)] In layperson's terms, a material fact is a fact of such importance that without it the outcome of the claim (payment) would be different.

Imagine that a physician saw one of her regular patients in the office for a five-minute follow-up examination. Though the visit was simple and brief, the physician billed Medicaid for a high-complexity office visit. (A complex visit would require approximately 40 minutes of face-to-face contact and pay more per claim than a simple, brief visit.) The physician had rendered a service, but in billing Medicaid the physician had misrepresented a material fact (the complexity of the visit). The physician could be charged with a violation under this statute.

It is important to note that both individuals and corporations can be charged under this statute. If, for example, a home health agency submitted 100 claims for services not rendered, both the corporation and the individuals involved could potentially be charged under a 100-count indictment. If convicted, the charges might be consolidated for judgment, or a person could be sentenced to consecutive terms, or multiples of the five-year imprisonment limitation, all of which are subject to sentencing guidelines.

Illegal Remunerations

Part (b) of this statute addresses bribes, kickbacks, rebates, and the like, including payments in cash, goods, or services. Part (b) states:

(1) Whoever knowingly and willfully solicits or receives any remuneration (including any kickback, bribe, or rebate) directly or indirectly, overtly or covertly, in cash or in kind -

    (A) in return for referring an individual to a person for the furnishing or arranging for the furnishing of any item or service for which payment may be made in whole or in part under a Federal health care program, or

    (B) in return for purchasing, leasing, ordering, or arranging for or recommending purchasing, leasing, or ordering any good, facility, service, or item for which payment may be made in whole or in part under a Federal health care program, shall be guilty of a felony and upon conviction thereof, shall be fined not more than $25,000 or imprisoned for not more than five years, or both.

(2) Whoever knowingly and willfully offers or pays any remuneration (including any kickback, bribe, or rebate) directly or indirectly, overtly or covertly, in cash or in kind to any person to induce such person -

(A) to refer an individual to a person for the furnishing or arranging for the furnishing of any item or service for which payment may be made in whole or in part under a Federal health care program, or

(B) to purchase, lease, order, or arrange for or recommend purchasing, leasing, or ordering any good, facility, service, or item for which payment may be made in whole or in part under a Federal health care program, shall be guilty of a felony and upon conviction thereof, shall be fined not more than $25,000 or imprisoned for not more than five years, or both.[7]

This portion of the statute is basically self-explanatory. The statute makes it a criminal offense to solicit or receive, offer or pay, any remuneration in return for either obtaining or recommending any Federal health care program. It should be noted that this portion of the statute lists several areas where this portion of the law does not apply. If the reader has specific questions as to exclusions, the complete cite should be read and the activity reviewed by legal counsel.

False Statements or Representations with Respect to Condition or Operation of Institutions

Part (c) of the statute states that:

Whoever knowingly and willfully makes or causes to be made, or induces or seeks to induce the making of, any false statement or representation of a material fact with respect to the conditions or operation of any institution, facility, or entity in order that such institution, facility, or entity may qualify (either upon initial certification or upon recertification) as a hospital, rural primary care hospital, skilled nursing facility, nursing facility, intermediate care facility for the mentally retarded, home health agency, or other entity . . . for which certification is required under subchapter XVIII of this chapter or a State health care program . . . or with respect to information required to be provided under section 1320a-3a of this title, shall be guilty of a felony and upon conviction thereof shall be fined not more than $25,000 or imprisoned for not more than five years, or both.[8]

Illegal Patient Admittance and Retention Practices

Part (d) states that:

Whoever knowingly and willfully -

(1) charges, for any service provided to a patient under a State plan approved under subchapter XIX of this chapter, money or other consideration at a rate in excess of the rates established by the State . . . or

(2) charges, solicits, accepts, or receives, in addition to any amount otherwise required to be paid under a State plan approved under subchapter XIX of this chapter, any gift, money, donation, or other consideration (other than a charitable, religious, or philanthropic contribution from an organization or from a person unrelated to the patient) -

> (A) as a precondition of admitting a patient to a hospital, nursing facility, or intermediate care facility for the mentally retarded, or

> (B) as a requirement for the patient's continued stay in such a facility,

> when the cost of the services provided therein to the patient is paid for (in whole or in part) under the State plan,

shall be guilty of a felony and upon conviction thereof shall be fined not more than $25,000 or imprisoned for not more than five years, or both.[9]

Violation of Assignment Terms

Part (e) states:

Whoever accepts assignments described in section 1395u(b)(3)(B)(ii) of this title or agrees to be a participating physician or supplier under section 1395u(h)(1) of this title and knowingly, willfully, and repeatedly violates the term of such assignments or agreement, shall be guilty of a misdemeanor and upon conviction thereof shall be fined not more than $2,000 or imprisoned for not more than six months, or both.[10]

False, Fictitious, or Fraudulent Claims

Title 18, Section 287 of the United States Code addresses false, fictitious, or fraudulent claims.

Whoever makes or presents to any person or officer in the civil, military, or naval service of the United States, or to any department or agency thereof, any claim upon or against the United States, or any department or agency thereof, knowing such claim to be false, fictitious, or fraudulent, shall be imprisoned not more than five years and shall be subject to a fine in the amount provided in this title.[11]

This is a general fraudulent claims statute, not one specific to federal health care programs.

Conspiracy

Conspiracy to commit offense or to defraud the United States is addressed in Title 18, Section 371, of the United States Code, which states the following:

> If two or more persons conspire either to commit any offense against the United States, or to defraud the United States, or any agency thereof in any manner or for any purpose, and one or more of such persons do any act to effect the object of the conspiracy, each shall be fined under this title or imprisoned not more than five years, or both.

> If, however, the offense, the commission of which is the object of the conspiracy, is a misdemeanor only, the punishment for such conspiracy shall not exceed the maximum punishment provided for such misdemeanor.[12]

Mail Fraud

If a health care fraud was perpetrated by using the United States Postal Service, another charge that may be appropriate is mail fraud, discussed in Title 18, Section 1341, of the United States Code.

> Whoever, having devised or intending to devise any scheme or artifice to defraud, or for obtaining money or property by means of false or fraudulent pretenses, representations, or promises, or to sell, dispose of, loan, exchange, alter, give away, distribute, supply, or furnish or procure for unlawful use any counterfeit or spurious coin, obligation, security, or other article, or anything represented to be or intimated or held out to be such counterfeit or spurious article, for the purpose of executing such scheme or artifice or attempting so to do, places in any post office or authorized depository for mail matter, any matter or thing whatever to be sent or delivered by the Postal Service, or deposits or causes to be deposited any matter or thing whatever to be sent or delivered by any private or commercial interstate carrier, or takes or receives therefrom, any such matter or thing, or knowingly causes to be delivered by mail or such carrier according to the direction thereon, or at the place at which it is directed to be delivered by the person to whom it is addressed, any such matter or thing, shall be fined under this title or imprisoned not more than five years, or both. If the violation affects a financial institution, such person shall be fined not more than $1,000,000 or imprisoned not more than 30 years, or both.[13]

Mail Fraud: Fraud by Wire, Radio, or Television

Section 1343 of Title 18 of the United States Code updated the older "mail fraud" statute above by including fraud perpetrated using more modern technology.

> Whoever, having devised or intending to devise any scheme or artifice to defraud, or for obtaining money or property by means of false or fraudulent pretenses, representations, or promises, transmits or causes to be transmitted by means of wire,

radio, or television communication in interstate or foreign commerce, any writings, signs, signals, pictures, or sounds for the purpose of executing such scheme or artifice, shall be fined under this title or imprisoned not more than five years, or both. If the violation affects a financial institution, such person shall be fined not more than $1,000,000 or imprisoned not more than 30 years, or both.[14]

The mail and wire fraud statutes have been used to prosecute numerous different types of health care fraud violations. Use of the mail and wire fraud statutes is common in these cases in that under the provisions of the statutes a district court may grant an injunction or restraining order to halt the fraud. The court may also order that all or a portion of the defendant's assets be seized.

The use of the mail and wire fraud statutes may also generate additional charges under the Racketeer Influenced and Corrupt Organizations Act or the money laundering statute(s).

Some other federal criminal laws that may apply to health care fraud include the following sections of the United States Code:

- Title 18, Section 495—Counterfeiting and Forgery
- Title 18, Section 641—Theft or Conversion of Public Property
- Title 18, Section 666—Theft or Bribery Concerning Programs Receiving Public Money
- Title 18, Section 1001—False Statement to Government Agency
- Title 18, Section 495—Obstruction of Proceedings Before Departments, Agencies and Committees
- Title 18, Section 1510—Obstruction of Criminal Investigations
- Title 18, Section 1516—Obstruction of Federal Audit

There are also numerous state statutes that address health care fraud.

CIVIL REMEDIES

This portion of the chapter discusses three primary civil remedies for health care fraud and abuse under federal law. The first section covers the procedure generally utilized by the federal government to make civil recovery of false claims made against the government. The second section presents specific civil penalties regarding health care fraud. The third section discusses civil actions for false claims, including qui tam actions, which are civil actions brought by citizens against a person for a violation of the false claims provisions under Section 3729 of Title 31 of the United States Code.

False Claims

Title 31, Section 3729, of the United States Code discusses false claims.

(a) Liability for Certain Acts. - Any person who -

(1) knowingly presents, or causes to be presented, to an officer or employee of the United States Government or a member of the Armed Forces of the United States a false or fraudulent claim for payment or approval;

(2) knowingly makes, uses, or causes to be made or used, a false record or statement to get a false or fraudulent claim paid or approved by the Government;

(3) conspires to defraud the Government by getting a false or fraudulent claim allowed or paid;

(4) has possession, custody, or control of property or money used, or to be used, by the Government and, intending to defraud the Government or willfully to conceal the property, delivers, or causes to be delivered, less property than the amount for which the person receives a certificate or receipt;

(5) authorized to make or deliver a document certifying receipt of property used, or to be used, by the Government and, intending to defraud the Government, makes or delivers the receipt without completely knowing that the information on the receipt is true;

(6) knowingly buys, or receives as a pledge of an obligation or debt, public property from an officer or employee of the Government, or a member of the Armed Forces, who lawfully may not sell or pledge the property; or

(7) knowingly makes, uses, or causes to be made or used, a false record or statement to conceal, avoid, or decrease an obligation to pay or transmit money or property to the Government,

is liable to the United States Government for a civil penalty of not less than $5,000 and not more than $10,000, plus 3 times the amount of damages which the Government sustains because of the act of that person, except that if the court finds that -

(A) the person committing the violation of this subsection furnished officials of the United States responsible for investigating false claims violation with all information known to such person about the violation within 30 days after the date on which the defendant first obtained the information;

(B) such person fully cooperated with any Government investigation of such violation; and

(C) at the time such person furnished the United States with the information about the violation, no criminal prosecution, civil action, or administrative action had commenced under this title with respect to such violation, and the person did not have actual knowledge of the existence of an investigation into such violation;

the court may assess not less than 2 times the amount of damages which the Government sustains because of the act of the person. A person violating this subsection shall also be liable to the United States Government for the costs of a civil action brought to recover any such penalty or damages.[15]

Civil Monetary Penalties

Under the provisions of Title 42, Section 1320a-7a, of the United States Code, certain penalties are established that apply directly to health care fraud. This is a lengthy section, and only a portion will be provided in this text.

(a) Improperly filed claims

Any person (including an organization, agency, or other entity, but excluding a beneficiary, as defined in subsection (i)(5) of this section) that -

(1) knowingly presents or causes to be presented to an officer, employee, or agent of the United States, or of any department or agency thereof, or of any State agency (as defined in subsection (i)(1) of this section), a claim (as defined in subsection (i)(2) of this section) that the Secretary determines -

(A) is for a medical or other item or service that the person knows or should know was not provided as claimed, including any person who engages in a pattern or practice of presenting or causing to be presented a claim for an item or service that is based on a code that the person knows or should know will result in a greater payment to the person than the code the person knows or should know is applicable to the item or service actually provided,

(B) is for a medical or other item or service and the person knows or should know the claim is false or fraudulent,

(C) is presented for a physician's service (or an item or service incident to a physician's service) by a person who knows or should know that the individual who furnished (or supervised the furnishing of) the service -

(i) was not licensed as a physician,

(ii) was licensed as a physician, but such license had been obtained through misrepresentation of material fact (including cheating on an examination required for licensing), or

(iii) represented to the patient at the time the service was furnished that the physician was certified in a medical specialty by a medical specialty board when the individual was not so certified,

(D) is for a medical or other item or service furnished during a period in which the person was excluded from the program under which the claim was made pursuant to a determination by the Secretary under this section or under section 1320a-7, 1320c-5, 1320c-9(b) (as in effect on September 2, 1982), 1395y(d) (as in effect on August, 18, 1987), or 1395cc(b) of this title or as a result of the application of the provisions of section 1395u(j)(2) of this title, or

(E) is for a pattern of medical or other items or services that a person knows or should know are not medically necessary;

(2) knowingly presents or causes to be presented to any person a request for payment which is in violation of the terms of (A) an assignment under section 1395u(b)(3)(B)(ii) of this title, or (B) an agreement with a State agency (or other requirement of a State plan under subchapter XIX of this chapter) not to charge a person for an item or service in excess of the amount permitted to be charged, or (C) an agreement to be a participating physician or supplier under section 1395u(h)(1) of this title, or (D) an agreement pursuant to section 1395cc(a)(1)(G) of this title;

(3) knowingly gives or causes to be given to any person, with respect to coverage under subchapter XVIII of this chapter of inpatient hospital services subject to the provisions of section 1395ww of this title, information that he knows or should know is false or misleading, and that could reasonably be expected to influence the decision when to discharge such person or another individual from the hospital;

(4) in the case of a person who is not an organization, agency, or other entity, is excluded from participating in a program under subchapter XVIII of this chapter or a State health care program in accordance with this subsection or under section 1320a-7 of this title and who, at the time of a violation of this subsection -

(A) retains a direct or indirect ownership or control interest in an entity that is participating in a program under subchapter XVIII of this chapter or a State health care program, and who knows or should know of the action constituting the basis for the exclusion; or

(B) is an officer or managing employee (as defined in section 1320a-5(b) of this title) of such an entity

(5) offers to or transfers remuneration to any individual eligible for benefits under subchapter XVIII of this chapter, or under a State health care program (as defined in section 1320a-7(h) of this title) that such person knows or should know is likely to influence such individual to order or receive from a particular provider, practitioner, or supplier any item or service for which payment may be made, in whole or in part, under subchapter XVIII of this chapter, or a State health care program (as so defined); shall be subject, in addition to any other penalties that may be pre-

scribed by law, to a civil money penalty of not more than $10,000 for each item or service (or, in cases under paragraph (3), $15,000 for each individual with respect to whom false or misleading information was given; in cases under paragraph (4), $10,000 for each day the prohibited relationship occurs). In addition, such a person shall be subject to an assessment of not more than 3 times the amount claimed for each such item or service in lieu of damages sustained by the United States or a State agency because of such claim. In addition, the Secretary may make a determination in the same proceeding to exclude the person from participation in the Federal health care programs (as defined in section 1320a–7b(f)(1) of this title) and to direct the appropriate State agency to exclude the person from participation in any State health care program.

(b) Payments to induce reduction or limitation of services

(1) If a hospital or rural primary care hospital knowingly makes a payment, directly or indirectly, to a physician as an inducement to reduce or limit services provided with respect to individuals who -

(A) are entitled to benefits under part A or part B of subchapter XVIII of this chapter or to medical assistance under a State plan approved under subchapter XIX of this chapter, and

(B) are under the direct care of a physician, the hospital or a rural primary care hospital shall be subject, in addition to any other penalties that may be prescribed by law, to a civil money penalty of not more than $2,000 for each such individual with respect to whom the payment is made.

(2) Any physician who knowingly accepts receipt of a payment described in paragraph (1) shall be subject, in addition to any other penalties that may be prescribed by law, to a civil money penalty of not more than $2,000 for each individual described in such paragraph with respect to whom the payment is made.

(3)(A) Any physician who executes a document described in subparagraph (B) with respect to an individual knowing that all of the requirements referred to in such subparagraph are not met with respect to the individual shall be subject to a civil monetary penalty of not more than the greater of -

(i) $5,000, or

(ii) three times the amount of the payments under subchapter XVIII of this chapter for home health services which are made pursuant to such certification.

(B) A document described in this subparagraph is any document that certifies, for the purposes of subchapter XVIII of this chapter, that an individual meets the requirements of section

1395f(a)(2)(C) or 1395n(a)(2)(A) of this title in the case of home health services furnished to the individual.[16]

This statute raises several issues that need to be discussed. First is the oft-repeated phrase "knows or should know." Obviously, if the government can show that a person "knows" he or she has submitted a fraudulent claim, the "ignorance" defense can be mitigated. But when the law adds the words "or should know" to the statute, the burden for the accuracy of the claims basically shifts to the health care provider. This is especially true since all providers are, or should be, given manuals that show proper billing methods. In addition, the providers are periodically given updates on the changes that occur. Most plans also provide either telephone-based or on-line services for questions about the plans. Whether the manuals are actually read or questions are actually asked is not the government's problem. As part of the provider agreements, the providers agree to follow the "rules" in the manuals. It is their choice to remain ignorant as to the contents of the manuals and updates.

The reader should also note how substantial the monetary penalties are. It does not take long to amass a huge monetary penalty when the multiple is $10,000 per item or service. The government can also add to that figure an assessment of up to three times of the total amount of the claim(s) themselves in lieu of damages. It is clear that the potential monetary risk for those who commit health care fraud is great.

One of the bigger hammers in the law is the ability of the government to exclude a provider. Federal and state health care programs have become a huge portion of the health care industry. When a provider is excluded from these programs, it can have a devastating effect on the provider's business.

Civil Actions for False Claims, Including Qui Tam Actions

Title 31, Section 3730, of the United States Code is a significant portion of the civil law. It details the provisions that allow a private citizen to bring an action for a violation of Section 3729 (false claims). The section is lengthy, but a clear understanding of how an individual can use this law should be part of the training of anyone involved in the health care field. The statute states:

(a) Responsibilities of the Attorney General. - The Attorney General diligently shall investigate a violation under section 3729. If the Attorney General finds that a person has violated or is violating section 3729, the Attorney General may bring a civil action under this section against the person.

(b) Actions by Private Persons. - (1) A person may bring a civil action for a violation of section 3729 for the person and for the United States Government. The action shall be brought in the name of the Government. The action may be dismissed only if the court and the Attorney General give written consent to the dismissal and their reasons for consenting.

(2) A copy of the complaint and written disclosure of substantially all material evidence and information the person possesses shall be served on the Government pursuant to Rule 4(d)(4) of the Federal Rules of Civil Procedure. The complaint shall be filed in camera, shall remain under seal

for at least 60 days, and shall not be served on the defendant until the court so orders. The Government may elect to intervene and proceed with the action within 60 days after it receives both the complaint and the material evidence and information.

(3) The Government may, for good cause shown, move the court for extensions of the time during which the complaint remains under seal under paragraph (2). Any such motions may be supported by affidavits or other submissions in camera. The defendant shall not be required to respond to any complaint filed under this section until 20 days after the complaint is unsealed and served upon the defendant pursuant to Rule 4 of the Federal Rules of Civil Procedure.

(4) Before the expiration of the 60-day period or any extensions obtained under paragraph (3), the Government shall -

   (A) proceed with the action, in which case the action shall be conducted by the Government; or

   (B) notify the court that it declines to take over the action, in which case the person bringing the action shall have the right to conduct the action.

   (5) When a person brings an action under this subsection, no person other than the Government may intervene or bring a related action based on the facts underlying the pending action.

(c) Rights of the Parties to Qui Tam Actions. - (1) If the Government proceeds with the action, it shall have the primary responsibility for prosecuting the action, and shall not be bound by an act of the person bringing the action. Such person shall have the right to continue as a party to the action, subject to the limitations set forth in paragraph (2).

   (2) (A) The Government may dismiss the action notwithstanding the objections of the person initiating the action if the person has been notified by the Government of the filing of the motion and the court has provided the person with an opportunity for a hearing on the motion.

   (B) The Government may settle the action with the defendant notwithstanding the objections of the person initiating the action if the court determines, after a hearing, that the proposed settlement is fair, adequate, and reasonable under all the circumstances. Upon a showing of good cause, such hearing may be held in camera.

   (C) Upon a showing by the Government that unrestricted participation during the course of the litigation by the person initiating the action would interfere with or unduly delay the Government's prosecution of the case, or would be repetitious, irrelevant, or for purposes of harassment, the court may, in its discretion, impose limitations on the person's participation, such as -

(i) limiting the number of witnesses the person may call;

(ii) limiting the length of the testimony of such witnesses;

(iii) limiting the person's cross-examination of witnesses; or

(iv) otherwise limiting the participation by the person in the litigation.

(D) Upon a showing by the defendant that unrestricted participation during the course of the litigation by the person initiating the action would be for purpose of harassment or would cause the defendant undue burden or unnecessary expense, the court may limit the participation by the person in the litigation.

(3) If the Government elects not to proceed with the action, the person who initiated the action shall have the right to conduct the action. If the Government so requests, it shall be served with copies of all pleadings filed in the action and shall be supplied with copies of all deposition transcripts (at the Government's expense). When a person proceeds with the action, the court, without limiting the status and rights of the person initiating the action, may nevertheless permit the Government to intervene at a later date upon a showing of good cause.

(4) Whether or not the Government proceeds with the action, upon a showing by the Government that certain actions of discovery by the person initiating the action would interfere with the Government's investigation or prosecution of a criminal or civil matter arising out of the same facts, the court may stay such discovery for a period of not more than 60 days. Such a showing shall be conducted in camera. The court may extend the 60-day period upon a further showing in camera that the Government has pursued the criminal or civil investigation or proceedings with reasonable diligence and any proposed discovery in the civil action will interfere with the ongoing criminal or civil investigation or proceedings.

(5) Notwithstanding subsection (b), the Government may elect to pursue its claim through any alternate remedy available to the Government, including any administrative proceeding to determine a civil money penalty. If any such alternate remedy is pursued in another proceeding, the person initiating the action shall have the same rights in such proceeding as such person would have had if the action had continued under this section. Any finding of fact or conclusion of law made in such other proceeding that

has become final shall be conclusive on all parties to an action under this section. For purposes of the preceding sentence, a finding or conclusion is final if it has been finally determined on appeal to the appropriate court of the United States, if all time for filing such an appeal with respect to the finding or conclusion has expired, or if the finding or conclusion is not subject to judicial review.

(d) Award to Qui Tam Plaintiff. - (1) If the Government proceeds with an action brought by a person under subsection (b), such person shall, subject to the second sentence of this paragraph, receive at least 15 percent but not more than 25 percent of the proceeds of the action or settlement of the claim, depending upon the extent to which the person substantially contributed to the prosecution of the action. Where the action is one which the court finds to be based primarily on disclosures of specific information (other than information provided by the person bringing the action) relating to allegations or transactions in a criminal, civil, or administrative hearing, in a congressional, administrative, or Government (FOOTNOTE 1) Accounting Office report, hearing, audit, or investigation, or from the news media, the court may award such sums as it considers appropriate, but in no case more than 10 percent of the proceeds, taking into account the significance of the information and the role of the person bringing the action in advancing the case to litigation. Any payment to a person under the first or second sentence of this paragraph shall be made from the proceeds. Any such person shall also receive an amount for reasonable expenses which the court finds to have been necessarily incurred, plus reasonable attorneys' fees and costs. All such expenses, fees, and costs shall be awarded against the defendant.

(FOOTNOTE 1) So in original. Probably should be "General."

(2) If the Government does not proceed with an action under this section, the person bringing the action or settling the claim shall receive an amount which the court decides is reasonable for collecting the civil penalty and damages. The amount shall be not less than 25 percent and not more than 30 percent of the proceeds of the action or settlement and shall be paid out of such proceeds. Such person shall also receive an amount for reasonable expenses which the court finds to have been necessarily incurred, plus reasonable attorneys' fees and costs. All such expenses, fees, and costs shall be awarded against the defendant.

(3) Whether or not the Government proceeds with the action, if the court finds that the action was brought by a person who planned and initiated the violation of section 3729 upon which the action was brought, then the court may, to the extent the court considers appropriate, reduce the share of the proceeds of the action which the person would otherwise receive under paragraph (1) or (2) of this subsection, taking into account the role of that person in advancing the case to litigation and any relevant circumstances pertaining to the violation. If the person bringing the action is

convicted of criminal conduct arising from his or her role in the violation of section 3729, that person shall be dismissed from the civil action and shall not receive any share of the proceeds of the action. Such dismissal shall not prejudice the right of the United States to continue the action, represented by the Department of Justice.

(4) If the Government does not proceed with the action and the person bringing the action conducts the action, the court may award to the defendant its reasonable attorneys' fees and expenses if the defendant prevails in the action and the court finds that the claim of the person bringing the action was clearly frivolous, clearly vexatious, or brought primarily for purposes of harassment.

(e) Certain Actions Barred. - (1) No court shall have jurisdiction over an action brought by a former or present member of the armed forces under subsection (b) of this section against a member of the armed forces arising out of such person's service in the armed forces.

(2) (A) No court shall have jurisdiction over an action brought under subsection (b) against a Member of Congress, a member of the judiciary, or a senior executive branch official if the action is based on evidence or information known to the Government when the action was brought.

(B) For purposes of this paragraph, "senior executive branch official" means any officer or employee listed in paragraphs (1) through (8) of section 101(f) of the Ethics in Government Act of 1978 (5 U.S.C. App.).

(3) In no event may a person bring an action under subsection (b) which is based upon allegations or transactions which are the subject of a civil suit or an administrative civil money penalty proceeding in which the Government is already a party.

(4) (A) No court shall have jurisdiction over an action under this section based upon the public disclosure of allegations or transactions in a criminal, civil, or administrative hearing, in a congressional, administrative, or Government (FOOTNOTE 2) Accounting Office report, hearing, audit, or investigation, or from the news media, unless the action is brought by the Attorney General or the person bringing the action is an original source of the information.

(FOOTNOTE 2) So in original. Probably should be "General."

(B) For purposes of this paragraph, "original source" means an individual who has direct and independent knowledge of the information on which the allegations are based and has voluntarily provided the information to the Government before filing an action under this section which is based on the information.

(f) Government Not Liable for Certain Expenses. - The Government is not liable for expenses which a person incurs in bringing an action under this section.

(g) Fees and Expenses to Prevailing Defendant. - In civil actions brought under this section by the United States, the provisions of section 2412(d) of title 28 shall apply.

(h) Any employee who is discharged, demoted, suspended, threatened, harassed, or in any other manner discriminated against in the terms and conditions of employment by his or her employer because of lawful acts done by the employee on behalf of the employee or others in furtherance of an action under this section, including investigation for, initiation of, testimony for, or assistance in an action filed or to be filed under this section, shall be entitled to all relief necessary to make the employee whole. Such relief shall include reinstatement with the same seniority status such employee would have had but for the discrimination, 2 times the amount of back pay, interest on the back pay, and compensation for any special damages sustained as a result of the discrimination, including litigation costs and reasonable attorneys' fees. An employee may bring an action in the appropriate district court of the United States for the relief provided in this subsection.[17]

In simple language, this statute states that if a private citizen has direct knowledge of a fraud, the private citizen may bring civil action on behalf of the federal government. The complaint must be filed in federal court, and the complaint and the documentation of the fraud will remain "under seal" for at least 60 days. During this period of time, and any extensions granted by the court, the Department of Justice will determine whether the government will adopt the case.

If the government decides to adopt the case, the government then assumes the responsibility to prosecute the action. If the government declines to intervene, it is up to the private party to continue with the action.

The law gives significant latitude in the amount the qui tam plaintiff is entitled to recover. The recovery amount is influenced by whether the government adopts the case, the nature of the information provided by the plaintiff, and other factors.

Several other areas of consideration should also be noted. While legal assistance is not specifically required to file the action, the assistance of an attorney is strongly recommended for several reasons. First, the attorney should review the information to determine the basis for the action and to ensure the completeness and accuracy of the motion. As a bonus, the attorney will also look after the plaintiff's interests if the government decides to intervene. An attorney's services should be considered an absolute necessity if the government does not intervene and the plaintiff decides to continue the action.

A person who has information that may yield a qui tam action should also be aware that many of these cases take years to reach a conclusion. The plaintiff should try not to become impatient with the process.

FRAUD SCHEMES

Some fraud schemes are simple, others very sophisticated. Because there are so many schemes and the schemes are constantly evolving, it is impossible to present an exhaustive list. This section discusses some of the most common schemes.

Services or Goods Not Provided

One of the most common forms of fraud is billing for services that were never rendered. Physicians may bill for patients they have not seen, pharmacists may bill for drugs never delivered to a recipient, and labs or hospitals may bill for tests never performed or X-rays never taken.

Consider a case investigated by the Texas Medicaid Fraud Control Unit in which a psychiatric home for youths was billing for psychiatric services allegedly being provided by a psychiatrist. There was a major problem with these billings. Not only had the services never been provided but the psychiatrist was living in Connecticut at the time the services were supposedly performed. It was determined that the home had billed $406,163 for services that had never been rendered.[18]

To understand how large this simple fraud can become, one only needs to review the case involving Sheldon Weinberg and members of his family. Weinberg set up a medical clinic in Brooklyn and began to systematically bill for phantom patients. During a span of approximately four years, the clinic billed for close to 400,000 visits that never occurred. These visits amounted to more than $16 million taken from the health care coffers.[19] Who said a simple scheme could not involve large sums of money?

Illegal Remuneration

Kickbacks and other forms of illegal remuneration are common in health care fraud and abuse cases. Examples of this type of fraud can include physicians receiving kickbacks for prescribing drugs, ordering lab tests, and authorizing the issuance of durable medical equipment and other types of goods and services. Health care businesses can offer any number of forms of illegal remuneration in order to secure an increase in business.

The kickbacks do not always have to be in cash. Other forms of payment could include vacations, use of leased vehicles, reduced rental costs, and the like. Remember, health care fraud and abuse is a white-collar crime, and kickbacks are common in this area.

An example of this type of crime was reported in Michigan. In this situation, a medical laboratory paid kickbacks to physicians in exchange for referrals. In one case, a physician was offered a limited partnership in the laboratory, and in other cases, the lab provided employees to the physicians. Over $250,000 was repaid to the state for the fraudulent Medicaid claims and the cost of the investigation.[20]

A New York podiatrist was the owner of five orthotic laboratories. The podiatrist paid kickbacks to other podiatrists for referral and increased his revenues from fraud by providing either cheap stock items or nothing at all to the patients while billing for expensive items. New York reported that this subject defrauded the health care system for $1.8 million.[21]

Falsification of Cost Reports

Cost reports are reports generated by a facility that show the costs associated with the care of patients. Facilities submit these cost reports, which are then used to calculate the rate of payment to the facilities. The frauds involving the falsification of cost reports primarily involve hospitals, long-term care facilities (nursing homes), home health agencies, and other similar types of businesses.

Once the initial projections of the costs of patient care are established, the facility will generally be paid on a prospective basis. At the end of the year, a settlement is reached between the facility and the government. This settlement is based on the actual costs for patient care versus the projections of this cost made by the facility. Typically, if the government overpaid during the year, the facility will be required to return the overpaid funds to the government.

If health care providers want to perpetrate the scheme on the initial phase of the operation, fraudulent costs are built into the initial projections. If costs are closely projected and the actual costs turn out to be less, fraud can be perpetrated to avoid settlement payouts by including fraudulent costs throughout the year.

> In Pennsylvania, a family operated a nursing home. By including everything from children's toys to personal home remodeling in the nursing home's cost report, the family defrauded the state out of more than $155,000.[22]

Other examples of this type of fraud are numerous. Perhaps one of the more notable is the Columbia/HCA case spoken of earlier in this chapter. In this situation, the allegations center around two sets of books. One set contained "aggressive" cost figures while the second contained more "conservative" cost figures. The allegations noted that the second, more conservative cost figures had been marked not to be disclosed to the federal health care program investigators.

Upcoding

Most, if not all, physician billings are directly related to codes that are submitted for payment. These codes define the amount of time spent with an individual patient or the complexity of the service provided. As the time spent with the patient or the complexity of the medical problem increases, so do the amounts paid to the physician for the service.

For example, if a 19-year-old patient sees a physician for a sore throat, fever, and fatigue and the physician sees the patient for approximately 10 minutes, the proper billing code would be 99212. If the same patient came in to see the physician complaining of regional enteritis, diarrhea, and a low-grade fever and the physician spent approximately 25 minutes with the patient, the proper billing code would be 99214. The physician would be paid more for the 99214 code than for the 99212 code. Similar codes apply to both outpatient and hospital visits.

Simply stated, upcoding means billing for codes of services that bring higher payments than the services actually provided. In the example noted above, if the physician billed code 99214 for the service that should have been billed 99212, the physician has upcoded.

Examples of this type of fraud abound. The Medicaid Fraud Unit Control in Nevada recently investigated a case involving a psychiatrist in Las Vegas. The investigation indicated the psychiatrist had both billed for services that had not been provided and inflated the amount of time that had actually been spent with the patients. The investigators determined that in some instances the psychiatrist had billed for more than 24 hours of therapy in a single day. The investigation resulted in the physician paying $300,000 in restitution, fines, and penalties.[23]

Unbundling

Many services covered by Medicare and Medicaid are "bundled" together for payment purposes. Examples of services that may be "bundled" together for billing include certain preadmission tests for hospital admissions, the preanesthesia evaluation prior to the administration of anesthesia, and certain laboratory analyses such as blood tests that are commonly run simultaneously.

Unbundling occurs when a provider fragments the billing of a "global" service to increase the payment. For instance, if an anesthesiologist sees a patient for a routine preanesthesia evaluation and then provides anesthesia to the patient, the anesthesiologist should bill only for the anesthesia service. The preanesthesia evaluation is considered to be a part of the "global" payment and cannot be charged for separately. If the anesthesiologist actually submits a bill that shows both an anesthesia consult and the actual anesthesia administration, that anesthesiologist has both "unbundled" the service and submitted a false claim.

If a laboratory runs a routine blood test in which 10 different items are measured, the laboratory should bill for the single test. If, however, the laboratory ran the same test and billed for two or three different tests, the billing for the service would have been "unbundled," and the laboratory would be paid a higher rate since the number of tests submitted for payment would be higher.

Unnecessary Services

In this type of fraud, the provider submits claims for goods or services that were not medically necessary. Providers may misrepresent the diagnosis and symptoms on patient records and billings in order to obtain payment for unnecessary treatments, tests, or medical supplies. This scheme can generate huge amounts of revenue.

Bruce C. Vladeck, the former administrator of the Health Care Financing Administration, cited several examples of this problem in a report submitted to the United States Senate in 1997. Perhaps the most blatant example given by Vladeck concerns inpatient mental health services. According to Vladeck,

> As the occupancy rates of psychiatric hospital inpatient beds have dropped, many hospitals have attempted to find ways to fill the void, often by hospitalizing patients who should be cared for in other, non-psychiatric, facilities. This is a temptation because diagnostic-related groups (DRGs) are not imposed on care in psychiatric hospitals, as they are in short-term acute care hospitals. Hospitalization of patients in psychiatric facilities can be extremely lucrative, with charges as high as $1000 per day. Also, patients hospitalized in psychiatric facilities are sometimes billed for unnecessary and unordered tests.[24]

Vladeck also noted significant problems in the billing of mental health services relating to nursing home residents. In the same report he states, "It has been estimated that as much as 32% of mental health services ordered for Medicare nursing home residents were unnecessary or inappropriate."[25]

Others commit fraud through billing for unnecessary goods and services related to home health care. Home health care clientele are often elderly or disabled. Many do not have the education or the capacity to understand what is really going on or to interpret the benefit reports they may receive. Recipients may not understand that they have been billed for goods (e.g., oxygen supplies, tube feeding supplies) or services (e.g., home visits) that were not needed or did not occur.

Suffice it to say that if a good or service can be billed as a medical necessity, it can also be billed when it is not a medical necessity. For many health care providers, profits increase as volume does. It is in their economic interest to generate a large amount of business. Dishonest health care providers increase their amount of business and profit without actually increasing the amount of work they do or supplies they use.

Double Billing

In double billing, the provider submits bills to both a federal health care program and another program or person, or the recipient of the service. For instance, a provider might submit a bill to the Medicaid program and to a private insurance company. Or two different providers might submit bills for the same service on the same day.

An example of double billing was recently uncovered in Washington State. A company that provided mental health counseling was engaged in several different fraud schemes. One involved the falsification of Medicaid provider applications and the forging of medical credentials. The other part of the scheme was the double billing of services to the Washington State Crime Victims Compensation Program for services that had already been paid by Medicaid.[26]

Billing Services

There are a large number of companies that provide billing services for physicians and other health care providers. These companies take the information and handle all of the billings for the provider. If they desire to, these companies can commit large-scale fraud.

Many of the more questionable billing companies offer their services for a percentage of the amount recovered for the providers. This practice is illegal but common. Since these services are competitive, many of these companies will market themselves to the various providers by indicating that their company can maximize payments from Medicare and Medicaid. This is an attractive offer to the provider, and a deal is struck.

In order to maximize profits, the billing companies may resort to a variety of different frauds, including upcoding, fragmentation, and other forms of false reporting. These false claims produce higher profits for both the provider and the billing company.

It is appropriate to point out that the provider is ultimately responsible for the billings submitted on his or her behalf. Ignorance of the activity may protect the provider from criminal prosecution, but the provider may still be held responsible for discrepancies in billing. For this reason, it is important for those providers using billing companies to have a clear understanding of how the bills are being submitted and to perform a review of the payments to ensure billing accuracy.

Pharmacy Fraud

The frauds perpetrated by pharmacies are being discussed as a separate issue because the system of payments is easily defrauded in several different ways. Basically, the fraud begins with a Medicaid recipient's number. From that point on, the game has many variations.

One way the fraud can be initiated is the construction of a fraudulent prescription. Here a pharmacy can bill for a professional service fee and the costs of drugs when no service was rendered and no medication was given to a recipient. Not only can the original prescription be billed, but the pharmacist may also create refills under this same prescription number and continue the fraud for an extended period of time.

Another method may be the substitution of a generic product when a brand-name product has been ordered by the physician. In this case, the pharmacy provides the recipient with a generic product and bills Medicaid for the brand-name drug, which is more expensive.

Another method employed is the resale of medication. Drugs can be returned to a pharmacy from nursing homes or rest homes for a number of different reasons. The pharmacy then must decide to either give a credit (if the drugs are packaged in a manner that would allow resale) or destroy the drugs. A pharmacy in this position may simply state that the drugs were destroyed when they were actually resold. This reselling may take place several times with a single drug. Since the pharmacy paid for the drug only once, the resale is pure profit!

More elaborate schemes have been found involving pharmacies. Some of these schemes have involved physicians who work in conjunction with one or more pharmacies to further the fraud. For example, Medicaid recipients could go to a physician's office for a brief visit and receive one or more prescriptions. The recipients would then be told where to have the prescriptions filled. The drugs received from the pharmacies would then be bought back from the recipients at a fraction of their cost.

In such a scenario, everybody but the government "gets well." The physicians are paid for an office visit that was not necessary or was not performed and are probably receiving a kickback from the pharmacies. The pharmacies are buying back medications for a significantly reduced rate and then reselling the drugs over and over. The recipients are receiving cash for doing little or nothing, so there is no incentive for them to become "whistle-blowers."

These types of schemes can also be utilized for the diversion of drugs. If diversion is taking place through these schemes, the government is financing the drug operation.

Many pharmacy frauds involve noncontrolled substances that must be prescribed, not just controlled substances. Sometimes the most money can be made by prescribing antibiotics, medications to treat cancer, newly released medications, and the like. Some of these prescriptions cost several hundred dollars each, so it does not take long before a large amount of money is involved.

INVESTIGATIVE AGENCIES

There are numerous different agencies involved in the investigation of health care fraud. On the federal level, two groups focus on the criminal investigation of fraud: investigators at the Federal Bureau of Investigation (FBI) and investigators at the Office of Inspector General (OIG) of the Department of Health and Human Services. The Department of Health and Human Services also has individuals who focus on auditing and aspects of controlling the health care system.

On the state level, 47 states have organizations specifically dedicated to the criminal investigation of Medicaid fraud. These agencies focus on Medicaid but routinely coordinate their efforts with the FBI and OIG and may conduct investigations involving Medicare. The states will also have various agencies that focus on system integrity.

CONCLUSION

Though this chapter has focused on Medicare- and Medicaid-related fraud, government-funded programs are not the only victims of health care fraud. Private insurance companies are suffering losses as well.

Once third-party payments became almost universal in the health care industry, health care recipients lost most of their interest in how health care is paid for. Sometimes benefit explanations or bills are not even read by the person who received the service. Even if health care recipients read the documents, they may not understand the documents. Those who commit fraud rely on this aspect of the health care industry. Public ignorance and apathy are their allies. With only overworked government investigators to worry about, the schemes roll on and the likelihood of detection remains small.

The investigation of fraud and abuse within the health care industry is a difficult task. Those responsible for detecting health care fraud do a good job and are dedicated. But limited resources and constantly changing fraud methodology leave the perpetrators with the advantage. Investigating health care fraud is like trying to scoop water with both hands. Each attempt will capture some water, but most will slip through the fingers. After one fraudulent practice is shut down by investigators, the dishonest parties always seem to find another way to illegally divert funds.

KEY POINTS

- The health care industry today is a particularly easy target for fraud and abuse, and the likelihood of getting caught is rather low.
- Many different federal and state statutes address illegal actions associated with health care fraud and abuse cases.
- Fraud schemes come in many varieties—many different perpetrators are using many different methods to abuse the health care system.
- Those charged with investigating health care fraud and abuse have an extremely difficult task. While investigators uncover certain forms of fraud and abuse, other new forms are popping up every day.

REFERENCES

1. Health Care Financing Administration, "Highlights National Health Expenditures, 1997," http://www.hcfa.gov/stats/nhe-oact/hilites.htn (accessed 28 December 1998).

2. M.K. Sparrow, *License to Steal* (Boulder, CO: Westview Press, 1996), 2.

3. "Highlights National Health Expenditures, 1997."

4. Sparrow, *License,* 50.

5. 42 U.S.C. § 1320a-7b(a).

6. H.C. Black, *Black's Law Dictionary* (St. Paul, MN: West Publishing, 1968), 1128.

7. 42 U.S.C. § 1320a-7b(b).

8. 42 U.S.C. § 1320a-7b(c).

9. 42 U.S.C. § 1320a-7b(d).

10. 42 U.S.C. § 1320a-7b(e).

11. 18 U.S.C. § 287.

12. 18 U.S.C. § 371.

13. 18 U.S.C. § 1341.

14. 18 U.S.C. § 1343.

15. 31 U.S.C. § 3729.

16. 42 U.S.C. § 1320a-7a.

17. 31 U.S.C. § 3730.

18. National Association of Medicaid Fraud Control Units, *A Review of the State Medicaid Fraud Control Unit Program* (Washington, DC: 1998), 14.

19. National Association of Medicaid Fraud Control Units, *A Review of the State Medicaid Fraud Control Unit Program,* 16.

20. National Association of Medicaid Fraud Control Units, *A Review of the State Medicaid Fraud Control Unit Program,* 17.

21. National Association of Medicaid Fraud Control Units, *A Review of the State Medicaid Fraud Control Unit Program,* 18.

22. National Association of Medicaid Fraud Control Units, *A Review of the State Medicaid Fraud Control Unit Program,* 19.

23. National Association of Medicaid Fraud Control Units, *A Review of the State Medicaid Fraud Control Unit Program,* 16–17.

24. Health Care Financing Administration, "Statement of Bruce C. Vladeck on 'Prevalence of Health Care Fraud and Abuse,'" http://www.hcfa.gov/testmony/fraud1.htm (accessed 28 December 1998).

25. "Statement of Bruce C. Vladeck."

26. National Association of Medicaid Fraud Control Units, *A Review of the State Medicaid Fraud Control Unit Program,* 23.

About the Author

David H. Sells, Jr., MC/CJ, CPP, CHPA, CSE, is the president of Sells & Co., an international consulting corporation. He is a recognized expert in security. He has written five books on security, hosted and produced his own television program, hosted a spot on personal security on a popular radio show, and been an expert witness in litigation.

Mr. Sells gives speeches throughout the world on various security matters. He was the keynote speaker for the National HealthCare Security Conferences in 1995 and 1996 in Australia, and was retained by the Hong Kong Hospital Authority to conduct training sessions for its more than 60 medical centers.

Mr. Sells was formerly the corporate director of security and public safety for a multifacility health care system in Charlotte, North Carolina. In his role as corporate director, Mr. Sells was responsible for the security of four hospitals with over 1,400 beds, 97 medical and commercial office complexes, and 400-student child development center, a 300-student school of nursing, and a 389-bed nursing home.

Mr. Sells serves as an adjunct professor at Central Piedmont Community College and is a member of the advisory board for the Security & Safety Program and the Criminal Justice Program at the college. In addition, he is the Director of the Security Management Institute which provides training, testing, and credentialing to security executives on an international basis.

Mr. Sells holds a Master's certificate in Criminal Justice, a Bachelor's of Science degree in Business, and two Associate of Science degrees, one in Management and the other in Paralegalism. He is a graduate of both the North Carolina and South Carolina Criminal Justice Academies.

Mr. Sells is a Certified Protection Professional, a Certified Health Care Protection Administrator, and a Certified Security Executive. He is a past president of the SouthEastern Safety & Security Health Care Council and served as the North Carolina chairman for the International Association for Healthcare Security and Safety.

About the Contributors

During my 25 years in the security business, I have formed friendships with many fellow professionals. In preparing this work, I was fortunate enough to be able to call on the following talented professionals and good friends for assistance.

James P. Finn, CHPA, CSE, CHSE, is currently the manager of Safety & Security Services for Gaston Memorial Hospital. He is a senior member with the International Association for Healthcare Security and Safety, a member of the American Society for Industrial Security, and past president of the Southeastern Safety/Security Healthcare Council. Mr. Finn has lectured to professionals on safety and security both in the United States and Australia.

Mr. Finn holds a Bachelor's degree in Criminal Justice and the following professional credentials: Certified Healthcare Protection Administrator, Certified Security Executive, and Certified Healthcare Security Executive.

Rick J. Flinn, RN, MSN, currently serves as the executive director of Emergency and Trauma Services for the North Broward Hospital District. Mr. Flinn has 20 years of experience in health care as a clinician, educator, and manager within the specialty of emergency care. Mr. Flinn has lectured nationally on the design and operations of security systems within the health care setting and the impact of gang violence on communities.

Mr. Flinn is a registered nurse and holds a Master of Science in Nursing.

W.P. "Butch" Gibbons III is currently an engineer with SFI Electronics in Charlotte, North Carolina. He has over 20 years of experience in electronic security applications, especially closed-circuit television. Mr. Gibbons is a recognized expert in the design and integration of security systems. His projects have gained him national recognition in the industry.

Mr. Gibbons holds professional licenses in Alarm Systems and Electrical Contracting.

John B. Rabun, Jr., BA, MSSW, has been the vice president and chief operating officer for the National Center for Missing and Exploited Children since its founding by the U.S. Department of Justice in 1984. John has made guest appearances on most national television and radio talk shows and news programs in the United States and United Kingdom. Since 1987, John has provided consultation and training for over 700 hospitals and 47,000 hospital staff on the subject of infant abduction, and since 1987, the number of infant abductions has declined dramatically. John is the author of many works, including *For Healthcare Professionals: Guidelines on Prevention of and Response to Infant Abductions*. This work is considered the definitive publication on the subject.

Mr. Rabun holds a Bachelor of Arts and a Master of Science in Social Work.

John T. Readling is a special agent with the North Carolina State Bureau of Investigation. He is currently assigned to the Medicaid Investigations Unit of the North Carolina Attorney General's office. Prior to his current assignment, Mr. Readling was assigned to the Drug Diversion Unit. While in the Drug Diversion Unit, Agent Readling investigated over 300 cases of diversion by physicians, pharmacists, nurses, and other health care professionals.

Mr. Readling has lectured nationally on health care security issues and is considered an expert in investigations related to health care. He is the coauthor of *Drug Diversion: An Investigative Guide for the HealthCare Professional*.

Mr. Readling holds a Bachelor of Arts degree in Politics and has completed significant work on a Master's in Public Administration.

Index

Fraud and abuse—*continued*
  conspiracy, 408
  criminal statutes, 404–409
  double billing, 423
  false claim, 407, 409–411
    civil actions, 414–419
    qui tam action, 414–419
  false statements or representations, 404–405
    condition or operation of institutions, 406
  falsification of cost reports, 420–421
  fictitious or fraudulent claims, 407
  illegal patient admittance and retention practices, 406–407
  illegal remuneration, 405–406, 420
  investigative agencies, 425
  mail fraud, 408
    fraud by wire, radio or television, 408–409
  pharmacy, 424
  schemes, 419–424
  services or goods not provided, 420
  unbundling, 422
  unnecessary services, 422–423
  upcoding, 421–422

G

Gang violence, 307–333
  affiliation identifiers, 331–333
  categories, 308
  characteristics, 307–308
  defined, 307
  gang categories, 309–310
  gang data, 308
  graffiti, 327–329
  hierarchical structure, 308
  prevention, 312
  reasons for joining gangs, 309, 311
  recognition, 310–312
  terminology, 315–325
Government leader, 370
Government-owned facility, 2
Graffiti, gang violence, 327–329

H

Handcuffs, 111
Handicapped parking, 88
Health care cost, 401–403
  fraud, 401–403
Health care facility, types, 1–8
Health maintenance organization, 395–396
High-visibility patrol, 13

Home care, 271–277
  carjacking, 275
  domestic dispute, 276
  employee misconduct, 272–273
  employment-related issues, 271–272
  external security issues, 274–277
  firearms, 276
  home safety, 276–277
  internal security issues, 271–274
  maternity center security, 146
  patient visit issues, 273
  prescreening, 273
  safety tips, 273–274
  scheduling, 273
  street safety, 275–276
  substance abuse, 276
Home health care agency, 272
Home health worker, screening, 271–272
Hospital
  characterized, 1–4
  geographic region served, 2
  ownership, 2
  population, 2–4
  primary security issues, 15–16
  rural, 2
  suburban, 2
  urban, 2
Hospital administrator, 3
Hospital staff, 3
Hospital watch program, 14, 96, 97–98
Hostage situation, 289–292
  criminal hostage taker, 290–292
  hostage guidelines, 292
  hostage taker profile, 289–291
  incident management plan, 295–297
  mentally ill hostage taker, 290
  response rules, 291–292
  responsibilities of security, 292–294
Hostile situation, 14
Human resources, 243–244
  background check, 243–244
  confidentiality, 243
  storage, 243

I

Identification
  identification badge, 144
  identification band, 159
  maternity center security, 143, 146
Illegal remuneration, fraud and abuse, 405–406, 420
Impaired driver, 171